Aortic Aneurysms: Vascular Remodeling and Repair

Aortic Aneurysms: Vascular Remodeling and Repair

Editor

Elena Kaschina

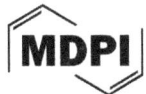

Basel • Beijing • Wuhan • Barcelona • Belgrade • Novi Sad • Cluj • Manchester

Editor
Elena Kaschina
Charité – Universitätsmedizin
Berlin
Berlin, Germany

Editorial Office
MDPI
St. Alban-Anlage 66
4052 Basel, Switzerland

This is a reprint of articles from the Special Issue published online in the open access journal *Biomedicines* (ISSN 2227-9059) (available at: https://www.mdpi.com/journal/biomedicines/special_issues/AAA_therapies).

For citation purposes, cite each article independently as indicated on the article page online and as indicated below:

Lastname, A.A.; Lastname, B.B. Article Title. *Journal Name* **Year**, *Volume Number*, Page Range.

ISBN 978-3-0365-8902-2 (Hbk)
ISBN 978-3-0365-8903-9 (PDF)
doi.org/10.3390/books978-3-0365-8903-9

© 2023 by the authors. Articles in this book are Open Access and distributed under the Creative Commons Attribution (CC BY) license. The book as a whole is distributed by MDPI under the terms and conditions of the Creative Commons Attribution-NonCommercial-NoDerivs (CC BY-NC-ND) license.

Contents

About the Editor . . . . **vii**

Elena Kaschina
Aortic Aneurysm: Finding the Right Target
Reprinted from: *Biomedicines* **2023**, *11*, 1345, doi:10.3390/biomedicines11051345 . . . . **1**

Veronika Kessler, Johannes Klopf, Wolf Eilenberg, Christoph Neumayer and Christine Brostjan
AAA Revisited: A Comprehensive Review of Risk Factors, Management, and Hallmarks of Pathogenesis
Reprinted from: *Biomedicines* **2022**, *10*, 94, doi:10.3390/biomedicines10010094 . . . . **5**

Maciej Jusko, Piotr Kasprzak, Alicja Majos and Waclaw Kuczmik
The Ratio of the Size of the Abdominal Aortic Aneurysm to That of the Unchanged Aorta as a Risk Factor for Its Rupture
Reprinted from: *Biomedicines* **2022**, *10*, 1997, doi:10.3390/biomedicines10081997 . . . . **41**

Matthias Buerger, Oliver Klein, Sebastian Kapahnke, Verena Mueller, Jan Paul Frese, Safwan Omran, et al.
Use of MALDI Mass Spectrometry Imaging to Identify Proteomic Signatures in Aortic Aneurysms after Endovascular Repair
Reprinted from: *Biomedicines* **2021**, *9*, 1088, doi:10.3390/biomedicines9091088 . . . . **55**

Lin Li, Kejia Kan, Prama Pallavi and Michael Keese
Identification of the Key Genes and Potential Therapeutic Compounds for Abdominal Aortic Aneurysm Based on a Weighted Correlation Network Analysis
Reprinted from: *Biomedicines* **2022**, *10*, 1052, doi:10.3390/biomedicines10051052 . . . . **71**

Ke-Jia Kan, Feng Guo, Lei Zhu, Prama Pallavi, Martin Sigl and Michael Keese
Weighted Gene Co-Expression Network Analysis Reveals Key Genes and Potential Drugs in Abdominal Aortic Aneurysm
Reprinted from: *Biomedicines* **2021**, *9*, 546, doi:10.3390/biomedicines9050546 . . . . **85**

Luca Piacentini, Mattia Chiesa and Gualtiero Ivanoe Colombo
Gene Regulatory Network Analysis of Perivascular Adipose Tissue of Abdominal Aortic Aneurysm Identifies Master Regulators of Key Pathogenetic Pathways
Reprinted from: *Biomedicines* **2020**, *8*, 288, doi:10.3390/biomedicines8080288 . . . . **103**

Jonathan Golledge, Shivshankar Thanigaimani and James Phie
A Systematic Review and Meta-Analysis of the Effect of Pentagalloyl Glucose Administration on Aortic Expansion in Animal Models
Reprinted from: *Biomedicines* **2021**, *9*, 1442, doi:10.3390/biomedicines9101442 . . . . **123**

Leander Gaarde Melin, Julie Husted Dall, Jes S. Lindholt, Lasse B. Steffensen, Hans Christian Beck, Sophie L. Elkrog, et al.
Cycloastragenol Inhibits Experimental Abdominal Aortic Aneurysm Progression
Reprinted from: *Biomedicines* **2022**, *10*, 359, doi:10.3390/biomedicines10020359 . . . . **139**

Shaiv Parikh, Berta Ganizada, Gijs Debeij, Ehsan Natour, Jos Maessen, Bart Spronck, et al.
Intra-Operative Video-Based Measurement of Biaxial Strains of the Ascending Thoracic Aorta
Reprinted from: *Biomedicines* **2021**, *9*, 670, doi:10.3390/biomedicines9060670 . . . . **161**

Stelia Ntika, Linda M. Tracy, Anders Franco-Cereceda, Hanna M. Björck and Camilla Krizhanovskii
Syndecan-1 Expression Is Increased in the Aortic Wall of Patients with Type 2 Diabetes but Is Unrelated to Elevated Fasting Plasma Glucagon-Like Peptide-1
Reprinted from: *Biomedicines* **2021**, *9*, 697, doi:10.3390/biomedicines9060697 . . . . **171**

About the Editor

Elena Kaschina

Elena Kaschina is a senior researcher and lecturer at the Max Rubner Center for Cardiovascular Metabolic Renal Research, Department of Pharmacology, Charité Universitätsmedizin Berlin, Germany. She studied Medicine and obtained an MD degree at Medical Academy St. Petersburg. She then carried out postdoctoral research at the University of Kiel, Germany, and the Department of Pharmacology at Charité—Universitätsmedizin, Berlin, where she received her habilitation PD in Pharmacology. Achievements include research in therapeutic effects of the components of the renin–angiotensin and kallikrein–kinin systems, especially angiotensin type 2 receptor stimulation, angiotensin type 1 receptor blockade in the models of heart failure and aneurysm formation. Recent research is also focused on cannabinoid receptor modulation and SGLT2 inhibition by cardiac and vascular remodeling, especially in the context of proteolysis and extracellular matrix turnover. Elena Kaschina has received several awards from the German Hypertension Foundation and European Council for Cardiovascular Research and successfully trained and mentored many young investigators. She has published numerous original articles, reviews and book chapters on cardiovascular pharmacology, including works in Circulation, Hypertension, Nature Communications and Pharmacological Reviews.

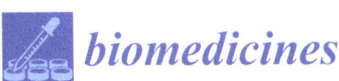

Editorial

Aortic Aneurysm: Finding the Right Target

Elena Kaschina

1. Cardiovascular-Metabolic-Renal (CMR)-Research Center, Institute of Pharmacology, Corporate Member of Freie Universität Berlin, Humboldt-Universität zu Berlin, Charité—Universitätsmedizin Berlin, 10115 Berlin, Germany; elena.kaschina@charite.de; Tel.: +49-30-450-525-024
2. DZHK (German Centre for Cardiovascular Research), Partner Site Berlin, 10115 Berlin, Germany

Citation: Kaschina, E. Aortic Aneurysm: Finding the Right Target. *Biomedicines* 2023, 11, 1345. https://doi.org/10.3390/biomedicines11051345

Received: 19 April 2023
Accepted: 27 April 2023
Published: 3 May 2023

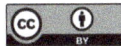

Copyright: © 2023 by the author. Licensee MDPI, Basel, Switzerland. This article is an open access article distributed under the terms and conditions of the Creative Commons Attribution (CC BY) license (https://creativecommons.org/licenses/by/4.0/).

This Special Issue of *Biomedicines* highlights many important scientific findings in aneurysm research. The issue publishes a systematic, up-to-date review on aortic aneurysms (AAs) and nine research articles on pathophysiology, gene expression, novel drug targets, clinical imaging, and prognostic methods. These investigations focus on different segments of the aorta, from the aortic root to the abdominal aorta, as well as on unruptured, ruptured, and repaired aneurysms. The issue also highlights the recent novel methods developed for the evaluation of aneurysm study outcomes. I would like to summarize and briefly discuss the articles in this Special Issue.

Abdominal AAs, being much more common than thoracic aneurysms and dissections [1], have also received a lot of attention in this issue. To begin with, the review by Kessler V. and co-authors [2] provides an appraisal of the literature on risk factors for abdominal AAs, their clinical manifestations, methods of diagnosis, and options for surgical interventions. The authors comprehensively describe the most relevant and up-to-date information on the key pathomechanisms of aneurysm formation, such as intraluminal thrombosis, increased proteolysis, and chronic inflammation, pointing to the role of activated monocytes, macrophages, and neutrophils. The authors also discuss the repurposing of the anti-diabetic drug metformin with anti-inflammatory pleiotropic properties, which may possibly be used for the prevention of aneurysm progression.

The aortic diameter of abdominal AA is a very important diagnostic parameter, as the risk of rupture increases with its size [1]. Jusko M., with co-authors [3], was looking for the diagnostic criteria, indicating the high risk of rupture. The diameters of the aneurysm and normal aorta were measured by computer tomography and compared in patients with ruptured and unruptured aneurysms. The authors found that in small aneurysms with a present neck segment, the ratio of the aneurysm sac to aorta diameter was a significant prognostic factor for aortic rupture. This work will help surgeons weigh the risk-to-benefit ratio of treating abdominal AA.

A secondary rupture may occur in patients after surgical treatment as well. A perfusion of the aneurysm after endovascular repair (EVAR), an endoleak, often triggers a secondary rupture. The special mechanisms that provoke this added complication and the ways of preventing it are unclear. Buerger M. et al. [4] investigated the structure of aortic tissues in patients after EVAR. The authors evaluated the peptide signature of the thoracic and abdominal aortas by using matrix-assisted laser desorption (MALDI) or ionization mass spectrometry imaging (MSI). Aortas after EVAR were characterized by decreased content of actin, tropomyosin, troponin, and collagen, as well as impaired respiratory chain function. These findings warrant further investigations into possible treatment options for patients with repaired aneurysms.

Knowledge of genetic architecture may advance understanding of the processes involved in aneurysm formation. Two in silico studies coming from the group of Michael Keese represent the key gene related to abdominal AA.

First, Li L. and co-authors [5] found the key modules, for example, the mitotic cell cycle, GTPase activity, and several metabolic processes, which may contribute to aneurysmal growth. Furthermore, the authors could identify seven key genes (CCR5, ADCY5, ADCY3, ACACB, LPIN1, ACSL1, and UCP3) that regulate disease progression and 35 compounds targeting these genes. These substances may be candidates for the prevention of aneurysm progression. Kan K.J. et al. [6] further identified significant genes in abdominal AA patients. Moreover, the authors could predict the potential therapeutic compounds for these genes. Weighted correlation network analysis (WGCNA) and text mining identified 3 hub modules and 144 hub genes. The most interesting hub genes were asparagine synthetase, axin-related protein 2, melanoma cell adhesion molecule, and testis-specific Y-encoded-like protein 1. Importantly, potential compounds targeting the genes were also defined: asparaginase, prednisolone, and abiraterone. Indeed, these novel candidates should be further tested in experimental models of aneurysms.

A genetic study by Piacentini L. and co-authors [7] focused on perivascular adipose tissue that is known to be involved in the pathogenesis of abdominal AA [8]. The authors identified the most relevant transcription factors NFKB1, SPIB, TBP, and the nuclear receptor RXRA, as well as the protein kinases MAPK1 and GSKB3. These factors are known to regulate gene subsets of immune response in the perivascular adipose tissue of abdominal AA.

The need for the development of effective novel drugs for abdominal AA remains urgent. Here, two studies analyze the effectiveness of new therapeutic approaches.

The first one is pentagalloyl glucose (PGG), a gallotannin, which prevents the degradation of elastin and collagen in blood vessels and restores the biomechanical properties of the arterial extracellular matrix [9]. Recent experimental studies investigated the effectiveness of this compound in abdominal AA. The work by Golledge J. and co-authors [10] performed a meta-analysis of eleven studies on the effects of PGG on abdominal AA expansion. Aortic expansion assessed by direct measurement was used as the primary outcome in this study. The authors additionally analyzed the effects of PGG delivery in specific forms and at different treatment regimes and tested them in different animal models. The authors concluded that the studies were inconsistent. Unfortunately, the evidence that PGG may be protective in patients with early-stage abdominal AA is of low quality. Thus, more information and qualitative research on PGG are needed.

Melin L.G. et al. [11] performed an experimental study in the rat using an elastase perfusion model of abdominal AA. The rats were treated with cycloastragenol, a compound from Astragalus, a Chinese medicinal herb, which improves the functioning of the immune and cardiovascular systems and boosts immunotherapy for some types of cancer [12]. The authors showed that treatment with cycloastragenol decreased aneurysm diameter, matrix metalloprotease-2 activity, reduced calcification, and preserved elastin content in the aorta. In view of these positive effects, cycloastragenol was suggested for a trial in abdominal AA patients.

Two further studies focused mainly on thoracic aneurysms. Parikh S. and co-authors [13] evaluated a new intra-operative video-based method to assess local biaxial strains of the ascending thoracic aorta. The authors performed repeated biaxial strain measurements on the patients undergoing open-chest surgery. Obtained data enable further investigations on the remodeling processes in the thoracic aorta and biomechanical modeling of aortic aneurysms.

Interestingly, diabetes mellitus is associated with a reduced risk of AA and dissection [14,15]. Therefore, Ntika S. and co-authors [16] were looking for the underlying mechanisms for the reduced risk of thoracic AA in diabetic patients. In aortic tissues from patients with type 2 diabetes, the authors found an increased expression of Syndecan-1 and a marker of macrophages. Syndecans are cell surface proteoglycans that interact with integrins, tyrosine kinase receptors, and extracellular matrix proteins [17]. The authors propose that increased aortic Syndecan-1 expression in humans may reduce the prevalence of thoracic AA in diabetes patients. Given that Syndecan-1 demonstrated protective anti-inflammatory function in aneurysm formation in animals [18], it needs further research as a promising drug candidate.

Altogether, genetic and basic science research presented in this issue identified novel pivotal cell signaling pathways in AAs and new drug targets to prevent aneurysmal growth. Cycloastragenol, Syndecan-1, and pentagalloyl glucose, being promising candidates, require further investigations. Perivascular adipose tissue remains an important source of gene subsets influencing innate and antigen-driven immune responses. Further identification of drug targets that could prevent distal and proximal aneurysmal extension following surgical correction is of great relevance. Moreover, modern scientific approaches described in this issue, such as biomechanical modeling, MALDI-MSI, and weighted correlation network analysis, may pave the way for the development of effective new treatments.

As the editor, I would like to take this opportunity to express my deep gratitude to all researchers for their great discoveries despite the challenges of COVID-19.

Conflicts of Interest: The author declares no conflict of interest.

References

1. Isselbacher, E.M. Thoracic and Abdominal Aortic Aneurysms. *Circulation* **2005**, *111*, 816–828. [CrossRef] [PubMed]
2. Kessler, V.; Klopf, J.; Eilenberg, W.; Neumayer, C.; Brostjan, C. AAA Revisited: A Comprehensive Review of Risk Factors, Management, and Hallmarks of Pathogenesis. *Biomedicines* **2022**, *10*, 94. [CrossRef]
3. Jusko, M.; Kasprzak, P.; Majos, A.; Kuczmik, W. The Ratio of the Size of the Abdominal Aortic Aneurysm to That of the Unchanged Aorta as a Risk Factor for Its Rupture. *Biomedicines* **2022**, *10*, 1997. [CrossRef]
4. Buerger, M.; Klein, O.; Kapahnke, S.; Mueller, V.; Frese, J.P.; Omran, S.; Greiner, A.; Sommerfeld, M.; Kaschina, E.; Jannasch, A.; et al. Use of MALDI Mass Spectrometry Imaging to Identify Proteomic Signatures in Aortic Aneurysms after Endovascular Repair. *Biomedicines* **2021**, *9*, 1088. [CrossRef] [PubMed]
5. Li, L.; Kan, K.; Pallavi, P.; Keese, M. Identification of the Key Genes and Potential Therapeutic Compounds for Abdominal Aortic Aneurysm Based on a Weighted Correlation Network Analysis. *Biomedicines* **2022**, *10*, 1052. [CrossRef] [PubMed]
6. Kan, K.-J.; Guo, F.; Zhu, L.; Pallavi, P.; Sigl, M.; Keese, M. Weighted Gene Co-Expression Network Analysis Reveals Key Genes and Potential Drugs in Abdominal Aortic Aneurysm. *Biomedicines* **2021**, *9*, 546. [CrossRef] [PubMed]
7. Piacentini, L.; Chiesa, M.; Colombo, G.I. Gene Regulatory Network Analysis of Perivascular Adipose Tissue of Abdominal Aortic Aneurysm Identifies Master Regulators of Key Pathogenetic Pathways. *Biomedicines* **2020**, *8*, 288. [CrossRef] [PubMed]
8. Krueger, F.; Kappert, K.; Foryst-Ludwig, A.; Kramer, F.; Clemenz, M.; Grzesiak, A.; Sommerfeld, M.; Frese, J.P.; Greiner, A.; Kintscher, U.; et al. AT1-receptor blockade attenuates outward aortic remodeling associated with diet-induced obesity in mice. *Clin. Sci.* **2017**, *131*, 1989–2005. [CrossRef] [PubMed]
9. Patnaik, S.S.; Piskin, S.; Pillalamarri, N.R.; Romero, G.; Escobar, G.P.; Sprague, E.; Finol, E.A. Biomechanical Restoration Potential of Pentagalloyl Glucose after Arterial Extracellular Matrix Degeneration. *Bioengineering* **2019**, *6*, 58. [CrossRef] [PubMed]
10. Golledge, J.; Thanigaimani, S.; Phie, J. A Systematic Review and Meta-Analysis of the Effect of Pentagalloyl Glucose Administration on Aortic Expansion in Animal Models. *Biomedicines* **2021**, *9*, 1442. [CrossRef] [PubMed]
11. Lederle, F.A. The strange relationship between diabetes and abdominal aortic aneurysm. *Eur. J. Vasc. Endovasc. Surg.* **2012**, *43*, 254–256. [CrossRef] [PubMed]
12. Nordness, M.J.; Baxter, B.T.; Matsumura, J.; Terrin, M.; Zhang, K.; Ye, F.; Webb, N.R.; Dalman, R.L.; Curci, J.A. The effect of diabetes on abdominal aortic aneurysm growth over 2 years. *J. Vasc. Surg.* **2022**, *75*, 1211–1222.e1. [CrossRef] [PubMed]
13. Yu, Y.; Zhou, L.; Yang, Y.; Liu, Y. Cycloastragenol: An exciting novel candidate for age-associated diseases. *Exp. Ther. Med.* **2018**, *16*, 2175–2182. [CrossRef] [PubMed]
14. Melin, L.G.; Dall, J.H.; Lindholt, J.S.; Steffensen, L.B.; Beck, H.C.; Elkrog, S.L.; Clausen, P.D.; Rasmussen, L.M.; Stubbe, J. Cycloastragenol Inhibits Experimental Abdominal Aortic Aneurysm Progression. *Biomedicines* **2022**, *10*, 359. [CrossRef] [PubMed]
15. Parikh, S.; Ganizada, B.; Debeij, G.; Natour, E.; Maessen, J.; Spronck, B.; Schurgers, L.; Delhaas, T.; Huberts, W.; Bidar, E.; et al. Intra-Operative Video-Based Measurement of Biaxial Strains of the Ascending Thoracic Aorta. *Biomedicines* **2021**, *9*, 670. [CrossRef] [PubMed]
16. Ntika, S.; Tracy, L.M.; Franco-Cereceda, A.; Björck, H.M.; Krizhanovskii, C. Syndecan-1 Expression Is Increased in the Aortic Wall of Patients with Type 2 Diabetes but Is Unrelated to Elevated Fasting Plasma Glucagon-Like Peptide-1. *Biomedicines* **2021**, *9*, 697. [CrossRef] [PubMed]
17. Afratis, N.A.; Nikitovic, D.; Multhaupt, H.A.B.; Theocharis, A.D.; Couchman, J.R.; Karamanos, N.K. Syndecans—Key regulators of cell signaling and biological functions. *FEBS J.* **2017**, *284*, 27–41. [CrossRef] [PubMed]
18. Xiao, J.; Angsana, J.; Wen, J.; Smith, S.V.; Park, P.W.; Ford, M.L.; Haller, C.A.; Chaikof, E.L. Syndecan-1 displays a protective role in aortic aneurysm formation by modulating T cell-mediated responses. *Arterioscler. Thromb. Vasc. Biol.* **2012**, *32*, 386–396. [CrossRef] [PubMed]

Disclaimer/Publisher's Note: The statements, opinions and data contained in all publications are solely those of the individual author(s) and contributor(s) and not of MDPI and/or the editor(s). MDPI and/or the editor(s) disclaim responsibility for any injury to people or property resulting from any ideas, methods, instructions or products referred to in the content.

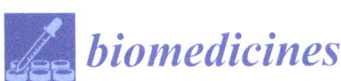

Review

AAA Revisited: A Comprehensive Review of Risk Factors, Management, and Hallmarks of Pathogenesis

Veronika Kessler, Johannes Klopf, Wolf Eilenberg, Christoph Neumayer and Christine Brostjan *

Department of General Surgery, Division of Vascular Surgery, Medical University of Vienna, Vienna General Hospital, 1090 Vienna, Austria; veronika.kessler@gmail.com (V.K.); johannes.klopf@meduniwien.ac.at (J.K.); wolf.eilenberg@meduniwien.ac.at (W.E.); christoph.neumayer@meduniwien.ac.at (C.N.)
* Correspondence: christine.brostjan@meduniwien.ac.at; Tel.: +43-1-40400-73514

Abstract: Despite declining incidence and mortality rates in many countries, the abdominal aortic aneurysm (AAA) continues to represent a life-threatening cardiovascular condition with an overall prevalence of about 2–3% in the industrialized world. While the risk of AAA development is considerably higher for men of advanced age with a history of smoking, screening programs serve to detect the often asymptomatic condition and prevent aortic rupture with an associated death rate of up to 80%. This review summarizes the current knowledge on identified risk factors, the multifactorial process of pathogenesis, as well as the latest advances in medical treatment and surgical repair to provide a perspective for AAA management.

Keywords: abdominal aortic aneurysm; risk factors; pathogenesis; review; treatment

1. Introduction

An aneurysm is a persistent and localized weakening and dilation of a blood vessel, typically an artery [1]. An abdominal aortic aneurysm (AAA) is, therefore, an irreversible dilation of the abdominal aorta between the diaphragm and the iliac bifurcation [2]. AAAs are typically 'true aneurysms', characterized by involvement and dilation of all three layers of the vascular wall. In contrast, a pseudoaneurysm or 'false aneurysm' caused by an arterial injury, such as a puncture or dissection, is hallmarked by blood infiltrating between the wall layers [2].

AAAs that are located below the renal arteries, i.e., infrarenally, account for about 80% of cases. The remainder are juxtarenal, pararenal, and suprarenal AAAs that involve the renal arteries or occur above them, respectively. Typically, the wall dilation in AAAs involves the whole circumference of the aorta ('fusiform'). Other morphological types such as saccular AAAs, where only part of the circumference is involved, are less common [3,4].

Clinically, no uniform definition of an AAA is universally accepted. The most commonly used definition is a maximum infrarenal abdominal aortic diameter of ≥30 mm, measured by ultrasonography or computed tomography angiography (CTA) [4,5]. This threshold is based on measurements of healthy infrarenal aortic diameters and is usually more than two standard deviations above the mean diameter of 17.9–19.3 mm for men [6,7]. However, this cutoff might not be appropriate for patients whose infrarenal aortic diameters differ from these dimensions, for instance, due to their height [5]. An alternative definition relates the maximum infrarenal aortic diameter to its expected normal value or to the diameter of the adjacent (i.e., the undilated suprarenal) aorta. Accordingly, a dilation should be considered aneurysmal when this ratio exceeds 1.5 [1,8]. This definition might be more useful for women, whose infrarenal aortic diameters measure a mean of 15.5–16.7 mm, as well as for distinct ethnic populations with deviating diameter values, and it can also be applied to other aneurysms [9,10].

2. Epidemiology

Lifetime risk of AAA is approximately 1 in 17 in the general population and up to 1 in 9 for current smokers [11]. A 2013 meta-analysis analyzing 56 studies of the years 1991–2013 found prevalence rates of 6.0% for men and 1.6% for women [12]. However, reported incidence and prevalence rates show a high degree of heterogeneity, owing to the specific definition of AAA used by the original studies and characteristics of the study populations, such as world region or population age [13]. Mortality of AAA patients is increased when compared to the general population, in both treated and untreated patient groups [14]. Rupture is the main and most often lethal complication of AAAs, but the most common causes of death for AAA patients are cardiovascular events [15,16]. Among AAA patients, women are more likely to die from an AAA-related death (i.e., rupture), while men die from cancer more often than from ruptures [17]. The mean time between a scan with no detected aortic abnormalities and AAA-related death is about 10 years (range 3.8–15.0) [18].

Analyses of historical data show a marked increase of AAA incidence, prevalence, and mortality during the 20th century. Over the past two decades, numbers have been on the decline in most countries, especially in Western Europe and North America [19,20]. Pooled prevalence rates have decreased from 5.7% in 1988–1998 to 2.8% in 2011–2013 [12]. AAA mortality has declined, as well, in most developed countries, with males and those under the age of 75 showing the greatest improvement [15,21]. The rise and fall of AAA-related mortality rates in developed countries correlate strongly with the changes in smoking prevalence [11,15]. Notably, AAA mortality in men is declining in many countries, particularly in the United States, the United Kingdom, and the Netherlands, while it seems to be on the rise among men and women in Hungary, Romania, and Japan [22].

3. Clinical Presentation and Course of Disease

AAAs are typically asymptomatic until they rupture. AAAs cause unspecific symptoms, if any, such as abdominal tenderness or pain radiating towards the back or to the genitals [23]. A pulsating abdominal mass may indicate the presence of an AAA, but abdominal palpation is inherently insensitive for detection of AAAs [24]. Symptoms may also be caused by complications such as compression of nearby organs or embolic events, but approximately half of patients have a ruptured aneurysm as their cause of primary presentation [25,26].

3.1. AAA Growth Rate

Disease progression is commonly non-linear with intermittent periods of aneurysm growth. The majority of AAAs enlarge over time and only a minority of patients show no detectable growth at all [27]. Mean growth rates range between 2.2 and 2.8 mm per year [28–31] and do not seem to have changed over the past 25 years [32]. Growth rates vary greatly between patients, however, and every second AAA never progresses to surgery or rupture [33]. A multicenter study found that in 0.9% of patients, the aorta progressed from a subaneurysmal aortic dilation (diameter 2.5–2.9 cm) to the threshold for elective surgical intervention of 5.5 cm in as little as five years, while another quarter of patients reached this size after 10–15 years [34].

Smoking is the most important modifiable risk factor influencing growth rates [28,30,31]. Current smoking increases growth rates by about 20%. Notably, large aneurysms are also known to grow faster: the baseline aneurysm diameter is strongly associated with growth. The mean estimated growth rate increases by 0.59 mm per year for every 0.5 cm increase in the baseline diameter. For instance, an aneurysm of 3.0 cm in diameter grows an average of 1.3 mm/year, while a 5.0 cm aneurysm grows 3.6 mm per year [35]. Other factors influencing growth rates will be further explored in the chapter on risk factors.

3.2. Aneurysm Rupture

Rupture is the main complication of AAAs and is associated with mortality rates of 65–80% overall [12,36]. Approximately 150,000–200,000 deaths per year worldwide can be attributed to AAA rupture [37,38]. Incidence and mortality rates of ruptured AAAs (rAAAs) have been declining over the past decades, while diagnoses of intact AAAs have increased [25,39]. These developments correspond with the decline in smoking rates among men, as well as the implementation of screening programs and subsequent uptake in elective repairs [15,20]. Less common complications of AAAs include aortoenteric or aortocaval fistulae and iliac vein compression resulting in deep vein thrombosis or emboli [40–42].

The clinical presentation of a ruptured AAA is usually dramatic with sudden-onset abdominal, chest, or back pain, and hypotension or hemorrhagic shock due to massive intra-abdominal bleeding [43]. However, the classic triad of abdominal or back pain, shock, and a palpable clinical mass is only present in about 50% of rAAA cases, causing frequent misdiagnosis as myocardial infarction, ureteric colic, or perforated gastrointestinal ulcer [44]. The rupture varies in location and extent, but if not surgically repaired immediately, it typically leads to fatal internal bleeding [26]. Retroperitoneal (posterolateral) rupture is observed most frequently, at about 80%, where bleeding may be temporarily restrained by a tamponade effect [40]. Around 20% of ruptures occur anteriorly, with mostly rapid intraperitoneal bleeding and patient death. Rupture in combination with the formation of an aortocaval fistula (3–4%) or a primary aortoduodenal fistula (<1%) are comparably rare events [40].

AAA diameter is the strongest predictor of rupture. The link between diameter and rupture is well established and provides the basis for surveillance intervals for patients with small AAAs [35]. A 2013 meta-analysis found that rupture rates doubled for every 0.5 cm increase in diameter [28]. Furthermore, rapid aneurysm growth of over 2 mm per year significantly predicts AAA-related clinical events [33]. Other factors associated with increased risk of rupture are increased age, female sex, current smoking, and untreated hypertension, as well as aneurysm morphology [30,45].

4. Risk Factors and Comorbidities

Besides age and male sex, the strongest predictors of AAA are smoking and atherosclerotic cardiovascular diseases. Notably, in contrast to its role in atherosclerotic disease, type II diabetes is associated negatively with AAA.

4.1. Influence of Age and Sex

Age is one of the most important risk factors for the development of an AAA. Compared to a 40–44-year-old man, the risk is increased almost 200-fold for a 75–79-year-old man (0.83 versus 164 per 100,000) [20]. Fewer data exist regarding AAA incidence in women, but meta-analyses of epidemiological data and population screenings indicate that the AAA risk increases with age for women in a similar fashion, albeit on a lower level [12,46]. AAA prevalence rates for women are approximated at around 0.74–1.6%. However, it is estimated that with an adapted threshold value of 26–27 mm for women, based on a 50% increase in size from the average baseline, the AAA prevalence in 70-year-old women would more than double [47,48].

As for men, increased age and current smoking are the strongest risk factors for women [49,50]. Women tend to develop AAAs later in life compared to men, but the disease progresses more aggressively [51]. Thus, AAAs in women grow faster and their rupture risk is about four times higher than in men [28,52,53]. Women's AAAs tend to rupture at smaller diameters than men's [30,54,55], and although prevalence is 4–6 times lower than in men, almost every third patient presenting to the hospital with a ruptured AAA is female [56].

4.2. Ethnicity and Socioeconomic Factors

AAA prevalence is higher among men of Caucasian descent than among African-American, Hispanic, and Asian men, and these differences persist even after adjusting for all other known risk factors [5,49,57,58]. While white men in the USA are more likely to develop an AAA, non-white ethnic groups exhibit worse outcomes [59–62]. A multitude of individual and environmental factors might help explain these differences, but the proportion of their respective impact is not without controversy [57,63]. It seems that, rather than anatomical or biological differences, disparities between different ethnicities' courses of disease and outcomes may be mediated by the level of education, socioeconomic status, and disposable income [64,65]. These factors have been shown to be associated with screening attendance and AAA prevalence [66,67], as well as with rupture rates [59,61,68], even after adjusting for sex, age, and comorbidities. Educational level influences how patients view and manage their own health. For instance, lower education reduces adherence to preventive medication and decreases the success rate of smoking cessation [69,70]. A low educational level does not affect survival after AAA repair, but low disposable household income is associated with increased mortality after AAA repair, both short-term and over one year, regardless of ethnicity [68,71]. On a nonindividual level, discrepancies in management of risk factors and medical management by health care personnel may hold a certain influence [60].

4.3. Family History and Genetic Influences

Individuals with a first-degree relative with an AAA (i.e., parent, sibling, or offspring) have an increased risk of developing an AAA themselves (odds ratio, OR 1.96–3.8) [72–74]. Familial AAA cases tend to present at a younger age, and are associated with an increased growth rate and higher rupture rate compared to sporadic cases, even though aneurysm morphology does not seem to be different [75,76].

About 6–20% of AAA patients have a positive family history [73,77–79], but except for rare hereditary diseases, such as Marfan syndrome or Ehlers–Danlos syndrome [80], no distinct inheritance patterns have been identified to help explain familial AAA clusters. Two large twin studies have concluded that genetic factors may contribute as much as 77% to development of an AAA, with the remaining 23% attributed to individual and environmental factors, such as smoking [81,82]. In recent years, efforts have been made to identify genetic and epigenetic factors (including microRNAs and long noncoding RNAs) that contribute to AAA pathogenesis [83–85]. With respect to single nucleotide polymorphisms, gene variations associated with AAA were found to be manifold and partly shared with cardiovascular disease [84,85]. Thus, polygenic effects are likely to contribute to AAA pathogenesis. As of yet, the identified factors explain but a fraction of the heritability of aneurysmal disease, but they may help to elucidate pathophysiological processes and potentially serve as biomarkers or therapeutic targets in the future [86,87].

4.4. Smoking

Smoking is widely accepted as the key modifiable risk factor for AAA, as it contributes significantly to development, growth, and rupture of AAAs. It is estimated that 75% of all AAAs larger than 4.0 cm in diameter can be attributed to smoking [88]. In a USA screening study with 3.1 million participants, 80.2% of all AAAs were diagnosed in smokers when they comprised 42.8% of the cohort [49]. The effect of smoking on AAA development seems to be even stronger in women [48,89,90]. While a 10-fold, as opposed to 3-fold, risk to develop AAA is reported for current versus past female smokers, risk factor exposure in the pre- and/or post-menopausal period is rarely discriminated in studies on women with aneurysmal disease, and might offer further pathomechanistic insight [89].

Reported ORs for AAA development between smokers and nonsmokers range between 2.3 and 13.72 [57,77,91,92], making the association even stronger than between smoking and coronary heart disease or chronic obstructive pulmonary disease (COPD) [93,94]. COPD itself has also been suggested to be positively associated with AAA [95,96], independently of smoking [97]. While COPD does not seem to increase AAA growth [98], it does increase the risk of rupture at smaller diameters [99–101]. Smoking increases AAA growth rate by 15–24% and is associated with an increased risk of rupture, regardless of diameter (hazard ratio (HR) 2.02) [28,30–32].

The effect of nicotine consumption on AAA development seems to be dose-dependent, i.e., both duration and amount of smoking matter [49,65,92]. Every year of smoking increases the relative risk (RR) of AAA by 4% [102] and a recent meta-analysis found a summary RR of 1.87 per 10 cigarettes per day [103]. Current smokers have a particularly high risk, with an HR of 5.55 compared to an HR of 1.91 for former smokers [57]. Smoking cessation reduces the risk of AAA formation, aneurysm growth, and lowers rupture rates [30,104]. Reports indicate that it may take about ten years for the excess risk for former smokers to be halved, and that it does not approach the risk of never-smokers until at least 25 years after quitting [90,94,103].

4.5. Atherosclerosis and Cardiovascular Diseases

Atherosclerotic cardiovascular diseases (CVDs) and AAAs often coincide, and their intricate relationship entails commonalities, as well as distinct aspects in risk factors and pathomechanisms. The most striking discrepancy in risk profiles is the contrasting role of diabetes mellitus [105]. Generally, CVDs and AAAs are considered distinct disease entities [41,106].

AAA patients often have cardiovascular comorbidities and vice versa. High coprevalence rates of AAA and coronary artery disease (CAD) [107], peripheral artery disease (PAD) [11,108], and cerebrovascular disease [109] are well established [16,110]. Prevalence rates of AAA in CVD patients are higher than among the general population, with a greater effect of PAD than CAD or carotid atherosclerosis [49,110]. In addition to mere coprevalence, it has been shown that a history of atherosclerotic disease increases the risk of developing an AAA about fourfold, and this risk is amplified by having multiple or severe CVDs [77,107]. It is estimated that up to two thirds of AAA patients have a relevant CAD, and AAA prevalence is higher in patients with three-vessel disease versus a lower-degree CAD [111,112]. An Italian population-based study found the highest AAA prevalence in the subgroups with high cardiovascular risk, previous myocardial infarction, and stroke [113].

No consistent and robust association between CAD or PAD and increased or reduced AAA growth or rupture rates has been found [27,99,114,115]. However, AAA patients seem to be prone to higher disease severity of atherothrombotic diseases and are at risk for cardiovascular events [110]. Polyvascular disease, i.e., atherothrombosis in multiple vascular beds, was found to be twice as common in AAA patients as in non-AAA patients with other CVDs or with at least three cardiovascular risk factors (31.6% versus 15.5%). In the same study, AAA patients were found at greater risk for newly diagnosed or worsening PAD and showed increased rates of hospitalization for atherothrombotic events and revascularization procedures at the 1-year follow-up [110]. A patient with a small AAA is about 1.5 times more likely to suffer a cardiovascular event than a patient without an aortic aneurysm, and has a 3% risk of cardiovascular death per year [16,116]. Thus, despite high mortality rates of AAA ruptures, cardiovascular events remain among the most common causes of death in AAA patients [117,118].

4.6. Arterial Hypertension and Dyslipidemia

Pre-existing arterial hypertension increases the risk of developing an AAA significantly, with a stronger effect on women than on men [119]. While hypertension does not seem to be associated with AAA growth, hypertensive AAA patients do show an increased rate of aneurysm rupture [28,31,120]. Reports indicate a dose-dependent relationship between blood pressure and AAA, both for formation and rupture [30,119], and diastolic blood pressure might have a more pronounced effect than systolic [31]. It is estimated that the risk of rupture increases 1.11-fold for every 10 mmHg increase in mean blood pressure [30].

Dysregulated serum levels of total cholesterol, triglycerides, and lipoproteins are major risk factors for atherosclerosis and CVDs. Regarding AAA development, high serum high-density lipoprotein (HDL) levels have an undisputed protective effect (OR 0.7–0.83) [11,121,122], while data are not as homogenous with regards to total cholesterol (TC), low-density lipoprotein (LDL), or triglyceride levels. An analysis of historical and current laboratory data of patients from 12 years before their initial AAA diagnoses found that prior elevated TC, LDL, and triglyceride levels were significantly associated with current AAA (ORs 1.9, 2.3, and 1.9, respectively) [77]. Two meta-analyses found conflicting results, with one confirming that increased LDL levels are associated with AAA presence [121], while the other found no such association for LDL, but found a significant effect on AAA development for elevated total cholesterol levels [122]. Dyslipidemia does not seem to influence AAA growth or rupture rates [27].

Methodological differences between clinical studies and interindividual variations in lipid metabolism could contribute to contradictory results [41]. Some authors suggest that the traditional classification of cholesterol and triglycerides could be insufficient to determine the true contribution of dyslipidemia to AAA development [41,123].

4.7. Obesity and Lifestyle Habits

Studies investigating the influence of obesity and high body surface area on AAA development and growth have yielded conflicting results [124]. Both waist circumference and waist-to-hip ratio as measures for intra-abdominal fat mass, i.e., visceral adiposity, have been reported to be associated with the risk of AAA [125,126]. This association was stronger in AAAs with a diameter above 40 mm, and seemed to increase linearly with waist circumference up to a certain point [127,128]. However, no clear association of visceral adiposity on AAA development or growth has been found [129]. A high body mass index may, however, be associated with reduced AAA mortality [15,20]. This phenomenon known as the 'obesity paradox', i.e., an association between cardiovascular risk factors and an improvement in clinical outcomes, has been observed in other diseases as well [130]. Obstructive sleep apnea, often associated with adiposity, is common in AAA patients and may be a risk factor for aneurysm growth, but further studies are required to elucidate this relationship [131,132].

Regular exercise is generally safe for, and well tolerated by, patients with small AAAs and does not influence growth rates, but may reduce the risk of AAA development [133–135]. A well-balanced diet may reduce the risk of AAA, but studies analyzing diet quality in AAA patients are scarce [136,137]. A deficiency of vitamin D has been associated with AAA presence [138], and a recent experimental study showed that vitamin D deficiency promoted AAA growth and rupture in mice [139], but further clinical studies are needed to resolve whether a putative antioxidant effect of vitamin D would benefit AAA patients [140].

4.8. The Role of Diabetes Mellitus

Although diabetes mellitus is a major risk factor for occlusive CVDs, type II diabetes is associated negatively with AAA. Multiple meta-analyses of numerous large-scale epidemiological and clinical studies show that the risk of developing AAA as a diabetic patient is about half that of a nondiabetic [141–143]. Furthermore, diabetics show lower AAA growth rates than nondiabetic AAA patients. It is estimated that type II diabetes slows the annual growth of an AAA by 0.51–0.60 mm or about 25% [28,30,144]. A meta-analysis investigating rupture risk found that diabetes was associated with significantly lower rates of rupture [145]. However, diabetic patients show increased mortality after AAA repair and lower survival rates over 2–5 years [141], which may be an indication of the higher overall cardiovascular burden of diabetic patients [146].

This curious relationship between diabetes and AAA may be mediated by the hyperglycemic environment and thickened aortic wall prevalent in diabetics exerting protective effects both biochemically and mechanically [147]. Experimental studies support a possible attenuation effect of hyperglycemia on AAA development and growth [148,149]. In recent years, evidence has emerged that indicates the beneficial effect of diabetes on AAA may in fact be mediated by the antidiabetic medication metformin [150–152]. This aspect will be explored further in the chapter on pharmacological approaches to limit AAA growth.

5. Diagnosis and Management

Most intact AAAs are diagnosed incidentally when patients undergo imaging of the abdominal region for an unrelated condition. Besides ultrasonography and computed tomography, imaging modalities that may detect an AAA are diverse and include spinal imaging and echocardiography [153,154], though analyses of sensitivity and specificity for these modalities are scarce [155,156]. In some countries, systematic screening programs by ultrasonography are in place [157]. After initial diagnosis, all patients should be referred to a vascular surgeon to determine further proceedings [158].

5.1. Screening Programs

Long-term follow-up studies of large randomized controlled trials (RCTs) from the 1990s revealed that screening all 65-year-old men by one-time ultrasonography reduces AAA-related mortality by 42–66% [159,160], with corresponding ORs in favor of screening of 0.53–0.60 in meta-analyses [161,162]. Nationwide screening programs have since been implemented in several countries such as the USA, UK, and Sweden [157]. Recent results from these programs and large population-based trials confirm the benefits of screening men with regard to AAA-specific mortality, though there are conflicting results regarding all-cause mortality [161,162]. It is estimated that 667 men need to be screened in order to prevent one premature AAA-related death [163]. Based on this calculation, screening of 65-year-old men for AAA is considered cost-effective and was implemented as a preventive health measure in Sweden [163]. This strategy has been proposed to remain cost-effective, even if AAA rates should drop by half [164]. Yet, the declining prevalence of disease is one of the major arguments for the decision of other governments against nationwide screening programs.

Despite possible overdiagnoses, the psychological consequences of an AAA diagnosis, and decreasing incidence and prevalence rates, the benefits of screening men are commonly considered to outweigh the drawbacks [164–166]. Analyses of cost-effectiveness of screening for men also raise the question of targeted screenings for other at-risk groups. It is estimated that screening only male smokers between the ages of 65 and 75 leads to an AAA detection rate of about 30% in the population aged 50–84 [49]. While most current guidelines do not recommend population screenings for women, again mainly due to low prevalence and cost-effectiveness considerations [10,157], Canada has recently challenged this notion and proposed one-time screening by ultrasonography for women of advanced age with a history of smoking or cardiovascular disease [167]. No assessments of feasibility and cost-effectiveness have yet been performed for other candidate groups, such as patients with other peripheral aneurysms [168], cardiovascular diseases [113,169], or a subaneurysmal aortic dilation (2.5–2.9 cm in diameter) [32,170]. Some authors aim to develop scoring tools for possible refinement of AAA screening strategies [171,172].

5.2. Imaging Techniques

Ultrasonography (US) and computed tomography angiography (CTA) are first-line imaging tools for detection and management of AAAs. CTA is the gold standard for the diagnosis of AAA rupture, therapeutic decision making, and treatment planning, as well as post-surgical assessment and follow-up [173,174]. It provides detailed anatomical information on the entire aorta and its adjacent vessels, allowing assessment of the extent of the AAA, and of possible acute and chronic comorbid pathologies and, thus, exact planning of surgical intervention [175]. Due to its wide availability, rapid image acquisition, and lower radiation burden, CTA has virtually rendered conventional invasive angiography for the evaluation of AAA obsolete.

Duplex US is the recommended modality for screening and diagnosis of asymptomatic patients [158,176], as it allows safe, noninvasive, and fast detection of AAAs with high sensitivity and specificity [7,177]. It can also be used in emergency settings for rapid assessment of symptomatic patients [178], but emergency conditions with possible active bleeding after rupture or endoleaks after endovascular aneurysm repair (EVAR) usually warrant an additional CTA due to inherent methodological limitations of US scans. For instance, adjacent vessels may be difficult to assess, and imaging methodology influences diameter measurements [179–181]. With both US and CTA, standardization of methodology and reporting standards are crucial to obtain reliable results and to reduce intra- and interobserver variability [182,183].

Magnetic resonance angiography (MRA) shares many of the advantages of CTA imaging, with the added plus of not exposing the patient to radiation or requiring iodinated contrast agents. These factors make MRA a viable alternative for patients with certain allergies or renal insufficiency [183,184]. However, contraindications for MR such as claustrophobia and some metal implants have to be considered, and MR imaging is not suitable in emergency situations, such as impending or suspected rupture [185].

Molecular imaging by positron emission tomography–computed tomography (PET–CT) is not routinely used in standard care for AAA, but may add valuable information for diagnosis and follow-up of specific pathologies, such as inflammatory or mycotic AAA and infected stent grafts [186,187]. In vivo visualization of functional activity by uptake of radiotracers enables quantification of metabolic activity of cells and, thus, may facilitate further understanding of AAA pathogenesis and, in the future, possibly provide a novel diagnostic tool for clinical risk stratification [188,189].

5.3. Management of Small AAAs

As no pharmacological therapy has been established yet to slow AAA growth or prevent rupture, surgical repair is the only curative treatment for AAAs. Thus, disease management requires careful assessment and gauging of the surgical risk versus the risk of aneurysm rupture. For as long as the risk of elective surgical repair exceeds the risk of rupture, conservative management, i.e., watchful waiting while following the current guidelines on cardiovascular disease control by best medical care, is indicated [35]. The safety of this course of action has been determined by several RCTs and large studies comparing early elective repair to surveillance [190–193]. For patents with small AAAs, early elective repair offers no advantage, and surveillance, coupled with best medical care and lifestyle modification, is considered safe and cost-effective [194].

Regular monitoring of aneurysm growth and symptoms is recommended at intervals between three years for aneurysms of 3.0–3.9 cm diameter, annually for aneurysms of 4.0–4.9 cm, and every 3–6 months for AAAs with a diameter ≥ 5.0 cm [158,176], but may be adapted according to individual patient factors, such as fast aneurysm growth or high peak wall stress [35,195]. Insufficient monitoring of incidentally detected AAAs is associated with increased mortality [196,197].

5.3.1. Control of Cardiovascular Risk

While aneurysm diameter is an important measure of disease progression, adequate control of cardiovascular risk factors is crucial to improve outcomes [198,199]. Control of cardiovascular risk factors can be accomplished by lifestyle modifications and auxiliary medication to manage aggravating conditions, such as hypertension or dyslipidemia.

Cessation of smoking is a key component of CVD prevention or reduction, and additionally, significantly lowers post-surgical pulmonary complications if achieved more than eight weeks before elective AAA repair versus quitting short-term [200,201]. A well-balanced diet reduces CVD events and improves outcomes, and was suggested to be even more effective in reducing obesity compared to exercising [202,203]. Nevertheless, physical activity can alleviate the CVD-associated health risks of excess weight and improve surgical outcomes [133,204,205].

When indicated, pharmaceutical management of cardiovascular risk factors is recommended for all AAA patients, unless contraindicated [158,176]. In line with CVD risk assessment, statins are applied to reduce LDL cholesterol to <110 mg/dL for low risk, to <70 mg/dL for intermediate risk, and to <55 mg/dL for high risk [206,207]. Systolic blood pressure should be maintained below 140 mmHg. The choice of specific antihypertensive drug depends on individual comorbidities and tolerability, though diuretics may be less beneficial than other antihypertensive drug classes [118]. Antiplatelet agents are another constituent to prevent cardiovascular events in AAA patients. A UK study examining medication regimens of AAA patients showed that patients taking statins, antiplatelet therapy, or antihypertensive medication had significantly improved five-year survival rates (68% vs 42%, 64% vs 40%, and 62% vs 39%, respectively) [118].

5.3.2. Pharmacological Approaches to Limit AAA Growth

A wide range of drug classes has been investigated for possible benefits in AAA treatment, as we have previously reviewed [208], but as of yet, no medical therapy has been found sufficiently effective in reducing AAA growth or in preventing rupture to be implemented in the treatment guidelines [158,209,210].

Betablockers were the first drug class to be examined in the context of AAA growth reduction. While initial results seemed encouraging, larger studies and RCTs found low tolerability of the drug regimen and no beneficial effect of propranolol treatment on AAA expansion [211–213]. For another class of antihypertensive drugs, inhibitors of angiotensin-converting enzyme (ACE), all but one study revealed no effect on AAA expansion either [214–217]. The deviating result originated from a prospective cohort study that intriguingly found increased growth rates in patients taking ACE inhibitors [218].

Antibiotics were thought to be another promising drug class, as chlamydia pneumoniae has been implicated in AAA pathogenesis [219,220]. Although doxycycline was shown to significantly reduce plasma markers of proteolytic activity [221,222], clinical studies obtained contradictory results and a recent RCT reported no decline in AAA growth [223–225]. Results for the macrolide antibiotics roxithromycin and azithromycin were similarly discouraging [226–228].

The influence of statins on AAA growth has been discussed controversially, as clinical studies were not able to consistently reproduce the promising results of experimental investigations but showed heterogeneity of outcome. Several meta-analyses tentatively support the ability of statins to reduce AAA growth [229–231], while others err on the side of caution [232]. Furthermore, ethical considerations and guidelines limit performing RCTs on statins, as they significantly increase 5-year survival rates in AAA patients [118,233].

Several other drug classes, such as nonsteroidal anti-inflammatory drugs [234], mast cell inhibitors [235], calcium channel blockers, diuretics, and angiotensin II receptor blockers [213,236] have been investigated clinically after showing promise in experimental studies, but none of these studies were able to show a reduction in AAA growth. Antiplatelet therapy by acetylsalicylic acid or ticagrelor seemed another auspicious treatment approach [237–239], but only one subanalysis of a small azithromycin RCT was able to detect a significant effect of acetylsalicylic acid on growth rate [228]. Currently, several RCTs are ongoing with hopes of finding a medical treatment for AAA [240–243].

An avenue of research that raises hope for successful AAA treatment in the future is a well-established antidiabetic medication. The previously observed protective effect of diabetes mellitus on AAA progression may not actually be inherent to the disease, but rather attributable to concurrent treatment with metformin [151,152,244]. Experimental studies were investigating a range of medications such as thiazolidinediones and dipeptidyl peptidase-4 inhibitors [245,246], but metformin seems to be the only drug consistently associated with reduced AAA growth in clinical studies [247]. Currently, two ongoing clinical trials [242,243] and a shortly upcoming study [248] are investigating whether metformin reduces AAA progression in nondiabetic patients, one of them at the Division of Vascular Surgery of the Medical University of Vienna [242].

Future perspectives of pharmacological approaches to limit AAA growth also include nucleic acid drugs that target mRNAs, microRNAs, or transcription factors in a sequence-specific manner to interfere with key molecules in AAA pathogenesis [249].

5.4. Surgical Treatment

Surgical repair is the only curative treatment for AAAs and is indicated when the risk of rupture exceeds the surgical risk. Nowadays, about 85% of AAA repairs are performed electively for intact aneurysms, though there are significant regional variations [250]. Naturally, a ruptured AAA is a surgical emergency that requires immediate repair, with a significant mortality of up to 85% [251,252].

Based on data from several RCTs comparing early elective repair to surveillance [194,253], current guidelines recommend elective AAA repair for asymptomatic fusiform AAAs at an aneurysm diameter of 5.5 cm in men and 5.0 cm in women, if the surgical risk is acceptable [158,176]. Some authors suggest reevaluation of the threshold for surgical repair for women in future guidelines [254], as the current cutoff diameters signify a larger relative rupture risk for women than for men [255,256]. Earlier elective repair should also be considered for saccular AAAs [257,258]. In the case of a rapid expansion rate of >10 mm/year or incident symptoms referable to the aneurysm, additional imaging for confirmation and then fast-track referral to a vascular surgeon is recommended, even at small diameters [259,260].

5.4.1. Open Surgical Repair

Open AAA repair aims to replace the aneurysmal wall by a synthetic vascular graft. The surgery involves a laparotomy, usually by midline incision, and transperitoneal or retroperitoneal exposure of the proximal abdominal aorta just below the renal arteries [261]. Depending on the aneurysm's morphology and size, either tube-shaped or bifurcated grafts can be used. After aortic cross clamping under full heparinization [262], the proximal end-to-end anastomosis is performed as close as possible to the renal arteries to counteract development of another aneurysm in the remaining infrarenal aortic portion [263]. The exact location of the distal dissection site depends on the individual's anatomy, the AAA's extent, and concomitant conditions, such as local atherosclerotic burden or an aneurysm of the iliac arteries. Finally, the aneurysm sac is closed over the graft.

Perioperative complications of open surgical repair (OSR) are mainly of cardiac, pulmonary, or renal nature, such as myocardial infarction, pneumonia, or renal insufficiency [264]. Postoperative wound complications can affect a patient's recovery severely [265], and midline laparotomy incisions are more prone to incisional hernias [266,267]. Long-term complications include graft infections, formation of secondary aorto-enteric fistulas, graft limb occlusion, or formation of a para-anastomotic aneurysm [268,269].

5.4.2. Endovascular Aneurysm Repair

EVAR does not aim to replace the aneurysmal sac, but excludes it from systemic circulation by minimally invasive implantation of a stent graft [270]. The stent graft is delivered to the abdominal aorta through the femoral artery, either by a percutaneous approach or by a surgical cut-down [271]. After confirmation of the exact vessel measurements by digital subtraction angiography, the delivery system is inserted over a stiff guidewire and then deployed and ballooned to expand and attach the stent graft to the aortic wall. Fixation and sealing of the stent grafts require certain morphological attributes, such as low angulation of the neck, and a certain length and diameter of the proximal and distal fixation sites [272]. Enhanced modular, fenestrated, bifurcated, or branched stent graft designs facilitate precise tailoring to individual anatomy, and allow for anatomical deviations such as accessory vessels, inadequate landing zones, or concomitant conditions [273,274].

Inadequate sizing or improper placement of the stent graft can cause various complications such as endoleaks from inadequate sealing or kinking of the stent graft with subsequent limb occlusion [275,276]. An endoleak is defined as persistent blood flow inside the aneurysm sac, resulting in a rise in pressure, renewed aneurysm growth, and eventual rupture. The various types of endoleaks are the most common complication of EVAR and often require reintervention [277]. Other complications of EVAR include problems related to the access site, especially when the iliac arteries are small, calcified or severely tortuous [271], and a systemic inflammatory response termed 'post-implantation syndrome' in the early postoperative phase [278]. Complex endovascular aortic repair should only be advised at tertiary university hospitals, due to the necessary case numbers for experience in both complex EVAR and OSR, in case of complication management [273,274].

Another novel concept, termed endovascular aneurysm sealing, relies on complete sealing of the aneurysm sac by way of surrounding the stent graft with polymer-filled endobags [279], but long-term durability is questionable [280–282].

5.4.3. Comparison of Surgical Methods

The choice of surgical technique depends on the aneurysm's morphology and on patient characteristics, such as comorbidities and functional capacity [283,284]. Another consideration is the patient's ability and willingness to adhere to necessary follow-up surveillance [285,286], as EVAR requires life-long surveillance with regular imaging, owing to the risk of late-onset endoleak, stent graft migration, or infection [287].

Exact assessment of anatomical and morphological attributes by pre-operative CT or MR angiography is crucial to ensure the best possible outcome [288]. With both OSR and EVAR, due care has to be exercised with regard to branch vessels to ensure adequate blood flow in renal, superior mesenteric, lumbar, and internal iliac supply zones to prevent postoperative sexual dysfunction and ischemic complications caused by inadequate pelvic circulation [289–291].

While initially intended for patients deemed unfit for OSR, EVAR has since become the method of choice if technically feasible, and nowadays, more than three quarters of elective AAA repairs are performed endovascularly [158,176]. With this dynamic change in the ratio of OSR to EVAR, a minimum of >30 cases annually per center is required in both techniques to achieve the required expertise [158,176]. A major advantage of EVAR over OSR is that it can be performed under local or epidural as well as general anesthesia, rendering it a possibility for patients with severe cardiac and pulmonary comorbidities [292,293]. However, the endovascular approach does not offer any long-term survival benefits in patients considered too physically frail for open AAA repair [294]. In patients currently unfit for elective surgery, optimization of functional capacity and overall cardiovascular health should be pursued before reassessment of surgical eligibility [294,295].

Open AAA repair is indicated for patients whose vessels do not meet the requirements of endovascular repair, for instance due to short landing zones or excessive thrombus formation [296]. OSR may also be required for treatment of certain EVAR-specific complications such as persistent endoleaks or aneurysm sac growth, as well as for patients with an inflammatory aneurysm or an infected graft.

5.4.4. Outcome of Elective AAA Repair

After the advent of EVAR in the 1990s, several RCTs aimed to evaluate outcomes of EVAR versus OSR for elective AAA repairs. A 2014 meta-analysis of these trials and more recent studies found that EVAR has better short-term outcomes than OSR in both morbidity and mortality [270]. Compared to OSR, cardiopulmonary complications are significantly lower in EVAR due to its minimally invasive approach. It is not surprising, therefore, that patients with EVAR benefit from a faster recovery and shorter length of hospital stay. EVAR's early benefits are offset against lower durability. Due to graft-related complications, the reintervention rates and AAA-related mortality are significantly higher for EVAR compared to OSR [264]. In the long term, outcomes balance out, and long-term return of functional level and health-related quality of life are similar between OSR and EVAR for elective AAA repair [297]. Despite the need for continuous follow-up and high rate of reinterventions, EVAR remains cost-effective when compared to OSR [298].

EVAR is associated with lower 30-day mortality (1.4% for EVAR, 4.2% for OSR) and a higher survival rate for up to one year after the repair [264,270,299]. However, this survival advantage is lost around the 2–4-year mark of follow-up, and long-term all-cause survival is similar for EVAR and OSR. Median survival after elective AAA repair is about 9 years, with cardiovascular and pulmonary diseases constituting the main causes of death [117,264,300]. Adequate management of cardiovascular risk factors improves long-term survival after AAA repair [301].

Besides advanced age and presence of cardiac, pulmonary, and renal comorbidities, frailty and preoperative functional status are predictors of postoperative morbidity and mortality [302–304]. Female sex, aneurysm diameter, and smoking habits are also associated with poor long-term survival. The worse outcomes for women may be due to a higher frequency of disadvantageous neck anatomy, but these anatomical differences do not seem to account for all differences in outcomes between men and women [56,305]. Increased cancer mortality rates in EVAR patients when compared to OSR have also raised concerns about long-term radiation exposure during EVAR follow-up [306].

5.4.5. Management of the Ruptured AAA

A ruptured AAA with acute hemorrhage into the intra- or retroperitoneal space is a surgical emergency. Depending on the hemodynamic situation, an immediate CTA, or alternatively, an intraoperative angiography is indicated to confirm the diagnosis and evaluate anatomical suitability for EVAR [307,308]. Both OSR and EVAR can be used for rAAA repair, with EVAR being the method of choice if anatomically feasible. EVAR and open surgery for rAAA have comparable morbidity rates and show no difference in cardiac or respiratory failure [251]. Reintervention rates are similar, as well, and EVAR is consistently associated with faster discharge and a gain in quality-adjusted life years, rendering it cost-effective [309].

As with elective AAA repairs, use of EVAR for rAAA repair has increased massively in the past two decades [251,252]. Analyses of earlier versus later cohorts show that outcomes have improved in recent years for both EVAR and OSR [310,311]. High mortality rates of unsuccessful EVAR for rAAA suggest that anatomical suitability and not hemodynamic condition should be the pivotal factor in choosing the surgical method for rAAA repair [251,312,313].

6. Pathogenesis

The development of an AAA is an intricate process of several pathomechanisms and is still not fully understood. Ignited by a possibly diverse initial trigger, a destructive process of oxidative stress, apoptosis of vascular smooth muscle cells (VSMCs), and proteolytic fragmentation of the extracellular matrix (ECM) are set in motion, potentiated by an inflammatory immune response. These key processes perturb the equilibrium between regenerative and degrading processes that normally ensures physiological tissue remodeling and injury repair. Now malfunctioning, the aortic wall becomes progressively eroded and weakened, dilates, and finally ruptures when it can no longer withstand the hemodynamic forces placed upon it.

6.1. Intraluminal Thrombosis and Biomechanical Aspects

The infrarenal portion of the aorta is especially prone to aneurysms, due to hemodynamic and mechanical characteristics. Due to the blood stream's impact on the iliac bifurcation, pressure-reflective waves within the blood are common in the infrarenal aorta. These disturbances lead to a higher number of collisions of circulating cells amongst each other and against the aortic wall. Endothelial injuries and atherosclerotic lesions often form at such locations, and the high wall stress and strain caused by the aortic blood stream likely contribute to the persistence of the endothelial injury at this location [314,315].

Historically, AAA was thought to be a particular, localized form of atherosclerosis, as most AAAs present with cholesterol and calcium deposits. The exact nature of the relationship between atherosclerosis and AAA is still a matter of discussion [106]. In both diseases, an atherosclerotic plaque may form on the basis of an intimal lesion and subsequently replace the subendothelium. In occlusive atherosclerotic diseases, inward remodeling of the aortic wall usually leads to a decrease in vessel lumen until either an erosion- or rupture-triggered thrombus itself or an embolus cause occlusion of the vessel to a hemodynamically relevant degree. Different theories have been proposed as to the role of the gradually forming intraluminal thrombus (ILT) in about 75% of AAA cases, such as a propensity of the aortic wall of AAA patients towards outwards remodeling in an attempt to maintain the vessel lumen [41,316,317].

Whether causally associated or a subsequent byproduct, the ILT provides the aneurysmal wall with a certain biomechanical protection against wall stress [318,319]. Permeation of the ILT with blood or contrast medium may announce the impending failure of the ILT as a protective layer. This distinguishing mark is visible as a 'crescent sign' in CTA [320] and is associated with AAA rupture [174,321,322]. However, clinical data support the notion that the ILT's active role in disruption of the wall's integrity exceeds its biomechanical protection. Indeed, presence of an ILT is associated with an increased rupture risk, especially in patients with small AAAs and when the thrombus encompasses the whole circumference of the aneurysm [45,323,324].

The ILT in AAA is a biologically active, dynamic component that contributes to the pivotal destruction and inflammation of the aortic wall's medial and adventitial layers [325–327]. The presence of an ILT in an AAA is associated with reduced thickness of the artery wall, greater elastolysis, lower VSMC content in the medial layer, and a higher level of inflammatory immune response in the adventitia [328]. Clinical data also show that the presence of an ILT is associated with faster AAA growth [329], which may be due to its biological activity [330,331], rather than size or volume [332–334].

The blood stream constantly replenishes the ILT's luminal side with fibrinogen and circulating cellular elements, such as platelets, erythrocytes, and immune cells [335]. The ILT entraps these cells, which release oxidative enzymes, proteases and proinflammatory cytokines [336–338]. Due to the high pressure gradient between the aortic blood flow and the interstitial tissue, the cells and released molecules are pushed outward towards the abluminal side through a canalicular system pervading the ILT [325]. Thus, the ILT contributes to the generation of a toxic environment that contributes to the decay and inflammation of the subjacent medial and adventitial layers of the aortic wall, as we have previously highlighted [339].

6.2. Oxidative Stress and VSMC Apoptosis

As mentioned above, the ILT accumulates blood cells, i.e., platelets, erythrocytes, and leukocytes. The adverse environment increases reactivity of entrapped cells, which in turn boost oxidative stress by mediating production of reactive nitrogen and oxygen species (ROS) [324,340,341]. These excess oxygen- and nitrogen-derived free radicals then activate proteolytic enzymes, trigger degradation processes, and induce apoptosis of VSMCs and mesenchymal progenitor cells [324,342]. This not only destabilizes the medial layer of the aortic wall, but also impedes its matrix-producing and -repairing capacities. Proinflammatory signals further stimulate VSMC apoptosis [343,344].

Excessive cell death and dedifferentiation ('phenotypic switch') of contractile VSMCs is characteristic of the aneurysmal aortic wall [345,346]. Loss of VSMCs puts additional hemodynamic stress on the weakened wall, which responds by stimulating angiogenesis in the medial layer [347,348]. Furthermore, the ILT in place of the endothelium causes localized hypoxia in the underlying AAA wall, which is an additional trigger for angiogenesis. However, medial neovascularization further instigates the destructive cycle because it facilitates infiltration of circulating inflammatory cells [349,350].

Clinical data support the importance of oxidative stress in AAA pathogenesis [351]. Excess levels of ROS have been detected in the blood of AAA patients and in AAA wall tissue, but not in the adjacent nonaneurysmal aorta or in healthy individuals [340,352].

These ROS stem from a variety of oxidative enzymes shown to be upregulated in expression and activity in aneurysmal aortic walls [353,354]. In mice, loss of antioxidants was found to increase AAA incidence and rupture rate [355]. Correspondingly, experimental activation of antioxidant enzymes, such as catalase, reduces AAA formation in mice [356–358], but a benefit of ROS-suppression in humans has not been shown yet [343].

6.3. Proteolysis

The destruction of the three-dimensional ECM network of the medial layer of the aortic wall is considered a key feature of AAA pathogenesis. Excessive dismantling of structure-bearing components reduces the wall's ability to withstand the hemodynamic load and leads to dilation of the aorta [359,360]. The physiological tissue remodeling process becomes unbalanced and tilts towards an overactivity of proteases that disintegrate the fibrillar ECM components, such as collagen and elastin [361–363]. Protease substrates also include cell adhesion molecules, thereby promoting VSMC detachment and apoptosis [344,364,365]. In addition, proteolytic enzymes augment AAA pathogenesis by activating ECM-contained, latent matrix metalloproteinases (MMPs), and by mediating inflammation and angiogenesis [366–369]. In turn, inflammatory conditions and oxidative stress boost production and activation of proteases, creating a destructive circle [370,371].

Several protease families have been implicated in the pathogenesis of AAAs. Clinical data show increased levels of MMPs, especially MMP-9 and MMP-2, cathepsins, and neutrophil elastase in blood and tissue samples of the aneurysmal wall of AAA patients, while their antagonists are reduced [122,372,373]. Population-based studies showed that high cathepsin levels are associated with higher AAA risk and a larger diameter [374,375]. MMP-9 plasma levels were reported to decrease after AAA repair [376,377]. In rodent studies, cathepsin deficiency was found to reduce aneurysm severity [378–380], and both MMP-2 and MMP-9 knockout mice were protected from AAA development compared to wild-type mice [381,382]. However, despite their central role in AAA development, unselective MMP inhibition by doxycycline has been unsuccessful in attenuating AAA growth in humans [223,224], illustrating that complex interactions and multiple mechanisms are at play.

6.4. Inflammation

Aneurysmal aortic wall tissue is characterized by infiltration of both innate and adaptive immune cells. At the luminal side, the ILT recruits circulating leukocytes, which then migrate towards the media. Diapedesis is facilitated by the medial layer's angiogenesis, hemodynamic factors, as well as by activation of the complement system [383–385]. Other entry points for immune cells to infiltrate the aortic wall are periadventitial lymph nodes and adventitial vasa vasorum. Development of tertiary lymphoid organs in the adventitia by a concerted collaboration of B-lymphocytes, follicular dendritic cells, and CD4+ T-helper-cells has been described [386,387]. Ectopic adipocytes in perivascular tissue promote recruitment and activity of immune cells by releasing proinflammatory cytokines, such as tumor necrosis factor alpha (TNF-α), IL-6, IL-8 [388,389], and may also mediate an autoimmune response [390].

Cytokines released by both innate and adaptive immune cells contribute to the inflammatory environment in the AAA wall. High levels of adventitial CD4+ T-helper-cells and macrophages mediate recruitment and activation of inflammatory cells, establishing a vicious circle of chronic inflammation of the aortic wall, while also boosting proteolysis and oxidative tissue injury [341,391]. Circulating levels of Th1- and Th2-secreted cytokines such as IFN-γ, TNF-α, IL-4, and IL-22 are consistently elevated in AAA patients [392,393]. IFN-γ and IL-17 secreted by CD8+ T-cells and Th17 CD4+ T-cells have also been implicated in AAA pathogenesis [394–396]. B-cell-derived immunoglobulins such as IgG4 and IgE drive macrophage and mast cell activation and degranulation [397,398]. Regulatory CD4+ T-cells have a protective function by releasing anti-inflammatory cytokines such as IL-10 and TGF-β [399–401], but both regulatory CD4+ cells and their mediators are reduced in AAA patients [402].

A prospective clinical study using enhanced MR imaging has shown that the degree of aortic wall inflammation predicts AAA growth and rupture [331]. The crucial role of inflammation is supported by a number of experimental rodent studies showing that depletion of immune cells, in particular myeloid cells, diminishes or abolishes AAA growth [41,403].

6.5. Myeloid cells in AAA

6.5.1. Monocytes and Macrophages in AAA

Monocytes and macrophages have been consistently detected in AAA tissue of both rodent disease models and humans [404–407]. These immune cells of myeloid origin infiltrate early in aneurysm development, and predominantly accumulate in the inner adventitial layer of the aneurysmal aortic wall [349]. Monocyte and macrophage chemoattractants and activation parameters (e.g., chemokine ligand [CCL] 2, also referred to as monocyte chemoattractant protein 1, MCP-1 [393,408], CCL3 alias macrophage inflammatory protein-1a, MIP-1a [408]), receptors (e.g., chemokine C-X-C receptor 4, CXCR4 [409], triggering receptor expressed on myeloid cells-1, TREM-1 [410]) have been shown to be significantly increased in rodent models, AAA patient plasma, and aneurysmal wall tissue. Blocking or depleting the involved ligands or pertaining receptors inhibits AAA formation and progression in animal models (e.g., C-C chemokine receptor type 2, CCR2 [404], CXCR4 [409], CCL5 [411]).

Monocytes and macrophages contribute to AAA pathogenesis in various ways, depending on the functional characteristics of their subtype. Monocytes can be classified into distinct subsets [412,413] that assume different roles in the elimination of pathogens and maintenance of vessel integrity [414–416]. For instance, CD16-expressing monocytes with tissue-remodeling and proangiogenic features are associated with AAA diameter, and have been reported to be significantly elevated in AAA patient plasma [408,417,418]. Similarly, macrophages exhibit two distinct phenotypes that have opposing functions in mediating inflammatory processes [419]. An imbalance between the two macrophage phenotypes can create either a chronic inflammatory milieu or impairment of wound healing and tissue homeostasis [420]. Although analyses of AAA tissue have not yielded conclusive results to such a disproportion [407,421], rodent studies indicate that proinflammatory, destructive M1 macrophages may predominate during early stages of AAA development [422]. The proteinases and proinflammatory mediators released by M1 macrophages in close collaboration with T-cells contribute to aneurysmal wall degradation [407,423]. New data suggest that the M2 macrophage may not be entirely protective [424], as experimental rodent studies investigating macrophage polarization from M1 to M2 have claimed that M2 polarization can either suppress or attenuate AAA development [425–427].

6.5.2. Neutrophils in AAA

Neutrophils pose a crucial first line of defense in the innate immune system, as they are the most numerous type of granulocytes (or 'polymorphonuclear leukocytes') and can employ several effector mechanisms to eliminate pathogens [428]. As we have recently reviewed [429,430], neutrophils are recruited to the aneurysm site by various chemotactic factors, such as IL-8, platelet-derived factors or complement components. These mediators are mainly released from the luminal ILT and have been shown to be increased in the blood of AAA patients [337,393,431]. In rodent models, blockage or depletion of neutrophil chemotactic factors can impede or completely abolish AAA development by suspending neutrophil recruitment [383,432]. For instance, dipeptidyl peptidase I (DPPI) regulates the activity of neutrophil-secreted proteases, but also mediates neutrophil recruitment to the aneurysm site. Functional deficiency of DDPI has been shown to cause impaired local production of a neutrophil chemotactic factor and thereby protect mice from elastase-induced AAA formation [432].

Elevated levels of activated neutrophils have been detected in AAA wall tissue [337,349], as well as in AAA patient plasma in comparison to healthy controls, even after adjustment for known confounders such as smoking [408,433]. Activation of neutrophils induces degranulation, i.e., the release of cytotoxic contents of the neutrophil's cytoplasmic granules into the phagosome or into the extracellular space [434]. Besides bactericidal peptides (e.g., lactoferrin), defensins, and proteinases (e.g., neutrophil elastase, collagenase, cathepsins), neutrophil granules release myeloperoxidase (MPO) and nicotinamide adenine dinucleotide phosphate oxidase (NADPH oxidase or NOX). MPO and NOX enzymes are major sources of ROS and have been detected at high levels in AAA tissue and AAA patient plasma, while antioxidants such as catalase are reduced [351,352,435].

ECM degradation is facilitated by several neutrophil-mediated mechanisms. MPO has been shown to inactivate tissue inhibitors of MMPs, thereby increasing MMP activity [436]. Furthermore, neutrophils release neutrophil-gelatinase-associated lipocalin (NGAL), which binds MMP-9 and inhibits its degradation [338]. High concentrations of NGAL-MMP-9-complexes are present especially in the luminal ILT [335,337], and are higher in aneurysmal aortic wall samples compared to healthy aortas [437]. Neutrophil-secreted proteases directly cleave stabilizing ECM components, but can also activate MMPs [366,438,439]. Fragments of the dismantled elastin and collagen fibers then promote inflammation further by serving as chemotactic factors themselves [440–442]. As mentioned above, DPPI is not only necessary for activation of neutrophil-secreted proteases, but also vitally mediates inflammation of the aneurysmal aortic wall [432].

A 2005 study showed neutrophil-depleted mice to be protected from AAA formation [403]. However, contrary to the expected, this was only in part mediated by a decrease in MMP activity, suggesting that neutrophils critically contribute to AAA pathogenesis by another, independent mechanism. A novel effector mechanism of neutrophils, the formation of neutrophil extracellular traps (or 'NETs'), has since been implicated in AAA pathogenesis [443–445], which is the current focus of our research efforts [430,446].

7. Conclusions

Even though world-wide changes in smoking habits and other lifestyle factors have contributed to declining incidence and mortality rates of AAA, its prevalence and high death rate upon vessel rupture remain a subject of concern. Progress has been made in unraveling the multifactorial process of pathogenesis, in particular the components of chronic inflammation. This has led to promising candidates for conservative treatment such as metformin, an antidiabetes drug with pleiotropic anti-inflammatory effects, which is currently being tested in several prospective clinical trials to prevent AAA progression. Yet to date, surgical repair remains the only curative approach, but is associated with a considerable morbidity and mortality. The rise in endovascular versus open surgical interventions has revealed the challenge of establishing sufficient institutional expertise in both procedures in order to appropriately address patient needs.

Author Contributions: Conceptualization, V.K. and C.B.; writing—original draft preparation, V.K.; writing—review and editing, V.K., J.K., W.E., C.N. and C.B.; supervision, W.E., C.N. and C.B.; project administration, W.E., C.N. and C.B.; funding acquisition, C.B. All authors have read and agreed to the published version of the manuscript.

Funding: This work was funded by the Austrian Science Fund FWF, grant number F 5409-B21.

Institutional Review Board Statement: Not applicable.

Informed Consent Statement: Not applicable.

Data Availability Statement: Not applicable.

Conflicts of Interest: The authors declare no conflict of interest.

References

1. Johnston, K.; Rutherford, R.B.; Tilson, M.; Shah, D.M.; Hollier, L.; Stanley, J.C. Suggested Standards for Reporting on Arterial Aneurysms. Subcommittee on Reporting Standards for Arterial Aneurysms, Ad Hoc Committee on Reporting Standards, Society for Vascular Surgery and North American Chapter, International Society for Cardiovascular Surgery. *J. Vasc. Surg.* **1991**, *13*, 452–458. [CrossRef] [PubMed]
2. Matsumoto, T. Anatomy and Physiology for the Abdominal Aortic Aneurysm Repair. *Ann. Vasc. Dis.* **2019**, *12*, 329–333. [CrossRef]
3. Takayama, T.; Yamanouchi, D. Aneurysmal Disease: The Abdominal Aorta. *Surg. Clin. North Am.* **2013**, *93*, 877–891. [CrossRef] [PubMed]
4. Golledge, J.; Muller, J.; Daugherty, A.; Norman, P. Abdominal Aortic Aneurysm: Pathogenesis and implications for management. *Arter. Thromb. Vasc. Biol.* **2006**, *26*, 2605–2613. [CrossRef]
5. Lederle, F.A.; Johnson, G.R.; Wilson, S.E.; Chute, E.P.; Littooy, F.N.; Bandyk, D.F.; Krupski, W.C.; Barone, G.W.; Acher, C.W.; Ballard, D.J. Prevalence and Associations of Abdominal Aortic Aneurysm Detected through Screening. Aneurysm Detection and Management (ADAM) Veterans Affairs Cooperative Study Group. *Ann. Intern. Med.* **1997**, *126*, 441–449. [CrossRef]
6. Rogers, I.S.; Massaro, J.; Truong, Q.A.; Mahabadi, A.A.; Kriegel, M.F.; Fox, C.S.; Thanassoulis, G.; Isselbacher, E.M.; Hoffmann, U.; O'Donnell, C.J. Distribution, Determinants, and Normal Reference Values of Thoracic and Abdominal Aortic Diameters by Computed Tomography (from the Framingham Heart Study). *Am. J. Cardiol.* **2013**, *111*, 1510–1516. [CrossRef] [PubMed]
7. Lindholt, J.; Vammen, S.; Juul, S.; Henneberg, E.; Fasting, H. The Validity of Ultrasonographic Scanning as Screening Method for Abdominal Aortic Aneurysm. *Eur. J. Vasc. Endovasc. Surg.* **1999**, *17*, 472–475. [CrossRef] [PubMed]
8. Steinberg, C.R.; Archer, M.; Steinberg, I. Measurement of the Abdominal Aorta after Intravenous Aortography in Health and Arteriosclerotic Peripheral Vascular Disease. *Am. J. Roentgenol. Radium Ther. Nucl. Med.* **1965**, *95*, 703–708. [CrossRef]
9. Li, K.; Zhang, K.; Li, T.; Zhai, S. Primary results of abdominal aortic aneurysm screening in the at-risk residents in middle China. *BMC Cardiovasc. Disord.* **2018**, *18*, 60. [CrossRef] [PubMed]
10. Sweeting, M.J.; Masconi, K.L.; Jones, E.; Ulug, P.; Glover, M.J.; Michaels, J.A.; Bown, M.J.; Powell, J.T.; Thompson, S.G. Analysis of clinical benefit, harms, and cost-effectiveness of screening women for abdominal aortic aneurysm. *Lancet* **2018**, *392*, 487–495. [CrossRef]
11. Tang, W.; Yao, L.; Roetker, N.S.; Alonso, A.; Lutsey, P.L.; Steenson, C.C.; Lederle, F.A.; Hunter, D.W.; Bengtson, L.G.; Guan, W.; et al. Lifetime Risk and Risk Factors for Abdominal Aortic Aneurysm in a 24-Year Prospective Study: The ARIC Study (Atherosclerosis Risk in Communities). *Arter. Thromb. Vasc. Biol.* **2016**, *36*, 2468–2477. [CrossRef]
12. Li, X.; Zhao, G.; Zhang, J.; Duan, Z.; Xin, S. Prevalence and Trends of the Abdominal Aortic Aneurysms Epidemic in General Population—A Meta-Analysis. *PLoS ONE* **2013**, *8*, e81260. [CrossRef]
13. Savji, N.; Rockman, C.; Skolnick, A.H.; Guo, Y.; Adelman, M.; Riles, T.; Berger, J.S. Association between Advanced Age and Vascular Disease in Different Arterial Territories: A Population Database of over 3.6 Million Subjects. *J. Am. Coll. Cardiol.* **2013**, *61*, 1736–1743. [CrossRef] [PubMed]
14. Stather, P.; Sidloff, D.; Rhema, I.; Choke, E.; Bown, M.; Sayers, R. A Review of Current Reporting of Abdominal Aortic Aneurysm Mortality and Prevalence in the Literature. *Eur. J. Vasc. Endovasc. Surg.* **2014**, *47*, 240–242. [CrossRef]
15. Sidloff, D.; Stather, P.; Dattani, N.; Bown, M.; Thompson, J.; Sayers, R.; Choke, E. Aneurysm Global Epidemiology Study: Public Health Measures Can Further Reduce Abdominal Aortic Aneurysm Mortality. *Circulation* **2014**, *129*, 747–753. [CrossRef]
16. Bath, M.F.; Gokani, V.J.; Sidloff, D.A.; Jones, L.R.; Choke, E.; Sayers, R.D.; Bown, M. Systematic review of cardiovascular disease and cardiovascular death in patients with a small abdominal aortic aneurysm. *BJS* **2015**, *102*, 866–872. [CrossRef]
17. Hultgren, R.; Granath, F.; Swedenborg, J. Different Disease Profiles for Women and Men with Abdominal Aortic Aneurysms. *Eur. J. Vasc. Endovasc. Surg.* **2007**, *33*, 556–560. [CrossRef] [PubMed]
18. Ashton, H.A.; Gao, L.; Kim, L.; Druce, P.S.; Thompson, S.G.; Scott, R.A.P. Fifteen-year follow-up of a randomized clinical trial of ultrasonographic screening for abdominal aortic aneurysms. *Br. J. Surg.* **2007**, *94*, 696–701. [CrossRef]
19. Lederle, F.A. The Rise and Fall of Abdominal Aortic Aneurysm. *Circulation* **2011**, *124*, 1097–1099. [CrossRef] [PubMed]
20. Sampson, U.K.; Norman, P.E.; Fowkes, F.G.R.; Aboyans, V.; Song, Y.; Harrell, F.E.H., Jr.; Forouzanfar, M.H.; Naghavi, M.; Denenberg, J.O.; McDermott, M.M.; et al. Estimation of Global and Regional Incidence and Prevalence of Abdominal Aortic Aneurysms 1990 to 2010. *Glob. Hear.* **2014**, *9*, 159–170. [CrossRef] [PubMed]
21. Anjum, A.; von Allmen, R.; Greenhalgh, R.; Powell, J.T. Explaining the decrease in mortality from abdominal aortic aneurysm rupture. *Br. J. Surg.* **2012**, *99*, 637–645. [CrossRef]
22. Png, C.M.; Wu, J.; Tang, T.Y.; Png, I.P.; Sheng, T.J.; Choke, E. Editor's Choice—Decrease in Mortality from Abdominal Aortic Aneurysms (2001 to 2015): Is it Decreasing Even Faster? *Eur. J. Vasc. Endovasc. Surg.* **2021**, *61*, 900–907. [CrossRef]
23. Karkos, C.; Mukhopadhyay, U.; Papakostas, I.; Ghosh, J.; Thomson, G.; Hughes, R. Abdominal Aortic Aneurysm: The Role of Clinical Examination and Opportunistic Detection. *Eur. J. Vasc. Endovasc. Surg.* **2000**, *19*, 299–303. [CrossRef]
24. Fink, H.A.; Lederle, F.A.; Roth, C.S.; Bowles, C.A.; Nelson, D.B.; Haas, M.A. The Accuracy of Physical Examination to Detect Abdominal Aortic Aneurysm. *Arch. Intern. Med.* **2000**, *160*, 833–836. [CrossRef] [PubMed]
25. Schermerhorn, M.L.; Bensley, R.P.; Giles, K.A.; Hurks, R.; O'Malley, A.J.; Cotterill, P.; Chaikof, E.; Landon, B.E. Changes in Abdominal Aortic Aneurysm Rupture and Short-Term Mortality, 1995–2008: A Retrospective Observational Study. *Ann. Surg.* **2012**, *256*, 651–658. [CrossRef]

26. Jeanmonod, D.; Yelamanchili, V.S.; Jeanmonod, R. Abdominal Aortic Aneurysm Rupture. *StatPearls* **2021**. Available online: https://www.ncbi.nlm.nih.gov/books/NBK459176/ (accessed on 28 November 2021).
27. Brady, A.R.; Thompson, S.G.; Fowkes, F.G.R.; Greenhalgh, R.M.; Powell, J.T. UK Small Aneurysm Trial Participants Abdominal Aortic Aneurysm Expansion: Risk Factors and Time Intervals for Surveillance. *Circulation* **2004**, *110*, 16–21. [CrossRef] [PubMed]
28. Thompson, S.G.; Brown, L.C.; Sweeting, M.; Bown, M.; Kim, L.; Glover, M.; Buxton, M.J.; Powell, J. Systematic review and meta-analysis of the growth and rupture rates of small abdominal aortic aneurysms: Implications for surveillance intervals and their cost-effectiveness. *Heal. Technol. Assess.* **2013**, *17*, 1–118. [CrossRef] [PubMed]
29. Mofidi, R.; Goldie, V.J.; Kelman, J.; Dawson, A.R.W.; Murie, J.A.; Chalmers, R.T.A. Influence of sex on expansion rate of abdominal aortic aneurysms. *Br. J. Surg.* **2007**, *94*, 310–314. [CrossRef] [PubMed]
30. Sweeting, M.; Thompson, S.G.; Brown, L.C.; Powell, J.T. Meta-analysis of individual patient data to examine factors affecting growth and rupture of small abdominal aortic aneurysms. *Br. J. Surg.* **2012**, *99*, 655–665. [CrossRef]
31. Bhak, R.H.; Lederle, F.A.; Messina, L.M.; Wilson, S.E.; Wininger, M.; Johnson, G.R.; Ballard, D.J. Factors Associated With Small Abdominal Aortic Aneurysm Expansion Rate. *JAMA Surg.* **2015**, *150*, 44–50. [CrossRef] [PubMed]
32. Oliver-Williams, C.; Sweeting, M.; Turton, G.; Parkin, D.; Cooper, D.; Rodd, C.; Thompson, S.G.; Earnshaw, J.J. Gloucestershire and Swindon Abdominal Aortic Aneurysm Screening Programme Lessons Learned about Prevalence and Growth Rates of Abdominal Aortic Aneurysms from a 25-Year Ultrasound Population Screening Programme. *BJS* **2018**, *105*, 68–74. [CrossRef]
33. Thompson, A.R.; Cooper, J.A.; Ashton, H.A.; Hafez, H. Growth rates of small abdominal aortic aneurysms correlate with clinical events. *BJS* **2010**, *97*, 37–44. [CrossRef]
34. Wild, J.; Stather, P.; Biancari, F.; Choke, E.; Earnshaw, J.; Grant, S.; Hafez, H.; Holdsworth, R.; Juvonen, T.; Lindholt, J.; et al. A Multicentre Observational Study of the Outcomes of Screening Detected Sub-aneurysmal Aortic Dilatation. *Eur. J. Vasc. Endovasc. Surg.* **2013**, *45*, 128–134. [CrossRef]
35. RESCAN Collaborators; Bown, M.J.; Sweeting, M.J.; Brown, L.C.; Powell, J.T.; Thompson, S.G. Surveillance Intervals for Small Abdominal Aortic Aneurysms: A Meta-Analysis. *JAMA* **2013**, *309*, 806–813. [CrossRef] [PubMed]
36. Laine, M.T.; Laukontaus, S.J.; Kantonen, I.; Venermo, M. Population-based study of ruptured abdominal aortic aneurysm. *BJS* **2016**, *103*, 1634–1639. [CrossRef] [PubMed]
37. GBD 2019 Diseases and Injuries Collaborators. Global burden of 369 diseases and injuries in 204 countries and territories, 1990–2019: A systematic analysis for the Global Burden of Disease Study 2019. *Lancet* **2020**, *396*, 1204–1222. [CrossRef]
38. Sampson, U.K.; Norman, P.E.; Fowkes, F.G.R.; Aboyans, V.; Song, Y.; Harrell, F.E.H., Jr.; Forouzanfar, M.H.; Naghavi, M.; Denenberg, J.O.; McDermott, M.M.; et al. Global and Regional Burden of Aortic Dissection and Aneurysms: Mortality Trends in 21 World Regions, 1990 to 2010. *Glob. Hear.* **2014**, *9*, 171–180.e10. [CrossRef]
39. Fredrik, L.; Anders, W.; Kevin, M. Changes in abdominal aortic aneurysm epidemiology. *J. Cardiovasc. Surg.* **2017**, *58*, 848–853. [CrossRef]
40. Assar, A.N.; Zarins, C.K. Ruptured abdominal aortic aneurysm: A surgical emergency with many clinical presentations. *Postgrad. Med, J.* **2009**, *85*, 268–273. [CrossRef]
41. Golledge, J. Abdominal aortic aneurysm: Update on pathogenesis and medical treatments. *Nat. Rev. Cardiol.* **2019**, *16*, 225–242. [CrossRef]
42. Lee, F.-Y.; Chen, W.-K.; Chiu, C.-H.; Lin, C.-L.; Kao, C.-H.; Chen, C.-H.; Yang, T.-Y.; Lai, C.-Y. Increased risk of deep vein thrombosis and pulmonary thromboembolism in patients with aortic aneurysms: A nationwide cohort study. *PLoS ONE* **2017**, *12*, e0178587. [CrossRef]
43. Lech, C.; Swaminathan, A. Abdominal Aortic Emergencies. *Emerg. Med. Clin. North Am.* **2017**, *35*, 847–867. [CrossRef] [PubMed]
44. Azhar, B.; Patel, S.R.; Holt, P.J.; Hinchliffe, R.J.; Thompson, M.M.; Karthikesalingam, A. Misdiagnosis of Ruptured Abdominal Aortic Aneurysm: Systematic Review and Meta-Analysis. *J. Endovasc. Ther.* **2014**, *21*, 568–575. [CrossRef] [PubMed]
45. Schmitz-Rixen, T.; Keese, M.; Hakimi, M.; Peters, A.; Böckler, D.; Nelson, K.; Grundmann, R.T. Ruptured abdominal aortic aneurysm—Epidemiology, predisposing factors, and biology. *Langenbeck's Arch. Surg.* **2016**, *401*, 275–288. [CrossRef] [PubMed]
46. Ulug, P.; Powell, J.T.; Sweeting, M.; Bown, M.; Thompson, S.G.; Jones, E.; Glover, M.J. Meta-analysis of the current prevalence of screen-detected abdominal aortic aneurysm in women. *BJS* **2016**, *103*, 1097–1104. [CrossRef]
47. Wanhainen, A.; Themudo, R.; Ahlström, H.; Lind, L.; Johansson, L. Thoracic and abdominal aortic dimension in 70-year-old men and women—A population-based whole-body magnetic resonance imaging (MRI) study. *J. Vasc. Surg.* **2008**, *47*, 504–512. [CrossRef] [PubMed]
48. Svensjö, S.; Björck, M.; Wanhainen, A. Current prevalence of abdominal aortic aneurysm in 70-year-old women. *BJS* **2012**, *100*, 367–372. [CrossRef]
49. Kent, K.C.; Zwolak, R.M.; Egorova, N.N.; Riles, T.S.; Manganaro, A.; Moskowitz, A.; Gelijns, A.C.; Greco, G. Analysis of risk factors for abdominal aortic aneurysm in a cohort of more than 3 million individuals. *J. Vasc. Surg.* **2010**, *52*, 539–548. [CrossRef]
50. Chabok, M.; Nicolaides, A.; Aslam, M.; Farahmandfar, M.; Humphries, K.; Kermani, N.Z.; Coltart, J.; Standfield, N. Risk factors associated with increased prevalence of abdominal aortic aneurysm in women. *BJS* **2016**, *103*, 1132–1138. [CrossRef]
51. Boese, A.C.; Chang, L.; Yin, K.-J.; Chen, Y.E.; Lee, J.-P.; Hamblin, M.H. Sex differences in abdominal aortic aneurysms. *Am. J. Physiol. Circ. Physiol.* **2018**, *314*, H1137–H1152. [CrossRef]

52. Lederle, F.A.; Larson, J.C.; Margolis, K.L.; Allison, M.A.; Freiberg, M.S.; Cochrane, B.B.; Graettinger, W.F.; Curb, J.D. Women's Health Initiative Cohort Study Abdominal Aortic Aneurysm Events in the Women's Health Initiative: Cohort Study. *BMJ* **2008**, *337*, a1724. [CrossRef]
53. Norman, P.; Powell, J. Abdominal Aortic Aneurysm: The Prognosis in Women Is Worse than in Men. *Circulation* **2007**, *115*, 2865–2869. [CrossRef]
54. McPhee, J.T.; Hill, J.S.; Eslami, M. The impact of gender on presentation, therapy, and mortality of abdominal aortic aneurysm in the United States, 2001–2004. *J. Vasc. Surg.* **2007**, *45*, 891–899. [CrossRef]
55. Skibba, A.A.; Evans, J.R.; Hopkins, S.P.; Yoon, H.R.; Katras, T.; Kalbfleisch, J.H.; Rush, D.S. Reconsidering gender relative to risk of rupture in the contemporary management of abdominal aortic aneurysms. *J. Vasc. Surg.* **2015**, *62*, 1429–1436. [CrossRef]
56. Ulug, P.; Sweeting, M.; von Allmen, R.; Thompson, S.G.; Powell, J.T.; Jones, E.; Bown, M.J.; Glover, M.; Michaels, J. Morphological suitability for endovascular repair, non-intervention rates, and operative mortality in women and men assessed for intact abdominal aortic aneurysm repair: Systematic reviews with meta-analysis. *Lancet* **2017**, *389*, 2482–2491. [CrossRef]
57. Jahangir, E.; Lipworth, L.; Edwards, T.L.; Kabagambe, E.K.; Mumma, M.T.; Mensah, G.A.; Fazio, S.; Blot, W.J.; Sampson, U.K.A. Smoking, sex, risk factors and abdominal aortic aneurysms: A prospective study of 18,782 persons aged above 65 years in the Southern Community Cohort Study. *J. Epidemiol. Community Heal.* **2015**, *69*, 481–488. [CrossRef] [PubMed]
58. Jacomelli, J.; Summers, L.; Stevenson, A.; Lees, T.; Earnshaw, J. Editor's Choice—Inequalities in Abdominal Aortic Aneurysm Screening in England: Effects of Social Deprivation and Ethnicity. *Eur. J. Vasc. Endovasc. Surg.* **2017**, *53*, 837–843. [CrossRef] [PubMed]
59. Perlstein, M.D.; Gupta, S.; Ma, X.; Rong, L.Q.; Askin, G.; White, R.S. Abdominal Aortic Aneurysm Repair Readmissions and Disparities of Socioeconomic Status: A Multistate Analysis, 2007–2014. *J. Cardiothorac. Vasc. Anesthesia* **2019**, *33*, 2737–2745. [CrossRef] [PubMed]
60. Soden, P.A.; Zettervall, S.L.; Deery, S.E.; Hughes, K.; Stoner, M.C.; Goodney, P.P.; Vouyouka, A.G.; Schermerhorn, M.L. Society for Vascular Surgery Vascular Quality Initiative Black Patients Present with More Severe Vascular Disease and a Greater Burden of Risk Factors than White Patients at Time of Major Vascular Intervention. *J. Vasc. Surg.* **2018**, *67*, 549–556.e3. [CrossRef]
61. Deery, S.E.; O'Donnell, T.F.; Shean, K.E.; Darling, J.D.; Soden, P.A.; Hughes, K.; Wang, G.J.; Schermerhorn, M.L. Society for Vascular Surgery Vascular Quality Initiative Racial Disparities in Outcomes after Intact Abdominal Aortic Aneurysm Repair. *J. Vasc. Surg.* **2018**, *67*, 1059–1067. [CrossRef]
62. Williams, T.K.; Schneider, E.B.; Black, J.H.; Lum, Y.W.; Freischlag, J.A.; Perler, B.A.; Abularrage, C.J. Disparities in Outcomes for Hispanic Patients Undergoing Endovascular and Open Abdominal Aortic Aneurysm Repair. *Ann. Vasc. Surg.* **2013**, *27*, 29–37. [CrossRef]
63. Pujades-Rodriguez, M.; Timmis, A.; Stogiannis, D.; Rapsomaniki, E.; Denaxas, S.; Shah, A.D.; Feder, G.; Kivimäki, M.; Hemingway, H. Socioeconomic Deprivation and the Incidence of 12 Cardiovascular Diseases in 1.9 Million Women and Men: Implications for Risk Prediction and Prevention. *PLoS ONE* **2014**, *9*, e104671. [CrossRef]
64. Zommorodi, S.; Leander, K.; Roy, J.; Steuer, J.; Hultgren, R. Understanding abdominal aortic aneurysm epidemiology: Socioeconomic position affects outcome. *J. Epidemiol. Commun. Heal.* **2018**, *72*, 904–910. [CrossRef]
65. Iribarren, C.; Darbinian, J.A.; Go, A.S.; Fireman, B.H.; Lee, C.D.; Grey, D.P. Traditional and Novel Risk Factors for Clinically Diagnosed Abdominal Aortic Aneurysm: The Kaiser Multiphasic Health Checkup Cohort Study. *Ann. Epidemiol.* **2007**, *17*, 669–678. [CrossRef]
66. Badger, S.A.; O'Donnell, M.E.; Sharif, M.A.; Boyd, C.S.; Hannon, R.J.; Lau, L.L.; Lee, B.; Soong, C.V. Risk Factors for Abdominal Aortic Aneurysm and the Influence of Social Deprivation. *Angiology* **2008**, *59*, 559–566. [CrossRef]
67. Zarrouk, M.; Holst, J.; Malina, M.; Lindblad, B.; Wann-Hansson, C.; Rosvall, M.; Gottsäter, A. The importance of socioeconomic factors for compliance and outcome at screening for abdominal aortic aneurysm in 65-year-old men. *J. Vasc. Surg.* **2013**, *58*, 50–55. [CrossRef] [PubMed]
68. Khashram, M.; Pitama, S.; Williman, J.A.; Jones, G.T.; Roake, J.A. Survival Disparity Following Abdominal Aortic Aneurysm Repair Highlights Inequality in Ethnic and Socio-economic Status. *Eur. J. Vasc. Endovasc. Surg.* **2017**, *54*, 689–696. [CrossRef] [PubMed]
69. Cavelaars, A.E.J.M.; Kunst, A.E.; Geurts, J.J.M.; Crialesi, R.; Grötvedt, L.; Helmert, U.; Lahelma, E.; Lundberg, O.; Matheson, J.; Mielck, A.; et al. Educational differences in smoking: International comparison. *BMJ* **2000**, *320*, 1102–1107. [CrossRef] [PubMed]
70. Wallach-Kildemoes, H.; Andersen, M.; Diderichsen, F.; Lange, T. Adherence to preventive statin therapy according to socioeconomic position. *Eur. J. Clin. Pharmacol.* **2013**, *69*, 1553–1563. [CrossRef]
71. Ultee, K.; Gonçalves, F.B.; Hoeks, S.; Rouwet, E.; Boersma, E.; Stolker, R.; Verhagen, H. Low Socioeconomic Status is an Independent Risk Factor for Survival After Abdominal Aortic Aneurysm Repair and Open Surgery for Peripheral Artery Disease. *Eur. J. Vasc. Endovasc. Surg.* **2015**, *50*, 615–622. [CrossRef]
72. Joergensen, T.; Houlind, K.; Green, A.; Lindholt, J. Abdominal Aortic Diameter Is Increased in Males with a Family History of Abdominal Aortic Aneurysms: Results from the Danish VIVA-trial. *Eur. J. Vasc. Endovasc. Surg.* **2014**, *48*, 669–675. [CrossRef] [PubMed]
73. Ogata, T.; MacKean, G.L.; Cole, C.W.; Arthur, C.; Andreou, P.; Tromp, G.; Kuivaniemi, H. The lifetime prevalence of abdominal aortic aneurysms among siblings of aneurysm patients is eightfold higher than among siblings of spouses: An analysis of 187 aneurysm families in Nova Scotia, Canada. *J. Vasc. Surg.* **2005**, *42*, 891–897. [CrossRef]

74. Larsson, E.; Granath, F.; Swedenborg, J.; Hultgren, R. A population-based case-control study of the familial risk of abdominal aortic aneurysm. *J. Vasc. Surg.* **2009**, *49*, 47–51. [CrossRef] [PubMed]
75. Akai, A.; Watanabe, Y.; Hoshina, K.; Obitsu, Y.; Deguchi, J.; Sato, O.; Shigematsu, K.; Miyata, T. Family history of aortic aneurysm is an independent risk factor for more rapid growth of small abdominal aortic aneurysms in Japan. *J. Vasc. Surg.* **2015**, *61*, 287–290. [CrossRef] [PubMed]
76. van de Luijtgaarden, K.M.; Gonçalves, F.B.; Hoeks, S.E.; Majoor-Krakauer, D.; Rouwet, E.V.; Stolker, R.J.; Verhagen, H.J. Familial abdominal aortic aneurysm is associated with more complications after endovascular aneurysm repair. *J. Vasc. Surg.* **2014**, *59*, 275–282. [CrossRef]
77. Wanhainen, A.; Bergqvist, D.; Boman, K.; Nilsson, T.K.; Rutegård, J.; Björck, M. Risk factors associated with abdominal aortic aneurysm: A population-based study with historical and current data. *J. Vasc. Surg.* **2005**, *41*, 390–396. [CrossRef]
78. Sakalihasan, N.; Defraigne, J.-O.; Kerstenne, M.-A.; Cheramy-Bien, J.-P.; Smelser, D.T.; Tromp, G.; Kuivaniemi, H. Family Members of Patients with Abdominal Aortic Aneurysms Are at Increased Risk for Aneurysms: Analysis of 618 Probands and Their Families from the Liège AAA Family Study. *Ann. Vasc. Surg.* **2014**, *28*, 787–797. [CrossRef]
79. Kuivaniemi, H.; Shibamura, H.; Arthur, C.; Berguer, R.; Cole, C.W.; Juvonen, T.; Kline, R.A.; Limet, R.; MacKean, G.; Norrgård, Ö.; et al. Familial abdominal aortic aneurysms: Collection of 233 multiplex families. *J. Vasc. Surg.* **2003**, *37*, 340–345. [CrossRef]
80. Meester, J.A.N.; Verstraeten, A.; Schepers, D.; Alaerts, M.; Van Laer, L.; Loeys, B.L. Differences in manifestations of Marfan syndrome, Ehlers-Danlos syndrome, and Loeys-Dietz syndrome. *Ann. Cardiothorac. Surg.* **2017**, *6*, 582–594. [CrossRef]
81. Wahlgren, C.M.; Larsson, E.; Magnusson, P.; Hultgren, R.; Swedenborg, J. Genetic and environmental contributions to abdominal aortic aneurysm development in a twin population. *J. Vasc. Surg.* **2010**, *51*, 3–7. [CrossRef] [PubMed]
82. Joergensen, T.; Christensen, K.; Lindholt, J.; Larsen, L.A.; Green, A.; Houlind, K. Editor's Choice—High Heritability of Liability to Abdominal Aortic Aneurysms: A Population Based Twin Study. *Eur. J. Vasc. Endovasc. Surg.* **2016**, *52*, 41–46. [CrossRef]
83. Mangum, K.D.; Farber, M.A. Genetic and epigenetic regulation of abdominal aortic aneurysms. *Clin. Genet.* **2020**, *97*, 815–826. [CrossRef]
84. Jones, G.T.; Tromp, G.; Kuivaniemi, H.; Gretarsdottir, S.; Baas, A.F.; Giusti, B.; Strauss, E.; Hof, F.N.V.; Webb, T.; Erdman, R.; et al. Meta-Analysis of Genome-Wide Association Studies for Abdominal Aortic Aneurysm Identifies Four New Disease-Specific Risk Loci. *Circ. Res.* **2017**, *120*, 341–353. [CrossRef]
85. Bradley, D.; Badger, S.; McFarland, M.; Hughes, A. Abdominal Aortic Aneurysm Genetic Associations: Mostly False? A Systematic Review and Meta-analysis. *Eur. J. Vasc. Endovasc. Surg.* **2016**, *51*, 64–75. [CrossRef]
86. Wu, Z.-Y.; Trenner, M.; Boon, R.A.; Spin, J.M.; Maegdefessel, L. Long noncoding RNAs in key cellular processes involved in aortic aneurysms. *Atherosclerosis* **2020**, *292*, 112–118. [CrossRef]
87. Zalewski, D.P.; Ruszel, K.P.; Stępniewski, A.; Gałkowski, D.; Bogucki, J.; Komsta, Ł.; Kołodziej, P.; Chmiel, P.; Zubilewicz, T.; Feldo, M.; et al. Dysregulation of microRNA Modulatory Network in Abdominal Aortic Aneurysm. *J. Clin. Med.* **2020**, *9*, 1974. [CrossRef] [PubMed]
88. Lederle, F.A.; Johnson, G.R.; Wilson, S.E.; Chute, E.P.; Hye, R.J.; Makaroun, M.S.; Barone, G.W.; Bandyk, D.; Moneta, G.L.; Makhoul, R.G. The Aneurysm Detection and Management Study Screening Program: Validation Cohort and Final Results. Aneurysm Detection and Management Veterans Affairs Cooperative Study Investigators. *Arch. Intern. Med.* **2000**, *160*, 1425–1430. [CrossRef] [PubMed]
89. Nyrønning, L.; Videm, V.; Romundstad, P.R.; Hultgren, R.; Mattsson, E. Female sex hormones and risk of incident abdominal aortic aneurysm in Norwegian women in the HUNT study. *J. Vasc. Surg.* **2019**, *70*, 1436–1445.e2. [CrossRef] [PubMed]
90. Stackelberg, O.; Björck, M.; Larsson, S.; Orsini, N.; Wolk, A. Sex differences in the association between smoking and abdominal aortic aneurysm. *BJS* **2014**, *101*, 1230–1237. [CrossRef]
91. Altobelli, E.; Rapacchietta, L.; Profeta, V.F.; Fagnano, R. Risk Factors for Abdominal Aortic Aneurysm in Population-Based Studies: A Systematic Review and Meta-Analysis. *Int. J. Environ. Res. Public Health* **2018**, *15*, 2805. [CrossRef]
92. Forsdahl, S.H.; Singh, K.; Solberg, S.; Jacobsen, B.K. Risk Factors for Abdominal Aortic Aneurysms: A 7-Year Prospective Study: The Tromsø Study, 1994–2001. *Circulation* **2009**, *119*, 2202–2208. [CrossRef] [PubMed]
93. Lederle, F.A.; Nelson, D.B.; Joseph, A.M. Smokers' Relative Risk for Aortic Aneurysm Compared with Other Smoking-Related Diseases: A Systematic Review. *J. Vasc. Surg.* **2003**, *38*, 329–334. [CrossRef]
94. Pujades-Rodriguez, M.; George, J.; Shah, A.D.; Rapsomaniki, E.; Denaxas, S.; West, R.; Smeeth, L.; Timmis, A.; Hemingway, H. Heterogeneous associations between smoking and a wide range of initial presentations of cardiovascular disease in 1 937 360 people in England: Lifetime risks and implications for risk prediction. *Int. J. Epidemiol.* **2014**, *44*, 129–141. [CrossRef] [PubMed]
95. Flessenkaemper, I.; Loddenkemper, R.; Roll, S.; Enke-Melzer, K.; Wurps, H.; Bauer, T. Screening of COPD patients for abdominal aortic aneurysm. *Int. J. Chronic Obstr. Pulm. Dis.* **2015**, *10*, 1085–1091. [CrossRef] [PubMed]
96. Takagi, H.; Umemoto, T. A Meta-Analysis of the Association of Chronic Obstructive Pulmonary Disease with Abdominal Aortic Aneurysm Presence. *Ann. Vasc. Surg.* **2016**, *34*, 84–94. [CrossRef] [PubMed]
97. Meijer, C.; Kokje, V.; van Tongeren, R.; Hamming, J.; van Bockel, J.; Möller, G.; Lindeman, J. An Association between Chronic Obstructive Pulmonary Disease and Abdominal Aortic Aneurysm beyond Smoking: Results from a Case-Control Study. *Eur. J. Vasc. Endovasc. Surg.* **2012**, *44*, 153–157. [CrossRef]

98. Takagi, H.; Umemoto, T. No association of chronic obstructive pulmonary disease with abdominal aortic aneurysm growth. *Hear. Vessel.* **2016**, *31*, 1806–1816. [CrossRef]
99. Takagi, H.; Umemoto, T. Association of Chronic Obstructive Pulmonary, Coronary Artery, or Peripheral Artery Disease with Abdominal Aortic Aneurysm Rupture. *Int. Angiol.* **2017**, *36*, 322–331. [CrossRef]
100. Siika, A.; Liljeqvist, M.L.; Zommorodi, S.; Nilsson, O.; Andersson, P.; Gasser, T.C.; Roy, J.; Hultgren, R. A large proportion of patients with small ruptured abdominal aortic aneurysms are women and have chronic obstructive pulmonary disease. *PLoS ONE* **2019**, *14*, e0216558. [CrossRef] [PubMed]
101. Crawford, J.D.; Chivukula, V.K.; Haller, S.; Vatankhah, N.; Bohannan, C.J.; Moneta, G.L.; Rugonyi, S.; Azarbal, A.F. Aortic outflow occlusion predicts rupture of abdominal aortic aneurysm. *J. Vasc. Surg.* **2016**, *64*, 1623–1628. [CrossRef]
102. Wilmink, T.B.; Quick, C.R.; Day, N.E. The association between cigarette smoking and abdominal aortic aneurysms. *J. Vasc. Surg.* **1999**, *30*, 1099–1105. [CrossRef]
103. Aune, D.; Schlesinger, S.; Norat, T.; Riboli, E. Tobacco smoking and the risk of abdominal aortic aneurysm: A systematic review and meta-analysis of prospective studies. *Sci. Rep.* **2018**, *8*, 14786. [CrossRef]
104. Norman, P.E.; Curci, J.A. Understanding the Effects of Tobacco Smoke on the Pathogenesis of Aortic Aneurysm. *Arter. Thromb. Vasc. Biol.* **2013**, *33*, 1473–1477. [CrossRef] [PubMed]
105. Palazzuoli, A.; Gallotta, M.; Guerrieri, G.; Quatrini, I.; Franci, B.; Campagna, M.S.; Neri, E.; Benvenuti, A.; Sassi, C.; Nuti, R. Prevalence of risk factors, coronary and systemic atherosclerosis in abdominal aortic aneurysm: Comparison with high cardiovascular risk population. *Vasc. Heal. Risk Manag.* **2008**, *ume 4*, 877–883. [CrossRef]
106. Toghill, B.J.; Saratzis, A.; Bown, M.J. Abdominal aortic aneurysm—An independent disease to atherosclerosis? *Cardiovasc. Pathol.* **2017**, *27*, 71–75. [CrossRef] [PubMed]
107. Elkalioubie, A.; Haulon, S.; Duhamel, A.; Rosa, M.; Rauch, A.; Staels, B.; Susen, S.; Van Belle, E.; Dupont, A. Meta-Analysis of Abdominal Aortic Aneurysm in Patients With Coronary Artery Disease. *Am. J. Cardiol.* **2015**, *116*, 1451–1456. [CrossRef]
108. Grøndal, N.; Søgaard, R.; Lindholt, J. Baseline prevalence of abdominal aortic aneurysm, peripheral arterial disease and hypertension in men aged 65–74 years from a population screening study (VIVA trial). *BJS* **2015**, *102*, 902–906. [CrossRef]
109. Yao, L.; Folsom, A.R.; Alonso, A.; Lutsey, P.L.; Pankow, J.; Guan, W.; Cheng, S.; Lederle, F.A.; Tang, W. Association of carotid atherosclerosis and stiffness with abdominal aortic aneurysm: The atherosclerosis risk in communities (ARIC) study. *Atherosclerosis* **2018**, *270*, 110–116. [CrossRef] [PubMed]
110. Baumgartner, I.; Hirsch, A.T.; Abola, M.T.B.; Cacoub, P.; Poldermans, D.; Steg, P.G.; Creager, M.A.; Bhatt, D.L. REACH Registry investigators Cardiovascular Risk Profile and Outcome of Patients with Abdominal Aortic Aneurysm in Out-Patients with Atherothrombosis: Data from the Reduction of Atherothrombosis for Continued Health (REACH) Registry. *J. Vasc. Surg.* **2008**, *48*, 808–814.e1. [CrossRef]
111. Hernesniemi, J.A.; Vänni, V.; Hakala, T. The prevalence of abdominal aortic aneurysm is consistently high among patients with coronary artery disease. *J. Vasc. Surg.* **2015**, *62*, 232–240.e3,. [CrossRef]
112. Durieux, R.; Van Damme, H.; Labropoulos, N.; Yazici, A.; Legrand, V.; Albert, A.; Defraigne, J.-O.; Sakalihasan, N. High Prevalence of Abdominal Aortic Aneurysm in Patients with Three-vessel Coronary Artery Disease. *Eur. J. Vasc. Endovasc. Surg.* **2014**, *47*, 273–278. [CrossRef]
113. Gianfagna, F.; Veronesi, G.; Tozzi, M.; Tarallo, A.; Borchini, R.; Ferrario, M.M.; Bertù, L.; Montonati, A.; Castelli, P.; Mara, L.; et al. RoCAV (Risk of Cardiovascular diseases and abdominal aortic Aneurysm in Varese) Project Investigators Prevalence of Abdominal Aortic Aneurysms in the General Population and in Subgroups at High Cardiovascular Risk in Italy. Results of the RoCAV Population Based Study. *Eur. J. Vasc. Endovasc. Surg.* **2018**, *55*, 633–639. [CrossRef] [PubMed]
114. Matthews, E.O.; Rowbotham, S.E.; Moxon, J.V.; Jones, R.E.; de Ceniga, M.V.; Golledge, J. Meta-analysis of the association between peripheral artery disease and growth of abdominal aortic aneurysms. *BJS* **2017**, *104*, 1765–1774. [CrossRef]
115. Takagi, H.; Umemoto, T. Associations of coronary and peripheral artery disease with presence, expansion, and rupture of abdominal aortic aneurysm—A grin without a cat! *Vasa* **2017**, *46*, 151–158. [CrossRef] [PubMed]
116. Freiberg, M.S.; Arnold, A.M.; Newman, A.B.; Edwards, M.S.; Kraemer, K.L.; Kuller, L.H. Abdominal Aortic Aneurysms, Increasing Infrarenal Aortic Diameter, and Risk of Total Mortality and Incident Cardiovascular Disease Events: 10-Year Follow-up Data from the Cardiovascular Health Study. *Circulation* **2008**, *117*, 1010–1017. [CrossRef]
117. Goodney, P.P.; Tavris, D.; Lucas, F.L.; Gross, T.; Fisher, E.S.; Finlayson, S.R.G. Causes of late mortality after endovascular and open surgical repair of infrarenal abdominal aortic aneurysms. *J. Vasc. Surg.* **2010**, *51*, 1340–1347.e1. [CrossRef] [PubMed]
118. Bahia, S.S.; Vidal-Diez, A.; Seshasai, S.R.K.; Shpitser, I.; Brownrigg, J.R.; Patterson, B.O.; Ray, K.K.; Holt, P.J.; Thompson, M.M.; Karthikesalingam, A. Cardiovascular risk prevention and all-cause mortality in primary care patients with an abdominal aortic aneurysm. *BJS* **2016**, *103*, 1626–1633. [CrossRef]
119. Kobeissi, E.; Hibino, M.; Pan, H.; Aune, D. Blood pressure, hypertension and the risk of abdominal aortic aneurysms: A systematic review and meta-analysis of cohort studies. *Eur. J. Epidemiol.* **2019**, *34*, 547–555. [CrossRef] [PubMed]
120. Takagi, H.; Umemoto, T. Association of Hypertension with Abdominal Aortic Aneurysm Expansion. *Ann. Vasc. Surg.* **2016**, *39*, 74–89. [CrossRef]
121. Takagi, H.; Manabe, H.; Kawai, N.; Goto, S.-N.; Umemoto, T. Serum High-Density and Low-Density Lipoprotein Cholesterol Is Associated with Abdominal Aortic Aneurysm Presence: A Systematic Review and Meta-Analysis. *Int. Angiol.* **2010**, *29*, 371–375. [PubMed]

122. Stather, P.W.; Sidloff, D.A.; Dattani, N.; Gokani, V.J.; Choke, E.; Sayers, R.D.; Bown, M. Meta-analysis and meta-regression analysis of biomarkers for abdominal aortic aneurysm. *BJS* **2014**, *101*, 1358–1372. [CrossRef]
123. Rizzo, M.; Krayenbühl, P.-A.; Pernice, V.; Frasheri, A.; Rini, G.B.; Berneis, K. LDL size and subclasses in patients with abdominal aortic aneurysm. *Int. J. Cardiol.* **2009**, *134*, 406–408. [CrossRef] [PubMed]
124. Takagi, H.; Umemoto, T.; Information, R. The association between body mass index and abdominal aortic aneurysm growth: A systematic review. *Vasa* **2016**, *45*, 119–124. [CrossRef]
125. Cronin, O.; Walker, P.J.; Golledge, J. The association of obesity with abdominal aortic aneurysm presence and growth. *Atherosclerosis* **2013**, *226*, 321–327. [CrossRef] [PubMed]
126. Apoloni, R.C.; Zerati, A.E.; Wolosker, N.; Saes, G.F.; Wolosker, M.; Curado, T.; Puech-Leão, P.; De Luccia, N. Analysis of the Correlation Between Central Obesity and Abdominal Aortic Diseases. *Ann. Vasc. Surg.* **2019**, *54*, 176–184. [CrossRef] [PubMed]
127. Stackelberg, O.; Björck, M.; Azodi, O.S.; Larsson, S.; Orsini, N.; Wolk, A. Obesity and abdominal aortic aneurysm. *BJS* **2013**, *100*, 360–366. [CrossRef] [PubMed]
128. Golledge, J.; Clancy, P.; Jamrozik, K.; Norman, P.E. Obesity, Adipokines, and Abdominal Aortic Aneurysm: Health in Men Study. *Circulation* **2007**, *116*, 2275–2279. [CrossRef]
129. Cronin, O.; Liu, D.; Bradshaw, B.; Iyer, V.; Buttner, P.; Cunningham, M.; Walker, P.J.; Golledge, J. Visceral adiposity is not associated with abdominal aortic aneurysm presence and growth. *Vasc. Med.* **2014**, *19*, 272–280. [CrossRef] [PubMed]
130. Elagizi, A.; Kachur, S.; Lavie, C.J.; Carbone, S.; Pandey, A.; Ortega, F.B.; Milani, R.V. An Overview and Update on Obesity and the Obesity Paradox in Cardiovascular Diseases. *Prog. Cardiovasc. Dis.* **2018**, *61*, 142–150. [CrossRef]
131. Mason, R.H.; Ruegg, G.; Perkins, J.; Hardinge, M.; Amann-Vesti, B.; Senn, O.; Stradling, J.R.; Kohler, M. Obstructive Sleep Apnea in Patients with Abdominal Aortic Aneurysms: Highly Prevalent and Associated with Aneurysm Expansion. *Am. J. Respir. Crit. Care Med.* **2011**, *183*, 668–674. [CrossRef] [PubMed]
132. Bianchi, V.; Herbert, W.G.; Myers, J.; Ribisl, P.M.; Miller, L.; Dalman, R.L. Relationship of obstructive sleep apnea and cardiometabolic risk factors in elderly patients with abdominal aortic aneurysm. *Sleep Breath.* **2015**, *19*, 593–598. [CrossRef]
133. Kato, M.; Kubo, A.; Green, F.N.; Takagi, H. Meta-analysis of randomized controlled trials on safety and efficacy of exercise training in patients with abdominal aortic aneurysm. *J. Vasc. Surg.* **2019**, *69*, 933–943. [CrossRef]
134. Niebauer, S.; Niebauer, J.; Dalman, R.; Myers, J. Effects of Exercise Training on Vascular Markers of Disease Progression in Patients with Small Abdominal Aortic Aneurysms. *Am. J. Med.* **2021**, *134*, 535–541. [CrossRef]
135. Aune, D.; Sen, A.; Kobeissi, E.; Hamer, M.; Norat, T.; Riboli, E. Physical activity and the risk of abdominal aortic aneurysm: A systematic review and meta-analysis of prospective studies. *Sci. Rep.* **2020**, *10*, 1–10. [CrossRef]
136. Stackelberg, O.; Wolk, A.; Eliasson, K.; Hellberg, A.; Bersztel, A.; Larsson, S.C.; Orsini, N.; Wanhainen, A.; Björck, M. Lifestyle and Risk of Screening-Detected Abdominal Aortic Aneurysm in Men. *J. Am. Hear. Assoc.* **2017**, *6*. [CrossRef]
137. Nordkvist, S.; Sonestedt, E.; Acosta, S. Adherence to diet recommendations and risk of abdominal aortic aneurysm in the Malmö Diet and Cancer Study. *Sci. Rep.* **2018**, *8*, 2017. [CrossRef]
138. Takagi, H.; Umemoto, T. Vitamins and Abdominal Aortic Aneurysm. *Int. Angiol.* **2017**, *36*, 21–30. [CrossRef] [PubMed]
139. Nsengiyumva, V.; Krishna, S.M.; Moran, C.S.; Moxon, J.V.; Morton, S.K.; Clarke, M.W.; Seto, S.-W.; Golledge, J. Vitamin D deficiency promotes large rupture-prone abdominal aortic aneurysms and cholecalciferol supplementation limits progression of aneurysms in a mouse model. *Clin. Sci.* **2020**, *134*, 2521–2534. [CrossRef] [PubMed]
140. Pincemail, J.; Defraigne, J.-O.; Courtois, A.; Albert, A.; Cheramy-Bien, J.-P.; Sakalihasan, N. Abdominal Aortic Aneurysm (AAA): Is There a Role for the Prevention and Therapy Using Antioxidants? *Curr. Drug Targets* **2018**, *19*, 1256–1264. [CrossRef]
141. De Rango, P.; Farchioni, L.; Fiorucci, B.; Lenti, M. Diabetes and Abdominal Aortic Aneurysms. *Eur. J. Vasc. Endovasc. Surg.* **2014**, *47*, 243–261. [CrossRef]
142. Xiong, J.; Wu, Z.; Chen, C.; Wei, Y.; Guo, W. Association between diabetes and prevalence and growth rate of abdominal aortic aneurysms: A meta-analysis. *Int. J. Cardiol.* **2016**, *221*, 484–495. [CrossRef] [PubMed]
143. Shantikumar, S.; Ajjan, R.; Porter, K.; Scott, D. Diabetes and the Abdominal Aortic Aneurysm. *Eur. J. Vasc. Endovasc. Surg.* **2010**, *39*, 200–207. [CrossRef] [PubMed]
144. Takagi, H.; Umemoto, T. Diabetes and Abdominal Aortic Aneurysm Growth. *Angiology* **2016**, *67*, 513–525. [CrossRef]
145. Takagi, H.; Umemoto, T. Negative Association of Diabetes with Rupture of Abdominal Aortic Aneurysm. *Diabetes Vasc. Dis. Res.* **2016**, *13*, 341–347. [CrossRef] [PubMed]
146. Canto, E.D.; Ceriello, A.; Rydén, L.; Ferrini, M.; Hansen, T.B.; Schnell, O.; Standl, E.; Beulens, J.W. Diabetes as a cardiovascular risk factor: An overview of global trends of macro and micro vascular complications. *Eur. J. Prev. Cardiol.* **2019**, *26*, 25–32. [CrossRef] [PubMed]
147. Climent, E.; Benaiges, D.; Chillarón, J.J.; Roux, J.A.F.-L.; Pedro-Botet, J. Diabetes mellitus as a protective factor of abdominal aortic aneurysm: Possible mechanisms. *Clin. Investig. Arterioscler.* **2018**, *30*, 181–187. [CrossRef]
148. Miyama, N.; Dua, M.M.; Yeung, J.; Schultz, G.M.; Asagami, T.; Sho, E.; Sho, M.; Dalman, R.L. Hyperglycemia limits experimental aortic aneurysm progression. *J. Vasc. Surg.* **2010**, *52*, 975–983. [CrossRef]
149. Dua, M.M.; Miyama, N.; Azuma, J.; Schultz, G.M.; Sho, M.; Morser, J.; Dalman, R.L. Hyperglycemia modulates plasminogen activator inhibitor-1 expression and aortic diameter in experimental aortic aneurysm disease. *Surgery* **2010**, *148*, 429–435. [CrossRef]

150. Thompson, A.; Cooper, J.A.; Fabricius, M.; Humphries, S.E.; Ashton, H.A.; Hafez, H. An analysis of drug modulation of abdominal aortic aneurysm growth through 25 years of surveillance. *J. Vasc. Surg.* **2010**, *52*, 55–61.e2. [CrossRef]
151. Fujimura, N.; Xiong, J.; Kettler, E.; Xuan, H.; Glover, K.J.; Mell, M.W.; Xu, B.; Dalman, R.L. Metformin treatment status and abdominal aortic aneurysm disease progression. *J. Vasc. Surg.* **2016**, *64*, 46–54.e8. [CrossRef] [PubMed]
152. Golledge, J.; Moxon, J.; Pinchbeck, J.; Anderson, G.; Rowbotham, S.; Jenkins, J.; Bourke, M.; Bourke, B.; Dear, A.; Buckenham, T.; et al. Association between metformin prescription and growth rates of abdominal aortic aneurysms. *Br. J. Surg.* **2017**, *104*, 1486–1493. [CrossRef]
153. Gouliamos, A.D.; Tsiganis, T.; Dimakakos, P.; Vlahos, L.J. Screening for abdominal aortic aneurysms during routine lumbar CT scan: Modification of the standard technique. *Clin. Imaging* **2004**, *28*, 353–355. [CrossRef]
154. Argyriou, C.; Georgiadis, G.S.; Kontopodis, N.; Pherwani, A.D.; Van Herwaarden, J.A.; Hazenberg, C.E.; Antoniou, G.A. Screening for Abdominal Aortic Aneurysm During Transthoracic Echocardiography: A Systematic Review and Meta-analysis. *Eur. J. Vasc. Endovasc. Surg.* **2018**, *55*, 475–491. [CrossRef]
155. Matsumura, Y.; Wada, M.; Hirakawa, D.; Yasuoka, Y.; Morimoto, N.; Takeuchi, H.; Kitaoka, H.; Orihashi, K.; Sugiura, T. Clinical utility of transthoracic echocardiography for screening abdominal aortic aneurysm: A prospective study in a Japanese population. *Cardiovasc. Ultrasound* **2015**, *14*, 8. [CrossRef] [PubMed]
156. Aboyans, V.; Bataille, V.; Bliscaux, P.; Ederhy, S.; Filliol, D.; Honton, B.; Kurtz, B.; Messas, E.; Mohty, D.; Brochet, E.; et al. Effectiveness of Screening for Abdominal Aortic Aneurysm During Echocardiography. *Am. J. Cardiol.* **2014**, *114*, 1100–1104. [CrossRef]
157. Stather, P.; Dattani, N.; Bown, M.; Earnshaw, J.; Lees, T. International Variations in AAA Screening. *Eur. J. Vasc. Endovasc. Surg.* **2013**, *45*, 231–234. [CrossRef]
158. Wanhainen, A.; Verzini, F.; Van Herzeele, I.; Allaire, E.; Bown, M.; Cohnert, T.; Dick, F.; van Herwaarden, J.; Karkos, C.; Koelemay, M.; et al. Editor's Choice—European Society for Vascular Surgery (ESVS) 2019 Clinical Practice Guidelines on the Management of Abdominal Aorto-iliac Artery Aneurysms. *Eur. J. Vasc. Endovasc. Surg.* **2019**, *57*, 8–93. [CrossRef] [PubMed]
159. Thompson, S.G.; Ashton, H.A.; Gao, L.; Buxton, M.J.; Scott, R.A.P. Multicentre Aneurysm Screening Study (MASS) Group Final Follow-up of the Multicentre Aneurysm Screening Study (MASS) Randomized Trial of Abdominal Aortic Aneurysm Screening. *Br. J. Surg.* **2012**, *99*, 1649–1656. [CrossRef]
160. Lindholt, J.S.; Sørensen, J.; Søgaard, R.; Henneberg, E.W. Long-term benefit and cost-effectiveness analysis of screening for abdominal aortic aneurysms from a randomized controlled trial. *BJS* **2010**, *97*, 826–834. [CrossRef] [PubMed]
161. Cosford, P.A.; Leng, G.C.; Thomas, J. Screening for Abdominal Aortic Aneurysm. *Cochrane Database Syst. Rev.* **2007**, CD002945. [CrossRef]
162. Guirguis-Blake, J.M.; Beil, T.L.; Senger, C.A.; Coppola, E.L. Primary Care Screening for Abdominal Aortic Aneurysm: Updated Evidence Report and Systematic Review for the US Preventive Services Task Force. *JAMA* **2019**, *322*, 2219–2238. [CrossRef] [PubMed]
163. Wanhainen, A.; Hultgren, R.; Linné, A.; Holst, J.; Gottsäter, A.; Langenskiöld, M.; Smidfelt, K.; Björck, M.; Svensjö, S.; Lyttkens, L.; et al. Swedish Aneurysm Screening Study Group (SASS) Outcome of the Swedish Nationwide Abdominal Aortic Aneurysm Screening Program. *Circulation* **2016**, *134*, 1141–1148. [CrossRef]
164. Svensjö, S.; Mani, K.; Björck, M.; Lundkvist, J.; Wanhainen, A. Screening for Abdominal Aortic Aneurysm in 65-Year-old Men Remains Cost-effective with Contemporary Epidemiology and Management. *Eur. J. Vasc. Endovasc. Surg.* **2014**, *47*, 357–365. [CrossRef] [PubMed]
165. Glover, M.J.; Kim, L.G.; Sweeting, M.J.; Thompson, S.G.; Buxton, M.J. Cost-effectiveness of the National Health Service abdominal aortic aneurysm screening programme in England. *BJS* **2014**, *101*, 976–982. [CrossRef]
166. Bath, M.F.; Sidloff, D.; Saratzis, A.; Bown, M.J.; Pathak, R.; Brooks, M.; Hayes, P.; Imray, C.; Quarmby, J.; Choksy, S.; et al. UK Aneurysm Growth Study investigators Impact of Abdominal Aortic Aneurysm Screening on Quality of Life. *BJS* **2018**, *105*, 203–208. [CrossRef] [PubMed]
167. Kapila, V.; Jetty, P.; Wooster, D.; Vucemilo, V.; Dubois, L. Canadian Society for Vascular Surgery Screening for Abdominal Aortic Aneurysms in Canada: 2020 Review and Position Statement of the Canadian Society for Vascular Surgery. *Can. J. Surg.* **2021**, *64*, E461–E466. [CrossRef]
168. Ravn, H.; Wanhainen, A.; Björck, M. Risk of new aneurysms after surgery for popliteal artery aneurysm. *BJS* **2008**, *95*, 571–575. [CrossRef] [PubMed]
169. Lindholt, J.; Juul, S.; Henneberg, E. High-risk and Low-risk Screening for Abdominal Aortic Aneurysm Both Reduce Aneurysm-related Mortality. A Stratified Analysis from a Single-centre Randomised Screening Trial. *Eur. J. Vasc. Endovasc. Surg.* **2007**, *34*, 53–58. [CrossRef]
170. Lindholt, J.; Vammen, S.; Juul, S.; Fasting, H.; Henneberg, E.W. Optimal Interval Screening and Surveillance of Abdominal Aortic Aneurysms. *Eur. J. Vasc. Endovasc. Surg.* **2000**, *20*, 369–373. [CrossRef]
171. Greco, G.; Egorova, N.N.; Gelijns, A.C.; Moskowitz, A.J.; Manganaro, A.J.; Zwolak, R.M.; Riles, T.S.; Kent, K.C. Development of a Novel Scoring Tool for the Identification of Large ≥5 cm Abdominal Aortic Aneurysms. *Ann. Surg.* **2010**, *252*, 675–682. [CrossRef]
172. Bobadilla, J.L.; Kent, K.C. Screening for Abdominal Aortic Aneurysms. *Adv. Surg.* **2012**, *46*, 101–109. [CrossRef] [PubMed]
173. Hallett, R.L.; Ullery, B.W.; Fleischmann, D. Abdominal aortic aneurysms: Pre- and post-procedural imaging. *Abdom. Radiol.* **2018**, *43*, 1044–1066. [CrossRef]

174. Sever, A.; Rheinboldt, M. Unstable abdominal aortic aneurysms: A review of MDCT imaging features. *Emerg. Radiol.* **2016**, *23*, 187–196. [CrossRef] [PubMed]
175. Kumar, Y.; Hooda, K.; Li, S.; Goyal, P.; Gupta, N.; Adeb, M. Abdominal aortic aneurysm: Pictorial review of common appearances and complications. *Ann. Transl. Med.* **2017**, *5*, 256. [CrossRef] [PubMed]
176. Chaikof, E.L.; Dalman, R.L.; Eskandari, M.K.; Jackson, B.M.; Lee, W.A.; Mansour, M.A.; Mastracci, T.M.; Mell, M.; Murad, M.H.; Nguyen, L.L.; et al. The Society for Vascular Surgery practice guidelines on the care of patients with an abdominal aortic aneurysm. *J. Vasc. Surg.* **2018**, *67*, 2–77.e2. [CrossRef]
177. Wilmink, A.; Forshaw, M.; Quick, C.; Hubbard, C.; Day, N. Accuracy of serial screening for abdominal aortic aneurysms by ultrasound. *J. Med Screen.* **2002**, *9*, 125–127. [CrossRef]
178. Rubano, E.; Mehta, N.; Caputo, W.; Paladino, L.; Sinert, R. Systematic Review: Emergency Department Bedside Ultrasonography for Diagnosing Suspected Abdominal Aortic Aneurysm. *Acad. Emerg. Med.* **2013**, *20*, 128–138. [CrossRef]
179. Gürtelschmid, M.; Björck, M.; Wanhainen, A. Comparison of three ultrasound methods of measuring the diameter of the abdominal aorta. *Br. J. Surg.* **2014**, *101*, 633–636. [CrossRef]
180. Grøndal, N.; Bramsen, M.; Thomsen, M.; Rasmussen, C.; Lindholt, J. The Cardiac Cycle is a Major Contributor to Variability in Size Measurements of Abdominal Aortic Aneurysms by Ultrasound. *Eur. J. Vasc. Endovasc. Surg.* **2012**, *43*, 30–33. [CrossRef]
181. Meecham, L.; Evans, R.; Buxton, P.; Allingham, K.; Hughes, M.; Rajagopalan, S.; Fairhead, J.; Asquith, J.; Pherwani, A. Abdominal Aortic Aneurysm Diameters: A Study on the Discrepancy between Inner to Inner and Outer to Outer Measurements. *Eur. J. Vasc. Endovasc. Surg.* **2015**, *49*, 28–32. [CrossRef] [PubMed]
182. Beales, L.; Wolstenhulme, S.; Evans, J.A.; West, R.; Scott, D.J.A. Reproducibility of ultrasound measurement of the abdominal aorta. *BJS* **2011**, *98*, 1517–1525. [CrossRef]
183. Long, A.; Rouet, L.; Lindholt, J.; Allaire, E. Measuring the Maximum Diameter of Native Abdominal Aortic Aneurysms: Review and Critical Analysis. *Eur. J. Vasc. Endovasc. Surg.* **2012**, *43*, 515–524. [CrossRef] [PubMed]
184. Brambilla, M.; Cerini, P.; Lizio, D.; Vigna, L.; Carriero, A.; Fossaceca, R. Cumulative Radiation Dose and Radiation Risk from Medical Imaging in Patients Subjected to Endovascular Aortic Aneurysm Repair. *Radiol. Med.* **2015**, *120*, 563–570. [CrossRef]
185. Ayache, J.B.; Collins, J.D. MR Angiography of the Abdomen and Pelvis. *Radiol. Clin. North Am.* **2014**, *52*, 839–859. [CrossRef]
186. Mitra, A.; Pencharz, D.; Davis, M.; Wagner, T. Determining the Diagnostic Value of 18F-Fluorodeoxyglucose Positron Emission/Computed Tomography in Detecting Prosthetic Aortic Graft Infection. *Ann. Vasc. Surg.* **2018**, *53*, 78–85. [CrossRef]
187. Husmann, L.; Huellner, M.W.; Ledergerber, B.; Eberhard, N.; Kaelin, M.B.; Anagnostopoulos, A.; Kudura, K.; Burger, I.A.; Mestres, C.-A.; Rancic, Z.; et al. Diagnostic Accuracy of PET/CT and Contrast Enhanced CT in Patients With Suspected Infected Aortic Aneurysms. *Eur. J. Vasc. Endovasc. Surg.* **2020**, *59*, 972–981. [CrossRef]
188. Syed, M.B.; Fletcher, A.J.; Dweck, M.R.; Forsythe, R.; Newby, D.E. Imaging aortic wall inflammation. *Trends Cardiovasc. Med.* **2019**, *29*, 440–448. [CrossRef]
189. Brangsch, J.; Reimann, C.; Collettini, F.; Buchert, R.; Botnar, R.; Makowski, M.R. Molecular Imaging of Abdominal Aortic Aneurysms. *Trends Mol. Med.* **2017**, *23*, 150–164. [CrossRef]
190. Powell, J.T.; Brown, L.C.; Forbes, J.F.; Fowkes, F.G.R.; Greenhalgh, R.M.; Ruckley, C.V.; Thompson, S.G. Final 12-Year Follow-up of Surgery versus Surveillance in the UK Small Aneurysm Trial. *Br. J. Surg.* **2007**, *94*, 702–708. [CrossRef] [PubMed]
191. Lederle, F.A.; Wilson, S.E.; Johnson, G.R.; Reinke, D.B.; Littooy, F.N.; Acher, C.W.; Ballard, D.J.; Messina, L.M.; Gordon, I.L.; Chute, E.P.; et al. Immediate Repair Compared with Surveillance of Small Abdominal Aortic Aneurysms. *N. Engl. J. Med.* **2002**, *346*, 1437–1444. [CrossRef]
192. Cao, P.; De Rango, P.; Verzini, F.; Parlani, G.; Romano, L.; Cieri, E. CAESAR Trial Group Comparison of Surveillance versus Aortic Endografting for Small Aneurysm Repair (CAESAR): Results from a Randomised Trial. *Eur. J. Vasc. Endovasc. Surg.* **2011**, *41*, 13–25. [CrossRef]
193. Ouriel, K.; Clair, D.G.; Kent, K.C.; Zarins, C.K. Positive Impact of Endovascular Options for treating Aneurysms Early (PIVOTAL) Investigators Endovascular Repair Compared with Surveillance for Patients with Small Abdominal Aortic Aneurysms. *J. Vasc. Surg.* **2010**, *51*, 1081–1087. [CrossRef] [PubMed]
194. Filardo, G.; Powell, J.; Martinez, M.A.-M.; Ballard, D.J. Surgery for small asymptomatic abdominal aortic aneurysms. *Cochrane Database Syst. Rev.* **2015**, *2015*, CD001835. [CrossRef] [PubMed]
195. Leemans, E.; Willems, T.P.; Van Der Laan, M.J.; Slump, C.H.; Zeebregts, C.J. Biomechanical Indices for Rupture Risk Estimation in Abdominal Aortic Aneurysms. *J. Endovasc. Ther.* **2016**, *24*, 254–261. [CrossRef]
196. van Walraven, C.; Wong, J.; Morant, K.; Jennings, A.; Austin, P.C.; Jetty, P.; Forster, A.J. The influence of incidental abdominal aortic aneurysm monitoring on patient outcomes. *J. Vasc. Surg.* **2011**, *54*, 1290–1297.e2. [CrossRef]
197. Chun, K.C.; Schmidt, A.S.; Bains, S.; Nguyen, A.T.; Samadzadeh, K.M.; Wilson, M.D.; Peters, J.H.; Lee, E.S. Surveillance outcomes of small abdominal aortic aneurysms identified from a large screening program. *J. Vasc. Surg.* **2016**, *63*, 55–61. [CrossRef]
198. Galiñanes, E.L.; Reynolds, S.; Dombrovskiy, V.Y.; Vogel, T.R. The impact of preoperative statin therapy on open and endovascular abdominal aortic aneurysm repair outcomes. *Vascular* **2015**, *23*, 344–349. [CrossRef] [PubMed]
199. Saratzis, A.; Dattani, N.; Brown, A.; Shalhoub, J.; Bosanquet, D.; Sidloff, D.; Stather, P. Vascular and Endovascular Research Network (VERN) Multi-Centre Study on Cardiovascular Risk Management on Patients Undergoing AAA Surveillance. *Eur. J. Vasc. Endovasc. Surg.* **2017**, *54*, 116–122. [CrossRef]

200. Rigotti, N.A.; Clair, C. Managing tobacco use: The neglected cardiovascular disease risk factor. *Eur. Hear. J.* **2013**, *34*, 3259–3267. [CrossRef]
201. Arinze, N.; Farber, A.; Levin, S.R.; Cheng, T.W.; Jones, D.W.; Siracuse, C.G.; Patel, V.I.; Rybin, D.; Doros, G.; Siracuse, J.J. The effect of the duration of preoperative smoking cessation timing on outcomes after elective open abdominal aortic aneurysm repair and lower extremity bypass. *J. Vasc. Surg.* **2019**, *70*, 1851–1861. [CrossRef]
202. Martínez-González, M.A.; Gea, A.; Ruiz-Canela, M. The Mediterranean Diet and Cardiovascular Health. *Circ. Res.* **2019**, *124*, 779–798. [CrossRef] [PubMed]
203. Hlebowicz, J.; Drake, I.; Gullberg, B.; Sonestedt, E.; Wallström, P.; Persson, M.; Nilsson, J.; Hedblad, B.; Wirfält, E. A High Diet Quality Is Associated with Lower Incidence of Cardiovascular Events in the Malmö Diet and Cancer Cohort. *PLoS ONE* **2013**, *8*, e71095. [CrossRef]
204. Fiuza-Luces, C.; Santos-Lozano, A.; Joyner, M.; Carrera-Bastos, P.; Picazo, O.; Zugaza, J.L.; Izquierdo, M.; Ruilope, L.M.; Lucia, A. Exercise benefits in cardiovascular disease: Beyond attenuation of traditional risk factors. *Nat. Rev. Cardiol.* **2018**, *15*, 731–743. [CrossRef] [PubMed]
205. Petridou, A.; Siopi, A.; Mougios, V. Exercise in the management of obesity. *Metabolism* **2019**, *92*, 163–169. [CrossRef]
206. Aboyans, V.; Ricco, J.-B.; Bartelink, M.-L.E.L.; Björck, M.; Brodmann, M.; Cohnert, T.; Collet, J.-P.; Czerny, M.; De Carlo, M.; Debus, S.; et al. 2017 ESC Guidelines on the Diagnosis and Treatment of Peripheral Arterial Diseases, in collaboration with the European Society for Vascular Surgery (ESVS): Document Covering Atherosclerotic Disease of Extracranial Carotid and Vertebral, Mesenteric, Renal, Upper and Lower Extremity Arteries Endorsed by: The European Stroke Organization (ESO) The Task Force for the Diagnosis and Treatment of Peripheral Arterial Diseases of the European Society of Cardiology (ESC) and of the European Society for Vascular Surgery (ESVS). *Eur. Heart J.* **2018**, *39*, 763–816. [CrossRef] [PubMed]
207. Piepoli, M.F.; Hoes, A.W.; Agewall, S.; Albus, C.; Brotons, C.; Catapano, A.L.; Cooney, M.T.; Corrà, U.; Cosyns, B.; Deaton, C.; et al. 2016 European Guidelines on Cardiovascular Disease Prevention in Clinical Practice: The Sixth Joint Task Force of the European Society of Cardiology and Other Societies on Cardiovascular Disease Prevention in Clinical Practice (Constituted by Representatives of 10 Societies and by Invited Experts) Developed with the Special Contribution of the European Association for Cardiovascular Prevention & Rehabilitation (EACPR). *Atherosclerosis* **2016**, *252*, 207–274. [CrossRef]
208. Klopf, J.; Scheuba, A.; Brostjan, C.; Neumayer, C.; Eilenberg, W. Bisherige Strategien und zukünftige Perspektive zur Reduzierung der Wachstumsraten bei abdominellen Aortenaneurysmen: Eine selektive Literaturrecherche sowie Erörterung des aktuellen Vienna MetAAA Trials. *Gefässchirurgie* **2020**, *25*, 446–449. [CrossRef]
209. Yoshimura, K.; Morikage, N.; Nishino-Fujimoto, S.; Furutani, A.; Shirasawa, B.; Hamano, K. Current Status and Perspectives on Pharmacologic Therapy for Abdominal Aortic Aneurysm. *Curr. Drug Targets* **2018**, *19*, 1265–1275. [CrossRef] [PubMed]
210. Kokje, V.; Hamming, J.; Lindeman, J. Editor's Choice—Pharmaceutical Management of Small Abdominal Aortic Aneurysms: A Systematic Review of the Clinical Evidence. *Eur. J. Vasc. Endovasc. Surg.* **2015**, *50*, 702–713. [CrossRef] [PubMed]
211. The Propranolol Aneurysm Trial Investigators Propranolol for small abdominal aortic aneurysms: Results of a randomized trial. *J. Vasc. Surg.* **2002**, *35*, 72–79. [CrossRef] [PubMed]
212. Lindholt, J.S.; Henneberg, E.W.; Juul, S.; Fasting, H. Impaired Results of a Randomised Double Blinded Clinical Trial of Propranolol versus Placebo on the Expansion Rate of Small Abdominal Aortic Aneurysms. *Int. Angiol.* **1999**, *18*, 52–57.
213. Wilmink, A.B.M.; Vardulaki, K.A.; Hubbard, C.S.F.; Day, N.E.; Ashton, H.A.; Scott, A.P.; Quick, C.R.G. Are Antihypertensive Drugs Associated with Abdominal Aortic Aneurysms? *J. Vasc. Surg.* **2002**, *36*, 751–757. [CrossRef]
214. Hackam, D.G.; Thiruchelvam, D.; Redelmeier, D.A. Angiotensin-converting enzyme inhibitors and aortic rupture: A population-based case-control study. *Lancet* **2006**, *368*, 659–665. [CrossRef]
215. Kortekaas, K.E.; Meijer, C.A.; Hinnen, J.W.; Dalman, R.L.; Xu, B.; Hamming, J.F.; Lindeman, J.H. ACE Inhibitors Potently Reduce Vascular Inflammation, Results of an Open Proof-Of-Concept Study in the Abdominal Aortic Aneurysm. *PLoS ONE* **2014**, *9*, e111952. [CrossRef]
216. Bicknell, C.D.; Kiru, G.; Falaschetti, E.; Powell, J.T.; Poulter, N.R. AARDVARK Collaborators An Evaluation of the Effect of an Angiotensin-Converting Enzyme Inhibitor on the Growth Rate of Small Abdominal Aortic Aneurysms: A Randomized Placebo-Controlled Trial (AARDVARK). *Eur. Hear. J.* **2016**, *37*, 3213–3221. [CrossRef] [PubMed]
217. Salata, K.; Syed, M.; Hussain, M.A.; Eikelboom, R.; de Mestral, C.; Verma, S.; Al-Omran, M. Renin-angiotensin system blockade does not attenuate abdominal aortic aneurysm growth, rupture rate, or perioperative mortality after elective repair. *J. Vasc. Surg.* **2018**, *67*, 629–636.e2. [CrossRef]
218. Sweeting, M.; Thompson, S.G.; Brown, L.C.; Greenhalgh, R.M.; Powell, J.T. Use of angiotensin converting enzyme inhibitors is associated with increased growth rate of abdominal aortic aneurysms. *J. Vasc. Surg.* **2010**, *52*, 1–4. [CrossRef] [PubMed]
219. Juvonen, J.; Juvonen, T.; Laurila, A.; Alakärppä, H.; Lounatmaa, K.; Surcel, H.-M.; Leinonen, M.; Kairaluoma, M.I.; Saikku, P. Demonstration of Chlamydia pneumoniae in the walls of abdominal aortic aneurysms. *J. Vasc. Surg.* **1997**, *25*, 499–505. [CrossRef]
220. Halme, S.; Juvonen, T.; Laurila, A.; Mosorin, M.; Saikku, P.; Surcel, H.-M. Chlamydia pneumoniaereactive T lymphocytes in the walls of abdominal aortic aneurysms. *Eur. J. Clin. Investig.* **1999**, *29*, 546–552. [CrossRef]
221. Baxter, B.; Pearce, W.H.; Waltke, E.A.; Littooy, F.N.; Hallett, J.W.; Kent, K.; Upchurch, G.R.; Chaikof, E.L.; Mills, J.; Fleckten, B.; et al. Prolonged administration of doxycycline in patients with small asymptomatic abdominal aortic aneurysms: Report of a prospective (Phase II) multicenter study. *J. Vasc. Surg.* **2002**, *36*, 1–12. [CrossRef] [PubMed]

222. Curci, J.A.; Mao, D.; Bohner, D.G.; Allen, B.T.; Rubin, B.G.; Reilly, J.M.; Sicard, G.A.; Thompson, R.W. Preoperative treatment with doxycycline reduces aortic wall expression and activation of matrix metalloproteinases in patients with abdominal aortic aneurysms. *J. Vasc. Surg.* **2000**, *31*, 325–342. [CrossRef]
223. Mosorin, M.; Juvonen, J.; Biancari, F.; Satta, J.; Surcel, H.-M.; Leinonen, M.; Saikku, P.; Juvonen, T. Use of doxycycline to decrease the growth rate of abdominal aortic aneurysms: A randomized, double-blind, placebo-controlled pilot study. *J. Vasc. Surg.* **2001**, *34*, 606–610. [CrossRef] [PubMed]
224. Meijer, A.; Stijnen, T.; Wasser, M.N.; Hamming, J.F.; Van Bockel, J.H.; Lindeman, J.H. Pharmaceutical Aneurysm Stabilisation Trial Study Group Doxycycline for Stabilization of Abdominal Aortic Aneurysms: A Randomized Trial. *Ann. Intern. Med.* **2013**, *159*, 815–823. [CrossRef] [PubMed]
225. Baxter, B.T.; Matsumura, J.; Curci, J.A.; McBride, R.; Larson, L.; Blackwelder, W.; Lam, D.; Wijesinha, M.; Terrin, M. N-TA3CT Investigators Effect of Doxycycline on Aneurysm Growth Among Patients With Small Infrarenal Abdominal Aortic Aneurysms: A Randomized Clinical Trial. *JAMA* **2020**, *323*, 2029–2038. [CrossRef]
226. Vammen, S.; Lindholt, J.; Østergaard, L.; Fasting, H.; Henneberg, E.W. Randomized double-blind controlled trial of roxithromycin for prevention of abdominal aortic aneurysm expansion. *Br. J. Surg.* **2001**, *88*, 1066–1072. [CrossRef] [PubMed]
227. Høgh, A.; Vammen, S.; Østergaard, L.; Joensen, J.B.; Henneberg, E.W.; Lindholt, J. Intermittent Roxithromycin for Preventing Progression of Small Abdominal Aortic Aneurysms: Long-Term Results of a Small Clinical Trial. *Vasc. Endovasc. Surg.* **2009**, *43*, 452–456. [CrossRef] [PubMed]
228. Karlsson, L.; Gnarpe, J.; Bergqvist, D.; Lindbäck, J.; Pärsson, H. The effect of azithromycin and Chlamydophilia pneumonia infection on expansion of small abdominal aortic aneurysms—A prospective randomized double-blind trial. *J. Vasc. Surg.* **2009**, *50*, 23–29. [CrossRef]
229. Takagi, H.; Yamamoto, H.; Iwata, K.; Goto, S.; Umemoto, T. ALICE (All-Literature Investigation of Cardiovascular Evidence) Group Effects of Statin Therapy on Abdominal Aortic Aneurysm Growth: A Meta-Analysis and Meta-Regression of Observational Comparative Studies. *Eur. J. Vasc. Endovasc. Surg.* **2012**, *44*, 287–292. [CrossRef]
230. Salata, K.; Syed, M.; Hussain, M.A.; de Mestral, C.; Greco, E.; Mamdani, M.; Tu, J.V.; Forbes, T.L.; Bhatt, D.L.; Verma, S.; et al. Statins Reduce Abdominal Aortic Aneurysm Growth, Rupture, and Perioperative Mortality: A Systematic Review and Meta-Analysis. *J. Am. Hear. Assoc.* **2018**, *7*, e008657. [CrossRef]
231. Pan, Z.; Cui, H.; Wu, N.; Zhang, H. Effect of Statin Therapy on Abdominal Aortic Aneurysm Growth Rate and Mortality: A Systematic Review and Meta-analysis. *Ann. Vasc. Surg.* **2020**, *67*, 503–510. [CrossRef]
232. Dunne, J.A.; Bailey, M.A.; Griffin, K.J.; Sohrabi, S.; Coughlin, P.A.; Scott, D.J.A. Statins: The Holy Grail of Abdominal Aortic Aneurysm (AAA) Growth Attenuation? A Systematic Review of the Literature. *Curr. Vasc. Pharmacol.* **2014**, *12*, 168–172. [CrossRef]
233. Golledge, J.; Norman, P.E.; Murphy, M.P.; Dalman, R.L. Challenges and opportunities in limiting abdominal aortic aneurysm growth. *J. Vasc. Surg.* **2016**, *65*, 225–233. [CrossRef]
234. Franklin, I.J.; Walton, L.J.; Brown, L.; Greenhalgh, R.N.; Powell, J.T. Vascular Surgical Society of Great Britain and Ireland: Non-Steroidal Anti-Inflammatory Drugs to Treat Abdominal Aortic Aneurysm. *BJS* **1999**, *86*, 707. [CrossRef] [PubMed]
235. Sillesen, H.; Eldrup, N.; Hultgren, R.; Lindeman, J.; Bredahl, K.; Thompson, M.; Wanhainen, A.; Wingren, U.; Swedenborg, J.; Janson, I.; et al. AORTA Trial Investigators Randomized Clinical Trial of Mast Cell Inhibition in Patients with a Medium-Sized Abdominal Aortic Aneurysm. *BJS* **2015**, *102*, 894–901. [CrossRef] [PubMed]
236. Golledge, J.; Pinchbeck, J.; Tomee, S.M.; Rowbotham, S.E.; Singh, T.; Moxon, J.V.; Jenkins, J.S.; Lindeman, J.H.; Dalman, R.L.; McDonnell, L.; et al. Efficacy of Telmisartan to Slow Growth of Small Abdominal Aortic Aneurysms: A Randomized Clinical Trial. *JAMA Cardiol.* **2020**, *5*, 1374. [CrossRef] [PubMed]
237. Lindholt, J.S.; Sorensen, H.T.; Michel, J.B.; Thomsen, H.F.; Henneberg, E.W. Low-Dose Aspirin May Prevent Growth and Later Surgical Repair of Medium-Sized Abdominal Aortic Aneurysms. *Vasc. Endovasc. Surg.* **2008**, *42*, 329–334. [CrossRef] [PubMed]
238. Wemmelund, H.; Jørgensen, T.M.; Høgh, A.; Behr-Rasmussen, C.; Johnsen, S.P.; Lindholt, J.S. Low-dose aspirin and rupture of abdominal aortic aneurysm. *J. Vasc. Surg.* **2017**, *65*, 616–625.e4. [CrossRef] [PubMed]
239. Wanhainen, A.; Mani, K.; Kullberg, J.; Svensjö, S.; Bersztel, A.; Karlsson, L.; Holst, J.; Gottsäter, A.; Linné, A.; Gillgren, P.; et al. The Effect of Ticagrelor on Growth of Small Abdominal Aortic Aneurysms-a Randomized Controlled Trial. *Cardiovasc. Res.* **2020**, *116*, 450–456. [CrossRef]
240. Clinical Trial Record: Eplerenone in the Management of Abdominal Aortic Aneurysms: A Proof-of-Concept Randomised Controlled Trial. Available online: https://clinicaltrials.gov/ct2/show/NCT02345590 (accessed on 28 November 2021).
241. Clinical Trial Record: Brief Administration of Cyclosporine a to Induce the Stabilisation of the Diameter of Small Diameter Abdominal Aortic Aneurysms. Available online: https://clinicaltrials.gov/ct2/show/NCT02225756 (accessed on 28 November 2021).
242. Clinical Trial Record: A Prospective Randomized, Double Blind, Placebo-Controlled, Safety and Efficacy Study of Metformin as Add-on Therapy in Non-Diabetic Patients with Abdominal Aortic Aneurysm (MetAAA Study). Available online: https://clinicaltrials.gov/ct2/show/NCT03507413 (accessed on 28 November 2021).
243. Clinical Trial Record: Metformin for Abdominal Aortic Aneurysm Growth Inhibition (MAAAGI). Available online: https://clinicaltrials.gov/ct2/show/NCT04224051 (accessed on 28 November 2021).

244. Golledge, J.; Morris, D.R.; Pinchbeck, J.; Rowbotham, S.; Jenkins, J.; Bourke, M.; Bourke, B.; Norman, P.E.; Jones, R.; Moxon, J.V. Editor's Choice—Metformin Prescription is Associated with a Reduction in the Combined Incidence of Surgical Repair and Rupture Related Mortality in Patients with Abdominal Aortic Aneurysm. *Eur. J. Vasc. Endovasc. Surg.* **2019**, *57*, 94–101. [CrossRef]
245. Raffort, J.; Chinetti, G.; Lareyre, F. Glucagon-Like peptide-1: A new therapeutic target to treat abdominal aortic aneurysm? *Biochimie* **2018**, *152*, 149–154. [CrossRef]
246. Pini, R.; Ciavarella, C.; Faggioli, G.; Gallitto, E.; Indelicato, G.; Fenelli, C.; Mascoli, C.; Vacirca, A.; Gargiulo, M.; Pasquinelli, G. Different Drugs Effect on Mesenchymal Stem Cells Isolated From Abdominal Aortic Aneurysm. *Ann. Vasc. Surg.* **2020**, *67*, 490–496. [CrossRef]
247. Raffort, J.; Hassen-Khodja, R.; Jean-Baptiste, E.; Lareyre, F. Relationship between metformin and abdominal aortic aneurysm. *J. Vasc. Surg.* **2020**, *71*, 1056–1062. [CrossRef] [PubMed]
248. Clinical Trial Record: Limiting AAA With Metformin (LIMIT) Trial (LIMIT). Available online: https://clinicaltrials.gov/ct2/show/NCT04500756 (accessed on 28 November 2021).
249. Miyake, T.; Miyake, T.; Kurashiki, T.; Morishita, R. Molecular Pharmacological Approaches for Treating Abdominal Aortic Aneurysm. *Ann. Vasc. Dis.* **2019**, *12*, 137–146. [CrossRef] [PubMed]
250. Beck, A.W.; Sedrakyan, A.; Mao, J.; Venermo, M.; Faizer, R.; Debus, S.; Behrendt, C.-A.; Scali, S.T.; Altreuther, M.; Schermerhorn, M.; et al. Variations in Abdominal Aortic Aneurysm Care: A Report From the International Consortium of Vascular Registries. *Circulation* **2016**, *134*, 1948–1958. [CrossRef]
251. Acher, C.; Ramirez, M.C.C.; Wynn, M. Operative Mortality and Morbidity in Ruptured Abdominal Aortic Aneurysms in the Endovascular Age. *Ann. Vasc. Surg.* **2020**, *66*, 70–76. [CrossRef]
252. D'Oria, M.; Hanson, K.T.; Shermerhorn, M.; Bower, T.C.; Mendes, B.C.; Shuja, F.; Oderich, G.S.; DeMartino, R.R. Editor's Choice—Short Term and Long Term Outcomes After Endovascular or Open Repair for Ruptured Infrarenal Abdominal Aortic Aneurysms in the Vascular Quality Initiative. *Eur. J. Vasc. Endovasc. Surg.* **2020**, *59*, 703–716. [CrossRef]
253. Ulug, P.; Powell, J.T.; Martinez, M.A.-M.; Ballard, D.J.; Filardo, G. Surgery for small asymptomatic abdominal aortic aneurysms. *Cochrane Database Syst. Rev.* **2020**, *2020*, CD001835. [CrossRef]
254. Powell, J.T.; Wanhainen, A. Analysis of the Differences Between the ESVS 2019 and NICE 2020 Guidelines for Abdominal Aortic Aneurysm. *Eur. J. Vasc. Endovasc. Surg.* **2020**, *60*, 7–15. [CrossRef]
255. Lo, R.C.; Lu, B.; Fokkema, M.T.; Conrad, M.; Patel, V.I.; Fillinger, M.; Matyal, R.; Schermerhorn, M.L. Vascular Study Group of New England, Relative Importance of Aneurysm Diameter and Body Size for Predicting Abdominal Aortic Aneurysm Rupture in Men and Women. *J. Vasc. Surg.* **2014**, *59*, 1209–1216. [CrossRef]
256. Deery, S.E.; Schermerhorn, M.L. Should Abdominal Aortic Aneurysms in Women be Repaired at a Lower Diameter Threshold? *Vasc. Endovasc. Surg.* **2018**, *52*, 543–547. [CrossRef] [PubMed]
257. Karthaus, E.G.; Tong, T.M.L.; Vahl, A.; Hamming, J.F. Dutch Society of Vascular Surgery, the Steering Committee of the Dutch Surgical Aneurysm Audit and the Dutch Institute for Clinical Auditing Saccular Abdominal Aortic Aneurysms: Patient Characteristics, Clinical Presentation, Treatment, and Outcomes in the Netherlands. *Ann. Surg.* **2019**, *270*, 852–858. [CrossRef]
258. Kristmundsson, T.; Dias, N.; Resch, T.; Sonesson, B. Morphology of Small Abdominal Aortic Aneurysms Should be Considered before Continued Ultrasound Surveillance. *Ann. Vasc. Surg.* **2016**, *31*, 18–22. [CrossRef]
259. Soden, P.A.; Zettervall, S.L.; Ultee, K.H.; Darling, J.D.; Buck, D.B.; Hile, C.N.; Hamdan, A.D.; Schermerhorn, M.L. Outcomes for symptomatic abdominal aortic aneurysms in the American College of Surgeons National Surgical Quality Improvement Program. *J. Vasc. Surg.* **2016**, *64*, 297–305. [CrossRef]
260. Ten Bosch, J.A.; Koning, S.W.; Willigendael, E.M.; VAN Sambeek, M.R.; Stokmans, R.A.; Prins, M.H.; Teijink, J.A. Symptomatic Abdominal Aortic Aneurysm Repair: To Wait or Not to Wait. *J. Cardiovasc. Surg.* **2016**, *57*, 830–838.
261. Ma, B.; Wang, Y.-N.; Chen, K.; Zhang, Y.; Pan, H.; Yang, K. Transperitoneal versus Retroperitoneal Approach for Elective Open Abdominal Aortic Aneurysm Repair. *Cochrane Database Syst. Rev.* **2016**, *2*, CD010373. [CrossRef] [PubMed]
262. Wiersema, A.M.; Jongkind, V.; Bruijninckx, C.M.A.; Reijnen, M.M.P.J.; Vos, J.A.; van Delden, O.M.; Zeebregts, C.J.; Moll, F.L. CAPPAStudy Group Consensus on Arterial PeriProcedural Anticoagulation Prophylactic Perioperative Anti-Thrombotics in Open and Endovascular Abdominal Aortic Aneurysm (AAA) Surgery: A Systematic Review. *Eur. J. Vasc. Endovasc. Surg.* **2012**, *44*, 359–367. [CrossRef] [PubMed]
263. Cao, P.; De Rango, P.; Parlani, G.; Verzini, F. Fate of Proximal Aorta Following Open Infrarenal Aneurysm Repair. *Semin. Vasc. Surg.* **2009**, *22*, 93–98. [CrossRef]
264. Salata, K.; Hussain, M.A.; De Mestral, C.; Greco, E.; Aljabri, B.A.; Mamdani, M.; Forbes, T.L.; Bhatt, D.L.; Verma, S.; Al-Omran, M. Comparison of Outcomes in Elective Endovascular Aortic Repair vs Open Surgical Repair of Abdominal Aortic Aneurysms. *JAMA Netw. Open* **2019**, *2*, e196578. [CrossRef]
265. Lee, S.Y.; Peacock, M.R.; Farber, A.; Shah, N.K.; Eslami, M.H.; Kalish, J.A.; Rybin, D.; Komshian, S.; Siracuse, J.J. Perioperative Infections after Open Abdominal Aortic Aneurysm Repair Lead to Increased Risk of Subsequent Complications. *Ann. Vasc. Surg.* **2017**, *44*, 203–210. [CrossRef]
266. Nicolajsen, C.W.; Eldrup, N. Abdominal Closure and the Risk of Incisional Hernia in Aneurysm Surgery—A Systematic Review and Meta-analysis. *Eur. J. Vasc. Endovasc. Surg.* **2020**, *59*, 227–236. [CrossRef]

267. Indrakusuma, R.; Jalalzadeh, H.; van der Meij, J.E.; Balm, R.; Koelemay, M.J. Prophylactic Mesh Reinforcement versus Sutured Closure to Prevent Incisional Hernias after Open Abdominal Aortic Aneurysm Repair via Midline Laparotomy: A Systematic Review and Meta-Analysis. *Eur. J. Vasc. Endovasc. Surg.* **2018**, *56*, 120–128. [CrossRef] [PubMed]
268. Biancari, F.; Ylönen, K.; Anttila, V.; Juvonen, J.; Romsi, P.; Satta, J.; Juvonen, T. Durability of open repair of infrarenal abdominal aortic aneurysm: A 15-year follow-up study. *J. Vasc. Surg.* **2002**, *35*, 87–93. [CrossRef]
269. Conrad, M.F.; Crawford, R.S.; Pedraza, J.D.; Brewster, D.C.; LaMuraglia, G.M.; Corey, M.; Abbara, S.; Cambria, R.P. Long-term durability of open abdominal aortic aneurysm repair. *J. Vasc. Surg.* **2007**, *46*, 669–675. [CrossRef] [PubMed]
270. Paravastu, S.C.V.; Jayarajasingam, R.; Cottam, R.; Palfreyman, S.J.; Michaels, J.A.; Thomas, S.M. Endovascular Repair of Abdominal Aortic Aneurysm. *Cochrane Database Syst. Rev.* **2014**, CD004178. [CrossRef]
271. Antoniou, G.A.; Antoniou, S.A. Editor's Choice—Percutaneous Access Does Not Confer Superior Clinical Outcomes Over Cutdown Access for Endovascular Aneurysm Repair: Meta-Analysis and Trial Sequential Analysis of Randomised Controlled Trials. *Eur. J. Vasc. Endovasc. Surg.* **2020**, *61*, 383–394. [CrossRef]
272. Belvroy, V.M.; Houben, I.B.; Trimarchi, S.; Patel, H.J.; Moll, F.L.; Van Herwaarden, J.A. Identifying and addressing the limitations of EVAR technology. *Expert Rev. Med. Devices* **2018**, *15*, 541–554. [CrossRef]
273. Kontopodis, N.; Galanakis, N.; Tzartzalou, I.; Tavlas, E.; Georgakarakos, E.; Dimopoulos, I.; Tsetis, D.; Ioannou, C.V. An update on the improvement of patient eligibility with the use of new generation endografts for the treatment of abdominal aortic aneurysms. *Expert Rev. Med. Devices* **2020**, *17*, 1231–1238. [CrossRef]
274. Gopal, M.; Lau, I.; Harris, J.; Berger, K.; Faries, P.; Marin, M.; Tadros, R. A Review of the Evolution of Abdominal Aortic Endografts and Future Directions. *Surg. Technol. Int.* **2020**, *37*, 193–201. [PubMed]
275. Daye, D.; Walker, T.G. Complications of endovascular aneurysm repair of the thoracic and abdominal aorta: Evaluation and management. *Cardiovasc. Diagn. Ther.* **2018**, *8*, S138–S156. [CrossRef]
276. Spanos, K.; Karathanos, C.; Saleptsis, V.; Giannoukas, A.D. Systematic review and meta-analysis of migration after endovascular abdominal aortic aneurysm repair. *Vascular* **2015**, *24*, 323–336. [CrossRef]
277. de la Motte, L.; Falkenberg, M.; Koelemay, M.J.; Lönn, L. Is EVAR a Durable Solution? Indications for Reinterventions. *J Cardiovasc Surg* **2018**, *59*, 201–212. [CrossRef]
278. Bradley, N.A.; Roxburgh, C.; Khan, F.; Guthrie, G. Postimplantation syndrome in endovascular aortic aneurysm repair—A systematic review. *Vasa* **2021**, *50*, 174–185. [CrossRef]
279. Holden, A. Aneurysm Repair with Endovascular Aneurysm Sealing: Technique, Patient Selection, and Management of Complications. *Tech. Vasc. Interv. Radiol.* **2018**, *21*, 181–187. [CrossRef] [PubMed]
280. Martinelli, O.; Alunno, A.; Gattuso, R.; Di Girolamo, A.; Irace, L. Nellix endovascular aneurysm-sealing system: A single-center experience and review of current evidence. *Futur. Cardiol.* **2021**, *17*, 875–884. [CrossRef] [PubMed]
281. Quaglino, S.; Mortola, L.; Ferrero, E.; Ferri, M.; Cirillo, S.; Lario, C.V.; Negro, G.; Ricotti, A.; Gaggiano, A. Long-Term Failure after EVAS in a Real-Life Single Center Experience with the Nellix Endograft. *J. Vasc. Surg.* **2020**, *73*, 1958–1965.e1. [CrossRef]
282. Singh, A.A.; Benaragama, K.S.; Pope, T.; Coughlin, P.A.; Winterbottom, A.P.; Harrison, S.C.; Boyle, J.R. Progressive Device Failure at Long Term Follow Up of the Nellix EndoVascular Aneurysm Sealing (EVAS) System. *Eur. J. Vasc. Endovasc. Surg.* **2020**, *61*, 211–218. [CrossRef]
283. Kristensen, S.D.; Knuuti, J.; Saraste, A.; Anker, S.D.; Bøtker, H.E.; De Hert, S.; Ford, I.; Gonzalez-Juanatey, J.R.; Gorenek, B.; Heyndrickx, G.R.; et al. 2014 ESC/ESA Guidelines on non-cardiac surgery: Cardiovascular assessment and management: The Joint Task Force on non-cardiac surgery: Cardiovascular assessment and management of the European Society of Cardiology (ESC) and the European Society of Anaesthesiology (ESA). *Eur. Hear. J.* **2014**, *35*, 2383–2431. [CrossRef]
284. Biagi, P.; de Donato, G.; Setacci, C. Cardiac Risk Stratification in Patients Undergoing Endovascular Aortic Repair. *Minerva Cardioangiol.* **2016**, *64*, 195–203.
285. Spanos, K.; Karathanos, C.; Athanasoulas, A.; Sapeltsis, V.; Giannoukas, A.D. Systematic Review of Follow-up Compliance after Endovascular Abdominal Aortic Aneurysm Repair. *J. Cardiovasc. Surg (Torino)* **2018**, *59*, 611–618. [CrossRef]
286. Grima, M.J.; Boufi, M.; Law, M.; Jackson, D.; Stenson, K.; Patterson, B.; Loftus, I.; Thompson, M.; Karthikesalingam, A.; Holt, P. Editor's Choice—The Implications of Non-compliance to Endovascular Aneurysm Repair Surveillance: A Systematic Review and Meta-analysis. *Eur. J. Vasc. Endovasc. Surg.* **2018**, *55*, 492–502. [CrossRef] [PubMed]
287. Kim, S.H.; Litt, H.I. Surveillance Imaging following Endovascular Aneurysm Repair: State of the Art. *Semin. Interv. Radiol.* **2020**, *37*, 356–364. [CrossRef] [PubMed]
288. Hu, D.K.; Pisimisis, G.T.; Sheth, R.A. Repair of abdominal aortic aneurysms: Preoperative imaging and evaluation. *Cardiovasc. Diagn. Ther.* **2018**, *8*, S157–S167. [CrossRef] [PubMed]
289. Kudo, T. Surgical Complications after Open Abdominal Aortic Aneurysm Repair: Intestinal Ischemia, Buttock Claudication and Sexual Dysfunction. *Ann. Vasc. Dis.* **2019**, *12*, 157–162. [CrossRef] [PubMed]
290. Kouvelos, G.; Katsargyris, A.; Antoniou, G.; Oikonomou, K.; Verhoeven, E. Outcome after Interruption or Preservation of Internal Iliac Artery Flow During Endovascular Repair of Abdominal Aorto-iliac Aneurysms. *Eur. J. Vasc. Endovasc. Surg.* **2016**, *52*, 621–634. [CrossRef] [PubMed]
291. Gaudric, J.; Tresson, P.; Derycke, L.; Du Montcel, S.T.; Couture, T.; Davaine, J.-M.; Kashi, M.; Lawton, J.; Chiche, L.; Koskas, F. Surgical internal iliac artery preservation associated with endovascular repair of infrarenal aortoiliac aneurysms to avoid buttock claudication and distal type I endoleaks. *J. Vasc. Surg.* **2018**, *68*, 1736–1743. [CrossRef] [PubMed]

292. Kalko, Y.; Ugurlucan, M.; Basaran, M.; Aydin, U.; Kafa, U.; Kosker, T.; Suren, M.; Yasar, T. Epidural anaesthesia and mini-laparotomy for the treatment of abdominal aortic aneurysms in patients with severe chronic obstructive pulmonary disease. *Acta Chir. Belg.* **2007**, *107*, 307–312. [CrossRef]
293. Hajibandeh, S.; Hajibandeh, S.; Adasonla, K.; Antoniou, S.A.; Barrie, J.; Madan, M.; Antoniou, G.A. Loco-regional versus general anaesthesia for elective endovascular aneurysm repair—Results of a cohort study and a meta-analysis. *Vasa* **2018**, *47*, 209–217. [CrossRef]
294. Sweeting, M.J.; Patel, R.; Powell, J.T.; Greenhalgh, R.M. EVAR Trial Investigators Endovascular Repair of Abdominal Aortic Aneurysm in Patients Physically Ineligible for Open Repair: Very Long-Term Follow-up in the EVAR-2 Randomized Controlled Trial. *Ann. Surg.* **2017**, *266*, 713–719. [CrossRef]
295. Sonesson, B.; Dias, N.; Resch, T. Is There an Age Limit for Abdominal Aortic Aneurysm Repair? *J. Cardiovasc. Surg.* **2018**, *59*, 190–194. [CrossRef]
296. Katsargyris, A.; Lenhardt Michael Florian, C.; Marques de Marino, P.; Botos, B.; Verhoeven, E.L. Reasons for and Outcomes of Open Abdominal Aortic Repair in the Endovascular Era. *Ann. Vasc. Surg.* **2020**, *73*, 417–422. [CrossRef] [PubMed]
297. Shan, L.; Saxena, A.; Goh, D.; Robinson, D. A systematic review on the quality of life and functional status after abdominal aortic aneurysm repair in elderly patients with an average age older than 75 years. *J. Vasc. Surg.* **2018**, *69*, 1268–1281. [CrossRef]
298. Nargesi, S.; Abutorabi, A.; Alipour, V.; Tajdini, M.; Salimi, J. Cost-Effectiveness of Endovascular Versus Open Repair of Abdominal Aortic Aneurysm: A Systematic Review. *Cardiovasc. Drugs Ther.* **2021**, *35*, 829–839. [CrossRef] [PubMed]
299. Yokoyama, Y.; Kuno, T.; Takagi, H. Meta-analysis of phase-specific survival after elective endovascular versus surgical repair of abdominal aortic aneurysm from randomized controlled trials and propensity score-matched studies. *J. Vasc. Surg.* **2020**, *72*, 1464–1472.e6. [CrossRef]
300. Bahia, S.; Holt, P.; Jackson, D.; Patterson, B.; Hinchliffe, R.; Thompson, M.; Karthikesalingam, A. Systematic Review and Meta-analysis of Long-term survival After Elective Infrarenal Abdominal Aortic Aneurysm Repair 1969–2011: 5 Year Survival Remains Poor Despite Advances in Medical Care and Treatment Strategies. *Eur. J. Vasc. Endovasc. Surg.* **2015**, *50*, 320–330. [CrossRef]
301. Khashram, M.; Williman, J.; Hider, P.N.; Jones, G.T.; Roake, J.A. Management of Modifiable Vascular Risk Factors Improves Late Survival following Abdominal Aortic Aneurysm Repair: A Systematic Review and Meta-Analysis. *Ann. Vasc. Surg.* **2017**, *39*, 301–311. [CrossRef] [PubMed]
302. Alberga, A.J.; Karthaus, E.G.; van Zwet, E.W.; de Bruin, J.L.; van Herwaarden, J.A.; Wever, J.J.; Verhagen, H.J.; Akker, P.V.D.; Akkersdijk, G.; Akkersdijk, W.; et al. Dutch Institute for Clinical Auditing Outcomes in Octogenarians and the Effect of Comorbidities After Intact Abdominal Aortic Aneurysm Repair in the Netherlands: A Nationwide Cohort Study. *Eur. J. Vasc. Endovasc. Surg.* **2021**, *61*, 920–928. [CrossRef]
303. Harris, D.G.; Bulatao, I.; Oates, C.P.; Kalsi, R.; Drucker, C.B.; Menon, N.; Flohr, T.R.; Crawford, R.S. Functional status predicts major complications and death after endovascular repair of abdominal aortic aneurysms. *J. Vasc. Surg.* **2017**, *66*, 743–750. [CrossRef]
304. Al Shakarchi, J.; Fairhead, J.; Rajagopalan, S.; Pherwani, A.; Jaipersad, A. Impact of Frailty on Outcomes in Patients Undergoing Open Abdominal Aortic Aneurysm Repair. *Ann. Vasc. Surg.* **2020**, *67*, 100–104. [CrossRef]
305. Liu, Y.; Yang, Y.; Zhao, J.; Chen, X.; Wang, J.; Ma, Y.; Huang, B.; Yuan, D.; Du, X. Systematic review and meta-analysis of sex differences in outcomes after endovascular aneurysm repair for infrarenal abdominal aortic aneurysm. *J. Vasc. Surg.* **2020**, *71*, 283–296.e4. [CrossRef]
306. Kalender, G.; Lisy, M.; Stock, U.; Endisch, A.; Kornberger, A. Long-term radiation exposure in patients undergoing EVAR: Reflecting clinical day-to-day practice to assess realistic radiation burden. *Clin. Hemorheol. Microcirc.* **2019**, *71*, 451–461. [CrossRef]
307. Lloyd, G.; Bown, M.; Norwood, M.; Deb, R.; Fishwick, G.; Bell, P.; Sayers, R. Feasibility of preoperative computer tomography in patients with ruptured abdominal aortic aneurysm: A time-to-death study in patients without operation. *J. Vasc. Surg.* **2004**, *39*, 788–791. [CrossRef]
308. Biancari, F.; Paone, R.; Venermo, M.; D'Andrea, V.; Perälä, J. Diagnostic Accuracy of Computed Tomography in Patients with Suspected Abdominal Aortic Aneurysm Rupture. *Eur. J. Vasc. Endovasc. Surg.* **2013**, *45*, 227–230. [CrossRef] [PubMed]
309. IMPROVE Trial Investigators. Comparative clinical effectiveness and cost effectiveness of endovascular strategy v open repair for ruptured abdominal aortic aneurysm: Three year results of the IMPROVE randomised trial. *BMJ* **2017**, *359*, j4859. [CrossRef]
310. Kontopodis, N.; Galanakis, N.; Antoniou, S.A.; Tsetis, D.; Ioannou, C.V.; Veith, F.J.; Powell, J.T.; Antoniou, G.A. Meta-Analysis and Meta-Regression Analysis of Outcomes of Endovascular and Open Repair for Ruptured Abdominal Aortic Aneurysm. *Eur. J. Vasc. Endovasc. Surg.* **2020**, *59*, 399–410. [CrossRef]
311. Varkevisser, R.R.; Swerdlow, N.J.; de Guerre, L.E.; Dansey, K.; Stangenberg, L.; Giles, K.A.; Verhagen, H.J.; Schermerhorn, M.L. Society for Vascular Surgery Vascular Quality Initiative Five-Year Survival Following Endovascular Repair of Ruptured Abdominal Aortic Aneurysms Is Improving. *J. Vasc. Surg.* **2020**, *72*, 105–113.e4. [CrossRef]
312. Li, Y.; Li, Z.; Wang, S.; Chang, G.; Wu, R.; Hu, Z.; Yin, H.; Wang, J.; Yao, C. Endovascular versus Open Surgery Repair of Ruptured Abdominal Aortic Aneurysms in Hemodynamically Unstable Patients: Literature Review and Meta-Analysis. *Ann. Vasc. Surg.* **2016**, *32*, 135–144. [CrossRef] [PubMed]
313. Kontopodis, N.; Tavlas, E.; Ioannou, C.V.; Giannoukas, A.D.; Geroulakos, G.; Antoniou, G.A. Systematic Review and Meta-Analysis of Outcomes of Open and Endovascular Repair of Ruptured Abdominal Aortic Aneurysm in Patients with Hostile vs. Friendly Aortic Anatomy. *Eur. J. Vasc. Endovasc. Surg.* **2020**, *59*, 717–728. [CrossRef] [PubMed]

314. Morbiducci, U.; Kok, A.M.; Kwak, B.; Stone, P.H.; Steinman, D.A.; Wentzel, J.J. Atherosclerosis at arterial bifurcations: Evidence for the role of haemodynamics and geometry. *Thromb. Haemost.* **2016**, *115*, 484–492. [CrossRef]
315. Chistiakov, D.A.; Orekhov, A.N.; Bobryshev, Y.V. Effects of shear stress on endothelial cells: Go with the flow. *Acta Physiol.* **2016**, *219*, 382–408. [CrossRef]
316. Golledge, J.; Norman, P.E. Atherosclerosis and Abdominal Aortic Aneurysm: Cause, Response, or Common Risk Factors? *Arter. Thromb. Vasc. Biol.* **2010**, *30*, 1075–1077. [CrossRef]
317. Johnsen, S.H.; Forsdahl, S.H.; Singh, K.; Jacobsen, B.K. Atherosclerosis in Abdominal Aortic Aneurysms: A Causal Event or a Process Running in Parallel? The Tromsø Study. *Arter. Thromb. Vasc. Biol.* **2010**, *30*, 1263–1268. [CrossRef] [PubMed]
318. Wang, D.H.; Makaroun, M.S.; Webster, M.W.; Vorp, D. Effect of intraluminal thrombus on wall stress in patient-specific models of abdominal aortic aneurysm. *J. Vasc. Surg.* **2002**, *36*, 598–604. [CrossRef]
319. Georgakarakos, E.; Ioannou, C.V.; Volanis, S.; Papaharilaou, Y.; Ekaterinaris, J.; Katsamouris, A.N. The Influence of Intraluminal Thrombus on Abdominal Aortic Aneurysm Wall Stress. *Int. Angiol.* **2009**, *28*, 325–333. [PubMed]
320. Gasser, T.C.; Görgülü, G.; Folkesson, M.; Swedenborg, J. Failure properties of intraluminal thrombus in abdominal aortic aneurysm under static and pulsating mechanical loads. *J. Vasc. Surg.* **2008**, *48*, 179–188. [CrossRef]
321. Roy, J.; Labruto, F.; Beckman, M.O.; Danielson, J.; Johansson, G.; Swedenborg, J. Bleeding into the intraluminal thrombus in abdominal aortic aneurysms is associated with rupture. *J. Vasc. Surg.* **2008**, *48*, 1108–1113. [CrossRef]
322. Talvitie, M.; Liljeqvist, M.L.; Siika, A.; Hultgren, R.; Roy, J. Localized Hyperattenuations in the Intraluminal Thrombus May Predict Rupture of Abdominal Aortic Aneurysms. *J. Vasc. Interv. Radiol.* **2018**, *29*, 144–145. [CrossRef]
323. Haller, S.J.; Crawford, J.D.; Courchaine, K.M.; Bohannan, C.J.; Landry, G.J.; Moneta, G.L.; Azarbal, A.F.; Rugonyi, S. Intraluminal thrombus is associated with early rupture of abdominal aortic aneurysm. *J. Vasc. Surg.* **2018**, *67*, 1051–1058.e1. [CrossRef] [PubMed]
324. Wiernicki, I.; Parafiniuk, M.; Kolasa-Wołosiuk, A.; Gutowska, I.; Kazimierczak, A.; Clark, J.; Baranowska-Bosiacka, I.; Szumilowicz, P.; Gutowski, P. Relationship between aortic wall oxidative stress/proteolytic enzyme expression and intraluminal thrombus thickness indicates a novel pathomechanism in the progression of human abdominal aortic aneurysm. *FASEB J.* **2019**, *33*, 885–895. [CrossRef]
325. Tong, J.; Holzapfel, G.A. Structure, Mechanics, and Histology of Intraluminal Thrombi in Abdominal Aortic Aneurysms. *Ann. Biomed. Eng.* **2015**, *43*, 1488–1501. [CrossRef] [PubMed]
326. Koole, D.; Zandvoort, H.J.; Schoneveld, A.; Vink, A.; Vos, J.A.; Hoogen, L.L.V.D.; de Vries, J.-P.P.; Pasterkamp, G.; Moll, F.L.; van Herwaarden, J.A. Intraluminal abdominal aortic aneurysm thrombus is associated with disruption of wall integrity. *J. Vasc. Surg.* **2013**, *57*, 77–83. [CrossRef]
327. Khan, J.A.; Rahman, M.A.; Mazari, F.; Shahin, Y.; Smith, G.; Madden, L.; Fagan, M.; Greenman, J.; McCollum, P.; Chetter, I. Intraluminal Thrombus has a Selective Influence on Matrix Metalloproteinases and Their Inhibitors (Tissue Inhibitors of Matrix Metalloproteinases) in the Wall of Abdominal Aortic Aneurysms. *Ann. Vasc. Surg.* **2012**, *26*, 322–329. [CrossRef]
328. Michel, J.-B.; Martin-Ventura, J.-L.; Egido, J.; Sakalihasan, N.; Treska, V.; Lindholt, J.; Allaire, E.; Thorsteinsdottir, U.; Cockerill, G.; Swedenborg, J. Novel aspects of the pathogenesis of aneurysms of the abdominal aorta in humans. *Cardiovasc. Res.* **2011**, *90*, 18–27. [CrossRef] [PubMed]
329. Zhu, C.; Leach, J.R.; Wang, Y.; Gasper, W.; Saloner, D.; Hope, M.D. Intraluminal Thrombus Predicts Rapid Growth of Abdominal Aortic Aneurysms. *Radiology* **2020**, *294*, 707–713. [CrossRef]
330. Nguyen, V.; Leiner, T.; Hellenthal, F.; Backes, W.; Wishaupt, M.; van der Geest, R.; Heeneman, S.; Kooi, M.; Schurink, G. Abdominal Aortic Aneurysms with High Thrombus Signal Intensity on Magnetic Resonance Imaging are Associated with High Growth Rate. *Eur. J. Vasc. Endovasc. Surg.* **2014**, *48*, 676–684. [CrossRef] [PubMed]
331. The MA^{3}RS Study Investigators. Aortic Wall Inflammation Predicts Abdominal Aortic Aneurysm Expansion, Rupture, and Need for Surgical Repair. *Circulation* **2017**, *136*, 787–797. [CrossRef] [PubMed]
332. Behr-Rasmussen, C.; Grøndal, N.; Bramsen, M.; Thomsen, M.; Lindholt, J. Mural Thrombus and the Progression of Abdominal Aortic Aneurysms: A Large Population-based Prospective Cohort Study. *Eur. J. Vasc. Endovasc. Surg.* **2014**, *48*, 301–307. [CrossRef] [PubMed]
333. Parr, A.; McCann, M.; Bradshaw, B.; Shahzad, A.; Buttner, P.; Golledge, J. Thrombus volume is associated with cardiovascular events and aneurysm growth in patients who have abdominal aortic aneurysms. *J. Vasc. Surg.* **2011**, *53*, 28–35. [CrossRef]
334. Golledge, J.; Iyer, V.; Jenkins, J.; Bradshaw, B.; Cronin, O.; Walker, P.J. Thrombus volume is similar in patients with ruptured and intact abdominal aortic aneurysms. *J. Vasc. Surg.* **2013**, *59*, 315–320. [CrossRef]
335. Folkesson, M.; Silveira, A.; Eriksson, P.; Swedenborg, J. Protease activity in the multi-layered intra-luminal thrombus of abdominal aortic aneurysms. *Atherosclerosis* **2011**, *218*, 294–299. [CrossRef]
336. Ramos-Mozo, P.; Madrigal-Matute, J.; de Ceniga, M.V.; Blanco-Colio, L.M.; Meilhac, O.; Feldman, L.; Michel, J.-B.; Clancy, P.; Golledge, J.; Norman, P.E.; et al. Increased plasma levels of NGAL, a marker of neutrophil activation, in patients with abdominal aortic aneurysm. *Atherosclerosis* **2012**, *220*, 552–556. [CrossRef] [PubMed]
337. Houard, X.; Touat, Z.; Ollivier, V.; Louedec, L.; Philippe, M.; Sebbag, U.; Meilhac, O.; Rossignol, P.; Michel, J.-B. Mediators of neutrophil recruitment in human abdominal aortic aneurysms. *Cardiovasc. Res.* **2009**, *82*, 532–541. [CrossRef]
338. Zhu, C.; Silveira, A.; Hemdahl, A.-L.; Hamsten, A.; Hedin, U.; Swedenborg, J.; Folkesson, M.; Kazil, M.; Eriksson, P. Presence of NGAL/MMP-9 complexes in human abdominal aortic aneurysms. *Thromb. Haemost.* **2007**, *98*, 427–433. [CrossRef]

339. Piechota-Polanczyk, A.; Ejózkowicz, A.; Nowak, W.; Eilenberg, W.; Eneumayer, C.; Emalinski, T.; Ehuk, I.; Ebrostjan, C. The Abdominal Aortic Aneurysm and Intraluminal Thrombus: Current Concepts of Development and Treatment. *Front. Cardiovasc. Med.* **2015**, *2*, 19. [CrossRef]
340. Sánchez-Infantes, D.; Nus, M.; Navas-Madroñal, M.; Fité, J.; Pérez, B.; Barros-Membrilla, A.; Soto, B.; Martínez-González, J.; Camacho, M.; Rodriguez, C.; et al. Oxidative Stress and Inflammatory Markers in Abdominal Aortic Aneurysm. *Antioxidants* **2021**, *10*, 602. [CrossRef]
341. Yuan, Z.; Lu, Y.; Wei, J.; Wu, J.; Yang, J.; Cai, Z. Abdominal Aortic Aneurysm: Roles of Inflammatory Cells. *Front. Immunol* **2020**, *11*, 609161. [CrossRef]
342. Cafueri, G.; Parodi, F.; Pistorio, A.; Bertolotto, M.B.; Ventura, F.; Gambini, C.; Bianco, P.; Dallegri, F.; Pistoia, V.; Pezzolo, A.; et al. Endothelial and Smooth Muscle Cells from Abdominal Aortic Aneurysm Have Increased Oxidative Stress and Telomere Attrition. *PLoS ONE* **2012**, *7*, e35312. [CrossRef]
343. Emeto, T.; Moxon, J.; Au, M.; Golledge, J. Oxidative stress and abdominal aortic aneurysm: Potential treatment targets. *Clin. Sci.* **2016**, *130*, 301–315. [CrossRef] [PubMed]
344. Morgan, S.; Yamanouchi, D.; Harberg, C.; Wang, Q.; Keller, M.; Si, Y.; Burlingham, W.; Seedial, S.; Lengfeld, J.; Liu, B. Elevated Protein Kinase C-δ Contributes to Aneurysm Pathogenesis Through Stimulation of Apoptosis and Inflammatory Signaling. *Arter. Thromb. Vasc. Biol.* **2012**, *32*, 2493–2502. [CrossRef] [PubMed]
345. Rowe, V.L.; Stevens, S.L.; Reddick, T.T.; Freeman, M.B.; Donnell, R.; Carroll, R.C.; Goldman, M.H. Vascular Smooth Muscle Cell Apoptosis in Aneurysmal, Occlusive, and Normal Human Aortas. *J. Vasc. Surg.* **2000**, *31*, 567–576. [CrossRef] [PubMed]
346. Zhang, J.; Schmidt, J.; Ryschich, E.; Schumacher, H.; Allenberg, J.R. Increased Apoptosis and Decreased Density of Medial Smooth Muscle Cells in Human Abdominal Aortic Aneurysms. *Chin. Med. J.* **2003**, *116*, 1549–1552. [PubMed]
347. Choke, E.; Thompson, M.M.; Dawson, J.; Wilson, W.R.W.; Sayed, S.; Loftus, I.M.; Cockerill, G.W. Abdominal Aortic Aneurysm Rupture Is Associated With Increased Medial Neovascularization and Overexpression of Proangiogenic Cytokines. *Arter. Thromb. Vasc. Biol.* **2006**, *26*, 2077–2082. [CrossRef]
348. Choke, E.; Cockerill, G.W.; Dawson, J.; Wilson, R.W.; Jones, A.; Loftus, I.M.; Thompson, M.M. Increased Angiogenesis at the Site of Abdominal Aortic Aneurysm Rupture. *Ann. New York Acad. Sci.* **2006**, *1085*, 315–319. [CrossRef]
349. Blassova, T.; Tonar, Z.; Tomasek, P.; Hosek, P.; Hollan, I.; Treska, V.; Molacek, J. Inflammatory cell infiltrates, hypoxia, vascularization, pentraxin 3 and osteoprotegerin in abdominal aortic aneurysms—A quantitative histological study. *PLoS ONE* **2019**, *14*, e0224818. [CrossRef]
350. Mäyränpää, M.I.; Trosien, J.A.; Fontaine, V.; Folkesson, M.; Kazi, M.; Eriksson, P.; Swedenborg, J.; Hedin, U. Mast cells associate with neovessels in the media and adventitia of abdominal aortic aneurysms. *J. Vasc. Surg.* **2009**, *50*, 388–395. [CrossRef]
351. Ramos-Mozo, P.; Madrigal-Matute, J.; Martinez-Pinna, R.; Blanco-Colio, L.M.; Lopez, J.A.; Camafeita, E.; Meilhac, O.; Michel, J.-B.; Aparicio, C.; de Ceniga, M.V.; et al. Proteomic Analysis of Polymorphonuclear Neutrophils Identifies Catalase as a Novel Biomarker of Abdominal Aortic Aneurysm: Potential Implication of Oxidative Stress in Abdominal Aortic Aneurysm Progression. *Arter. Thromb. Vasc. Biol.* **2011**, *31*, 3011–3019. [CrossRef] [PubMed]
352. Lucas, M.L.; Carraro, C.C.; Belló-Klein, A.; Kalil, A.N.; Aerts, N.R.; Carvalho, F.B.; Fernandes, M.C.; Zettler, C.G. Oxidative Stress in Aortas of Patients with Advanced Occlusive and Aneurysmal Diseases. *Ann. Vasc. Surg.* **2018**, *52*, 216–224. [CrossRef] [PubMed]
353. Guzik, B.; Sagan, A.; Ludew, D.; Mrowiecki, W.; Chwała, M.; Bujak-Gizycka, B.; Filip, G.; Grudzien, G.; Kapelak, B.; Żmudka, K.; et al. Mechanisms of oxidative stress in human aortic aneurysms—Association with clinical risk factors for atherosclerosis and disease severity. *Int. J. Cardiol.* **2013**, *168*, 2389–2396. [CrossRef] [PubMed]
354. Zhang, J.; Schmidt, J.; Ryschich, E.; Mueller-Schilling, M.; Schumacher, H.; Allenberg, J.R. Inducible nitric oxide synthase is present in human abdominal aortic aneurysm and promotes oxidative vascular injury. *J. Vasc. Surg.* **2003**, *38*, 360–367. [CrossRef]
355. Ho, Y.; Wu, M.-L.; Gung, P.-Y.; Chen, C.-H.; Kuo, C.-C.; Yet, S.-F. Heme oxygenase-1 deficiency exacerbates angiotensin II-induced aortic aneurysm in mice. *Oncotarget* **2016**, *7*, 67760–67776. [CrossRef] [PubMed]
356. Parastatidis, I.; Weiss, D.; Joseph, G.; Taylor, W.R. Overexpression of Catalase in Vascular Smooth Muscle Cells Prevents the Formation of Abdominal Aortic Aneurysms. *Arter. Thromb. Vasc. Biol.* **2013**, *33*, 2389–2396. [CrossRef] [PubMed]
357. Yu, Z.; Morimoto, K.; Yu, J.; Bao, W.; Okita, Y.; Okada, K. Endogenous superoxide dismutase activation by oral administration of riboflavin reduces abdominal aortic aneurysm formation in rats. *J. Vasc. Surg.* **2015**, *64*, 737–745. [CrossRef]
358. Xiong, W.; Mactaggart, J.; Knispel, R.; Worth, J.; Zhu, Z.; Li, Y.; Sun, Y.; Baxter, B.T.; Johanning, J. Inhibition of reactive oxygen species attenuates aneurysm formation in a murine model. *Atherosclerosis* **2009**, *202*, 128–134. [CrossRef]
359. Jones, B.; Tonniges, J.R.; Debski, A.; Albert, B.; Yeung, D.A.; Gadde, N.; Mahajan, A.; Sharma, N.; Calomeni, E.P.; Go, M.R.; et al. Collagen fibril abnormalities in human and mice abdominal aortic aneurysm. *Acta Biomater.* **2020**, *110*, 129–140. [CrossRef] [PubMed]
360. Niestrawska, J.A.; Regitnig, P.; Viertler, C.; Cohnert, T.U.; Babu, A.R.; Holzapfel, G.A. The role of tissue remodeling in mechanics and pathogenesis of abdominal aortic aneurysms. *Acta Biomater.* **2019**, *88*, 149–161. [CrossRef] [PubMed]
361. Krishna, S.M.; Seto, S.W.; Jose, R.; Li, J.; Moxon, J.; Clancy, P.; Crossman, D.J.; Norman, P.; Emeto, T.I.; Golledge, J. High serum thrombospondin-1 concentration is associated with slower abdominal aortic aneurysm growth and deficiency of thrombospondin-1 promotes angiotensin II induced aortic aneurysm in mice. *Clin. Sci.* **2017**, *131*, 1261–1281. [CrossRef]

362. Mordi, I.R.; Forsythe, R.O.; Gellatly, C.; Iskandar, Z.; McBride, O.M.; Saratzis, A.; Chalmers, R.; Chin, C.; Bown, M.J.; Newby, D.E.; et al. Plasma Desmosine and Abdominal Aortic Aneurysm Disease. *J. Am. Hear. Assoc.* **2019**, *8*, e013743. [CrossRef] [PubMed]
363. Holsti, M.; Wanhainen, A.; Lundin, C.; Björck, M.; Tegler, G.; Svensson, J.; Sund, M. Circulating Vascular Basement Membrane Fragments are Associated with the Diameter of the Abdominal Aorta and Their Expression Pattern is Altered in AAA Tissue. *Eur. J. Vasc. Endovasc. Surg.* **2018**, *56*, 110–118. [CrossRef]
364. Williams, H.; Johnson, J.L.; Jackson, C.L.; White, S.J.; George, S.J. MMP-7 mediates cleavage of N-cadherin and promotes smooth muscle cell apoptosis. *Cardiovasc. Res.* **2010**, *87*, 137–146. [CrossRef]
365. Lyon, C.A.; Williams, H.; Bianco, R.; Simmonds, S.; Brown, B.A.; Wadey, K.S.; Smith, F.C.T.; Johnson, J.L.; George, S.J. Aneurysm Severity is Increased by Combined Mmp-7 Deletion and N-cadherin Mimetic (EC4-Fc) Over-Expression. *Sci. Rep.* **2017**, *7*, 17342. [CrossRef]
366. Geraghty, P.; Rogan, M.P.; Greene, C.M.; Boxio, R.M.M.; Poiriert, T.; O'Mahony, M.; Belaaouaj, A.; O'Neill, S.J.; Taggart, C.C.; McElvaney, N.G. Neutrophil elastase up-regulates cathepsin B and matrix metalloprotease-2 expression. *J. Immunol.* **2007**, *178*, 5871–5878. [CrossRef]
367. Tchougounova, E.; Lundequist, A.; Fajardo, I.; Winberg, J.-O.; Åbrink, M.; Pejler, G. A Key Role for Mast Cell Chymase in the Activation of Pro-matrix Metalloprotease-9 and Pro-matrix Metalloprotease-2. *J. Biol. Chem.* **2005**, *280*, 9291–9296. [CrossRef] [PubMed]
368. Krotova, K.; Khodayari, N.; Oshins, R.; Aslanidi, G.; Brantly, M.L. Neutrophil elastase promotes macrophage cell adhesion and cytokine production through the integrin-Src kinases pathway. *Sci. Rep.* **2020**, *10*, 1–10. [CrossRef]
369. Chamberlain, C.M.; Ang, L.S.; Boivin, W.A.; Cooper, D.M.; Williams, S.J.; Zhao, H.; Hendel, A.; Folkesson, M.; Swedenborg, J.; Allard, M.F.; et al. Perforin-Independent Extracellular Granzyme B Activity Contributes to Abdominal Aortic Aneurysm. *Am. J. Pathol.* **2010**, *176*, 1038–1049. [CrossRef] [PubMed]
370. Erdozain, O.J.; Pegrum, S.; Winrow, V.R.; Horrocks, M.; Stevens, C.R. Hypoxia in Abdominal Aortic Aneurysm Supports a Role for HIF-1α and Ets-1 as Drivers of Matrix Metalloproteinase Upregulation in Human Aortic Smooth Muscle Cells. *J. Vasc. Res.* **2011**, *48*, 163–170. [CrossRef]
371. Tsai, S.-H.; Huang, P.-H.; Hsu, Y.-J.; Peng, Y.-J.; Lee, C.-H.; Wang, J.-C.; Chen, J.-W.; Lin, S.-J. Inhibition of hypoxia inducible factor-1α attenuates abdominal aortic aneurysm progression through the down-regulation of matrix metalloproteinases. *Sci. Rep.* **2016**, *6*, 28612. [CrossRef]
372. Rabkin, S.W. The Role Matrix Metalloproteinases in the Production of Aortic Aneurysm. *Progress Mol. Biol. Transl. Sci.* **2017**, *147*, 239–265. [CrossRef]
373. Kurianiuk, A.; Socha, K.; Gacko, M.; Blachnio-Zabielska, A.; Karwowska, A. The Relationship between the Concentration of Cathepsin A, D, and E and the Concentration of Copper and Zinc, and the Size of the Aneurysmal Enlargement in the Wall of the Abdominal Aortic Aneurysm. *Ann. Vasc. Surg.* **2018**, *55*, 182–188. [CrossRef]
374. Lv, B.-J.; Lindholt, J.S.; Wang, J.; Cheng, X.; Shi, G.-P. Plasma levels of cathepsins L, K, and V and risks of abdominal aortic aneurysms: A randomized population-based study. *Atherosclerosis* **2013**, *230*, 100–105. [CrossRef] [PubMed]
375. Lv, B.-J.; Lindholt, J.S.; Cheng, X.; Wang, J.; Shi, G.-P. Plasma Cathepsin S and Cystatin C Levels and Risk of Abdominal Aortic Aneurysm: A Randomized Population–Based Study. *PLoS ONE* **2012**, *7*, e41813. [CrossRef]
376. Lorelli, D.R.; Jean-Claude, J.M.; Fox, C.J.; Clyne, J.; Cambria, R.A.; Seabrook, G.R.; Towne, J.B. Response of plasma matrix metalloproteinase-9 to conventional abdominal aortic aneurysm repair or endovascular exclusion: Implications for endoleak. *J. Vasc. Surg.* **2002**, *35*, 916–922. [CrossRef] [PubMed]
377. Watanabe, T.; Sato, A.; Sawai, T.; Uzuki, M.; Goto, H.; Yamashita, H.; Akamatsu, D.; Sato, H.; Shimizu, T.; Miyama, N.; et al. The Elevated Level of Circulating Matrix Metalloproteinase-9 in Patients with Abdominal Aortic Aneurysms Decreased to Levels Equal to Those of Healthy Controls after an Aortic Repair. *Ann. Vasc. Surg.* **2006**, *20*, 317–321. [CrossRef] [PubMed]
378. Qin, Y.; Cao, X.; Guo, J.; Zhang, Y.; Pan, L.; Zhang, H.; Li, H.; Tang, C.; Du, J.; Shi, G.-P. Deficiency of cathepsin S attenuates angiotensin II-induced abdominal aortic aneurysm formation in apolipoprotein E-deficient mice. *Cardiovasc. Res.* **2012**, *96*, 401–410. [CrossRef]
379. Sun, J.; Sukhova, G.K.; Zhang, J.; Chen, H.; Sjöberg, S.; Libby, P.; Xia, M.; Xiong, N.; Gelb, B.D.; Shi, G.-P. Cathepsin K Deficiency Reduces Elastase Perfusion–Induced Abdominal Aortic Aneurysms in Mice. *Arter. Thromb. Vasc. Biol.* **2012**, *32*, 15–23. [CrossRef]
380. Sun, J.; Sukhova, G.K.; Zhang, J.; Chen, H.; Sjöberg, S.; Libby, P.; Xiang, M.; Wang, J.; Peters, C.; Reinheckel, T.; et al. Cathepsin L Activity Is Essential to Elastase Perfusion–Induced Abdominal Aortic Aneurysms in Mice. *Arter. Thromb. Vasc. Biol.* **2011**, *31*, 2500–2508. [CrossRef]
381. Pyo, R.; Lee, J.K.; Shipley, J.M.; Curci, J.A.; Mao, D.; Ziporin, S.J.; Ennis, T.L.; Shapiro, S.D.; Senior, R.M.; Thompson, R.W. Targeted gene disruption of matrix metalloproteinase-9 (gelatinase B) suppresses development of experimental abdominal aortic aneurysms. *J. Clin. Investig.* **2000**, *105*, 1641–1649. [CrossRef]
382. Longo, G.M.; Xiong, W.; Greiner, T.C.; Zhao, Y.; Fiotti, N.; Baxter, B.T. Matrix metalloproteinases 2 and 9 work in concert to produce aortic aneurysms. *J. Clin. Investig.* **2002**, *110*, 625–632. [CrossRef]
383. Pagano, M.B.; Zhou, H.-F.; Ennis, T.L.; Wu, X.; Lambris, J.; Atkinson, J.P.; Thompson, R.W.; Hourcade, D.E.; Pham, C.T. Complement-Dependent Neutrophil Recruitment Is Critical for the Development of Elastase-Induced Abdominal Aortic Aneurysm. *Circulation* **2009**, *119*, 1805–1813. [CrossRef]

384. Martinez-Pinna, R.; Madrigal-Matute, J.; Tarin, C.; Burillo, E.; Esteban-Salan, M.; Pastor-Vargas, C.; Lindholt, J.S.; Lopez, J.A.; Calvo, E.; de Ceniga, M.V.; et al. Proteomic Analysis of Intraluminal Thrombus Highlights Complement Activation in Human Abdominal Aortic Aneurysms. *Arter. Thromb. Vasc. Biol.* **2013**, *33*, 2013–2020. [CrossRef]
385. Martin-Ventura, J.L.; Martinez-Lopez, D.; Roldan-Montero, R.; Gomez-Guerrero, C.; Blanco-Colio, L.M. Role of complement system in pathological remodeling of the vascular wall. *Mol. Immunol.* **2019**, *114*, 207–215. [CrossRef] [PubMed]
386. Bobryshev, Y.Y.V.; Lord, R.S. Vascular-Associated Lymphoid Tissue (VALT) Involvement in Aortic Aneurysm. *Atherosclerosis* **2001**, *154*, 15–21. [CrossRef]
387. Spear, R.; Boytard, L.; Blervaque, R.; Chwastyniak, M.; Hot, D.; Vanhoutte, J.; Staels, B.; Lemoine, Y.; Lamblin, N.; Pruvot, F.-R.; et al. Adventitial Tertiary Lymphoid Organs as Potential Source of MicroRNA Biomarkers for Abdominal Aortic Aneurysm. *Int. J. Mol. Sci.* **2015**, *16*, 11276–11293. [CrossRef]
388. Kugo, H.; Moriyama, T.; Zaima, N. Adipocytes and Abdominal Aortic Aneurysm: Putative Potential Role of Adipocytes in the Process of AAA Development. *Curr. Drug Targets* **2018**, *19*, 1228–1232. [CrossRef] [PubMed]
389. Folkesson, M.; Vorkapic, E.; Gulbins, E.; Japtok, L.; Kleuser, B.; Welander, M.; Länne, T.; Wågsäter, D. Inflammatory cells, ceramides, and expression of proteases in perivascular adipose tissue adjacent to human abdominal aortic aneurysms. *J. Vasc. Surg.* **2017**, *65*, 1171–1179.e1. [CrossRef] [PubMed]
390. Piacentini, L.; Werba, J.P.; Bono, E.; Saccu, C.; Tremoli, E.; Spirito, R.; Colombo, G. Genome-Wide Expression Profiling Unveils Autoimmune Response Signatures in the Perivascular Adipose Tissue of Abdominal Aortic Aneurysm. *Arter. Thromb. Vasc. Biol.* **2019**, *39*, 237–249. [CrossRef]
391. Teo, F.H.; de Oliveira, R.T.D.; Villarejos, L.; Mamoni, R.L.; Altemani, A.; Menezes, F.H.; Blotta, M.H.S.L. Characterization of CD4+ T Cell Subsets in Patients with Abdominal Aortic Aneurysms. *Mediat. Inflamm.* **2018**, *2018*, 6967310. [CrossRef] [PubMed]
392. Eagleton, M.J. Inflammation in abdominal aortic aneurysms: Cellular infiltrate and cytokine profiles. *Vascular* **2012**, *20*, 278–283. [CrossRef]
393. Middleton, R.K.; Lloyd, G.M.; Bown, M.; Cooper, N.J.; London, N.J.; Sayers, R.D. The pro-inflammatory and chemotactic cytokine microenvironment of the abdominal aortic aneurysm wall: A protein array study. *J. Vasc. Surg.* **2007**, *45*, 574–580. [CrossRef]
394. Zhou, H.-F.; Yan, H.; Cannon, J.L.; Springer, L.E.; Green, J.M.; Pham, C.T.N. CD43-mediated IFN-γ production by CD8+ T cells promotes abdominal aortic aneurysm in mice. *J. Immunol.* **2013**, *190*, 5078–5085. [CrossRef]
395. Sharma, A.K.; Lu, G.; Jester, A.; Johnston, W.; Zhao, Y.; Hajzus, V.A.; Saadatzadeh, M.R.; Su, G.; Bhamidipati, C.M.; Mehta, G.S.; et al. Experimental Abdominal Aortic Aneurysm Formation Is Mediated by IL-17 and Attenuated by Mesenchymal Stem Cell Treatment. *Circulation* **2012**, *126*, S38–S45. [CrossRef]
396. Wei, Z.; Wang, Y.; Zhang, K.; Liao, Y.; Ye, P.; Wu, J.; Wang, Y.; Li, F.; Yao, Y.; Zhou, Y.; et al. Inhibiting the Th17/IL-17A–Related Inflammatory Responses with Digoxin Confers Protection Against Experimental Abdominal Aortic Aneurysm. *Arter. Thromb. Vasc. Biol.* **2014**, *34*, 2429–2438. [CrossRef] [PubMed]
397. Prucha, M.; Sedivy, P.; Stadler, P.; Zdrahal, P.; Prokopova, P.; Voska, L.; Sedlackova, L. Abdominal aortic aneurysm as an IgG4-related disease. *Clin. Exp. Immunol.* **2019**, *197*, 361–365. [CrossRef]
398. Li, J.; Deng, Z.; Zhang, X.; Liu, F.; Yang, C.; Shi, G. Deficiency of immunoglobulin E protects mice from experimental abdominal aortic aneurysms. *FASEB J.* **2020**, *34*, 3091–3104. [CrossRef] [PubMed]
399. Ait-Oufella, H.; Wang, Y.; Herbin, O.; Bourcier, S.; Potteaux, S.; Joffre, J.; Loyer, X.; Ponnuswamy, P.; Esposito, B.; Dalloz, M.; et al. Natural Regulatory T Cells Limit Angiotensin II–Induced Aneurysm Formation and Rupture in Mice. *Arter. Thromb. Vasc. Biol.* **2013**, *33*, 2374–2379. [CrossRef]
400. Zhou, Y.; Wu, W.; Lindholt, J.S.; Sukhova, G.K.; Libby, P.; Yu, X.; Shi, G.-P. Regulatory T cells in human and angiotensin II-induced mouse abdominal aortic aneurysms. *Cardiovasc. Res.* **2015**, *107*, 98–107. [CrossRef]
401. Zhu, H.; Qu, X.; Zhang, C.; Yu, Y. Interleukin-10 Promotes Proliferation of Vascular Smooth Muscle Cells by Inhibiting Inflammation in Rabbit Abdominal Aortic Aneurysm. *Int. J. Clin. Exp. Pathol.* **2019**, *12*, 1260–1271.
402. Meng, X.; Yang, J.; Dong, M.; Zhang, K.; Tu, E.; Gao, Q.; Chen, W.; Zhang, C.; Zhang, Y. Regulatory T cells in cardiovascular diseases. *Nat. Rev. Cardiol.* **2015**, *13*, 167–179. [CrossRef] [PubMed]
403. Eliason, J.L.; Hannawa, K.K.; Ailawadi, G.; Sinha, I.; Ford, J.W.; Deogracias, M.P.; Roelofs, K.J.; Woodrum, D.T.; Ennis, T.L.; Henke, P.K.; et al. Neutrophil Depletion Inhibits Experimental Abdominal Aortic Aneurysm Formation. *Circulation* **2005**, *112*, 232–240. [CrossRef]
404. Daugherty, A.; Rateri, D.L.; Charo, I.F.; Owens, A.P.; Howatt, D.A.; Cassis, L.A. Angiotensin II infusion promotes ascending aortic aneurysms: Attenuation by CCR2 deficiency in apoE−/− mice. *Clin. Sci.* **2010**, *118*, 681–689. [CrossRef] [PubMed]
405. Xiong, W.; Knispel, R.; MacTaggart, J.; Greiner, T.C.; Weiss, S.J.; Baxter, B.T. Membrane-type 1 Matrix Metalloproteinase Regulates Macrophage-dependent Elastolytic Activity and Aneurysm Formation in Vivo. *J. Biol. Chem.* **2009**, *284*, 1765–1771. [CrossRef]
406. Blomkalns, A.L.; Gavrila, D.; Thomas, M.; Neltner, B.S.; Blanco, V.M.; Benjamin, S.B.; McCormick, M.L.; Stoll, L.L.; Denning, G.M.; Collins, S.P.; et al. CD14 Directs Adventitial Macrophage Precursor Recruitment: Role in Early Abdominal Aortic Aneurysm Formation. *J. Am. Hear. Assoc.* **2013**, *2*, e000065. [CrossRef]
407. Boytard, L.; Spear, R.; Chinetti-Gbaguidi, G.; Acosta-Martin, A.E.; Vanhoutte, J.; Lamblin, N.; Staels, B.; Amouyel, P.; Haulon, S.; Pinet, F. Role of Proinflammatory CD68 + Mannose Receptor—Macrophages in Peroxiredoxin-1 Expression and in Abdominal Aortic Aneurysms in Humans. *Arter. Thromb. Vasc. Biol.* **2013**, *33*, 431–438. [CrossRef] [PubMed]

408. Zagrapan, B.; Eilenberg, W.; Prausmueller, S.; Nawrozi, P.; Muench, K.; Hetzer, S.; Elleder, V.; Rajic, R.; Juster, F.; Martelanz, L.; et al. A Novel Diagnostic and Prognostic Score for Abdominal Aortic Aneurysms Based on D-Dimer and a Comprehensive Analysis of Myeloid Cell Parameters. *Thromb. Haemost.* **2019**, *119*, 807–820. [CrossRef] [PubMed]
409. Michineau, S.; Franck, G.; Wagner-Ballon, O.; Dai, J.; Allaire, E.; Gervais, M. Chemokine (C-X-C Motif) Receptor 4 Blockade by AMD3100 Inhibits Experimental Abdominal Aortic Aneurysm Expansion Through Anti-Inflammatory Effects. *Arter. Thromb. Vasc. Biol.* **2014**, *34*, 1747–1755. [CrossRef]
410. Vandestienne, M.; Zhang, Y.; Santos-Zas, I.; Al-Rifai, R.; Joffre, J.; Giraud, A.; Laurans, L.; Esposito, B.; Pinet, F.; Bruneval, P.; et al. TREM-1 orchestrates angiotensin II–induced monocyte trafficking and promotes experimental abdominal aortic aneurysm. *J. Clin. Investig.* **2021**, *131*. [CrossRef] [PubMed]
411. Iida, Y.; Xu, B.; Xuan, H.; Glover, K.J.; Tanaka, H.; Hu, X.; Fujimura, N.; Wang, W.; Schultz, J.R.; Turner, C.R.; et al. Peptide Inhibitor of CXCL4–CCL5 Heterodimer Formation, MKEY, Inhibits Experimental Aortic Aneurysm Initiation and Progression. *Arter. Thromb. Vasc. Biol.* **2013**, *33*, 718–726. [CrossRef]
412. Wong, K.L.; Tai, J.J.-Y.; Wong, W.-C.; Han, H.; Sem, X.; Yeap, W.-H.; Kourilsky, P.; Wong, S.-C. Gene expression profiling reveals the defining features of the classical, intermediate, and nonclassical human monocyte subsets. *Blood* **2011**, *118*, e16–e31. [CrossRef]
413. Zawada, A.M.; Rogacev, K.S.; Rotter, B.; Winter, P.; Marell, R.-R.; Fliser, D.; Heine, G.H. SuperSAGE evidence for CD14++CD16+ monocytes as a third monocyte subset. *Blood* **2011**, *118*, e50–e61. [CrossRef]
414. Chimen, M.; Yates, C.M.; McGettrick, H.M.; Ward, L.S.C.; Harrison, M.J.; Apta, B.; Dib, L.H.; Imhof, B.A.; Harrison, P.; Nash, G.B.; et al. Monocyte Subsets Coregulate Inflammatory Responses by Integrated Signaling through TNF and IL-6 at the Endothelial Cell Interface. *J. Immunol.* **2017**, *198*, 2834–2843. [CrossRef]
415. Auffray, C.; Fogg, D.; Garfa, M.; Elain, G.; Join-Lambert, O.; Kayal, S.; Sarnacki, S.; Cumano, A.; Lauvau, G.; Geissmann, F. Monitoring of Blood Vessels and Tissues by a Population of Monocytes with Patrolling Behavior. *Science* **2007**, *317*, 666–670. [CrossRef] [PubMed]
416. Cros, J.; Cagnard, N.; Woollard, K.; Patey, N.; Zhang, S.-Y.; Senechal, B.; Puel, A.; Biswas, S.K.; Moshous, D.; Picard, C.; et al. Human CD14dim Monocytes Patrol and Sense Nucleic Acids and Viruses via TLR7 and TLR8 Receptors. *Immunity* **2010**, *33*, 375–386. [CrossRef] [PubMed]
417. Ghigliotti, G.; Barisione, C.; Garibaldi, S.; Brunelli, C.; Palmieri, D.; Spinella, G.; Pane, B.; Spallarossa, P.; Altieri, P.; Fabbi, P.; et al. CD16+Monocyte Subsets Are Increased in Large Abdominal Aortic Aneurysms and Are Differentially Related with Circulating and Cell-Associated Biochemical and Inflammatory Biomarkers. *Dis. Markers* **2013**, *34*, 131–142. [CrossRef] [PubMed]
418. Samadzadeh, K.M.; Chun, K.C.; Nguyen, A.T.; Baker, P.M.; Bains, S.; Lee, E.S. Monocyte activity is linked with abdominal aortic aneurysm diameter. *J. Surg. Res.* **2014**, *190*, 328–334. [CrossRef] [PubMed]
419. Dale, M.A.; Ruhlman, M.K.; Baxter, B.T. Inflammatory Cell Phenotypes in AAAs: Their Role and Potential as Targets for Therapy. *Arter. Thromb. Vasc. Biol.* **2015**, *35*, 1746–1755. [CrossRef]
420. Knappich, C.; Spin, J.M.; Eckstein, H.-H.; Tsao, P.S.; Maegdefessel, L. Involvement of Myeloid Cells and Noncoding RNA in Abdominal Aortic Aneurysm Disease. *Antioxidants Redox Signal.* **2020**, *33*, 602–620. [CrossRef]
421. Dutertre, C.-A.; Clement, M.; Morvan, M.; Schäkel, K.; Castier, Y.; Alsac, J.-M.; Michel, J.-B.; Nicoletti, A. Deciphering the Stromal and Hematopoietic Cell Network of the Adventitia from Non-Aneurysmal and Aneurysmal Human Aorta. *PLoS ONE* **2014**, *9*, e89983. [CrossRef]
422. Qin, Z.; Bagley, J.; Sukhova, G.; Baur, W.E.; Park, H.-J.; Beasley, D.; Libby, P.; Zhang, Y.; Galper, J.B. Angiotensin II-induced TLR4 mediated abdominal aortic aneurysm in apolipoprotein E knockout mice is dependent on STAT3. *J. Mol. Cell. Cardiol.* **2015**, *87*, 160–170. [CrossRef]
423. Hadi, T.; Boytard, L.; Silvestro, M.; Alebrahim, D.; Jacob, S.; Feinstein, J.; Barone, K.; Spiro, W.; Hutchison, S.; Simon, R.; et al. Macrophage-derived netrin-1 promotes abdominal aortic aneurysm formation by activating MMP3 in vascular smooth muscle cells. *Nat. Commun.* **2018**, *9*, 1–16. [CrossRef]
424. Guo, L.; Akahori, H.; Harari, E.; Smith, S.L.; Polavarapu, R.; Karmali, V.; Otsuka, F.; Gannon, R.L.; Braumann, R.E.; Dickinson, M.H.; et al. CD163+ macrophages promote angiogenesis and vascular permeability accompanied by inflammation in atherosclerosis. *J. Clin. Investig.* **2018**, *128*, 1106–1124. [CrossRef]
425. Li, J.; Xia, N.; Wen, S.; Li, D.; Lu, Y.; Gu, M.; Tang, T.; Jiao, J.; Lv, B.; Nie, S.; et al. IL (Interleukin)-33 Suppresses Abdominal Aortic Aneurysm by Enhancing Regulatory T-Cell Expansion and Activity. *Arter. Thromb. Vasc. Biol.* **2019**, *39*, 446–458. [CrossRef]
426. Zhang, Z.; Xu, J.; Liu, Y.; Wang, T.; Pei, J.; Cheng, L.; Hao, D.; Zhao, X.; Chen, H.-Z.; Liu, D.-P. Mouse macrophage specific knockout of SIRT1 influences macrophage polarization and promotes angiotensin II-induced abdominal aortic aneurysm formation. *J. Genet. Genom.* **2018**, *45*, 25–32. [CrossRef]
427. Chen, X.; Li, Y.; Xiao, J.; Zhang, H.; Yang, C.; Wei, Z.; Chen, W.; Du, X.; Liu, J. Modulating Neuro-Immune-Induced Macrophage Polarization With Topiramate Attenuates Experimental Abdominal Aortic Aneurysm. *Front. Pharmacol.* **2020**, *11*, 565461. [CrossRef] [PubMed]
428. Malech, H.L.; DeLeo, F.R.; Quinn, M.T. The Role of Neutrophils in the Immune System: An Overview. *Neutrophil* **2019**, *2087*, 3–10. [CrossRef]
429. Klopf, J.; Brostjan, C.; Neumayer, C.; Eilenberg, W. Neutrophils as Regulators and Biomarkers of Cardiovascular Inflammation in the Context of Abdominal Aortic Aneurysms. *Biomedicines* **2021**, *9*, 1236. [CrossRef]

430. Klopf, J.; Brostjan, C.; Eilenberg, W.; Neumayer, C. Neutrophil Extracellular Traps and Their Implications in Cardiovascular and Inflammatory Disease. *Int. J. Mol. Sci.* **2021**, *22*, 559. [CrossRef]
431. Zagrapan, B.; Eilenberg, W.; Scheuba, A.; Klopf, J.; Brandau, A.; Story, J.; Dosch, K.; Hayden, H.; Domenig, C.M.; Fuchs, L.; et al. Complement Factor C5a Is Increased in Blood of Patients with Abdominal Aortic Aneurysm and Has Prognostic Potential for Aneurysm Growth. *J. Cardiovasc. Transl. Res.* **2020**, *14*, 761–769. [CrossRef] [PubMed]
432. Pagano, M.B.; Bartoli, M.; Ennis, T.L.; Mao, D.; Simmons, P.M.; Thompson, R.W.; Pham, C.T.N. Critical role of dipeptidyl peptidase I in neutrophil recruitment during the development of experimental abdominal aortic aneurysms. *Proc. Natl. Acad. Sci. USA* **2007**, *104*, 2855–2860. [CrossRef] [PubMed]
433. Langenskiöld, M.; Smidfelt, K.; Nordanstig, J.; Bergström, G.; Tivesten, A. Leukocyte subsets and abdominal aortic aneurysms detected by screening in men. *J. Intern. Med.* **2020**, *288*, 345–355. [CrossRef] [PubMed]
434. Yang, P.; Li, Y.; Xie, Y.; Liu, Y. Different Faces for Different Places: Heterogeneity of Neutrophil Phenotype and Function. *J. Immunol. Res.* **2019**, *2019*, 8016254. [CrossRef]
435. Memon, A.; Zarrouk, M.; Ågren-Witteschus, S.; Sundquist, J.; Gottsäter, A.; Sundquist, K. Identification of novel diagnostic and prognostic biomarkers for abdominal aortic aneurysm. *Eur. J. Prev. Cardiol.* **2019**, *27*, 132–142. [CrossRef] [PubMed]
436. Wang, Y.; Rosen, H.; Madtes, D.K.; Shao, B.; Martin, T.R.; Heinecke, J.W.; Fu, X. Myeloperoxidase Inactivates TIMP-1 by Oxidizing Its N-Terminal Cysteine Residue: An Oxidative Mechanism for Regulating Proteolysis during Inflammation. *J. Biol. Chem.* **2007**, *282*, 31826–31834. [CrossRef]
437. Groeneveld, M.E.; Struik, J.A.; Musters, R.J.; Tangelder, G.J.; Koolwijk, P.; Niessen, H.; Hoksbergen, A.W.; Wisselink, W.; Yeung, K.K. The Potential Role of Neutrophil Gelatinase-Associated Lipocalin in the Development of Abdominal Aortic Aneurysms. *Ann. Vasc. Surg.* **2019**, *57*, 210–219. [CrossRef]
438. Adkison, A.M.; Raptis, S.Z.; Kelley, D.G.; Pham, C.T. Dipeptidyl peptidase I activates neutrophil-derived serine proteases and regulates the development of acute experimental arthritis. *J. Clin. Investig.* **2002**, *109*, 363–371. [CrossRef] [PubMed]
439. Abisi, S.; Burnand, K.G.; Waltham, M.; Humphries, J.; Taylor, P.R.; Smith, A. Cysteine protease activity in the wall of abdominal aortic aneurysms. *J. Vasc. Surg.* **2007**, *46*, 1260–1266. [CrossRef]
440. Dale, M.A.; Xiong, W.; Carson, J.S.; Suh, M.K.; Karpisek, A.D.; Meisinger, T.M.; Casale, G.P.; Baxter, B.T. Elastin-Derived Peptides Promote Abdominal Aortic Aneurysm Formation by Modulating M1/M2 Macrophage Polarization. *J. Immunol.* **2016**, *196*, 4536–4543. [CrossRef] [PubMed]
441. Tachieda, R.; Niinuma, H.; Ohira, A.; Endoh, S.; Hiramori, K.; Makita, S.; Nakamura, M. Circulating biochemical marker levels of collagen metabolism are abnormal in patients with abdominal aortic aneurysm. *Angiology* **2000**, *51*, 385–392. [CrossRef]
442. Hance, K.A.; Tataria, M.; Ziporin, S.J.; Lee, J.K.; Thompson, R.W. Monocyte chemotactic activity in human abdominal aortic aneurysms: Role of elastin degradation peptides and the 67–kD cell surface elastin receptor. *J. Vasc. Surg.* **2002**, *35*, 254–261. [CrossRef] [PubMed]
443. Delbosc, S.; Alsac, J.-M.; Journé, C.; Louedec, L.; Castier, Y.; Bonnaure-Mallet, M.; Ruimy, R.; Rossignol, P.; Bouchard, P.; Michel, J.-B.; et al. Porphyromonas gingivalis Participates in Pathogenesis of Human Abdominal Aortic Aneurysm by Neutrophil Activation. Proof of Concept in Rats. *PLoS ONE* **2011**, *6*, e18679. [CrossRef]
444. Meher, A.K.; Spinosa, M.; Davis, J.P.; Pope, N.; Laubach, V.E.; Su, G.; Serbulea, V.; Leitinger, N.; Ailawadi, G.; Upchurch, G.R. Novel Role of IL (Interleukin)-1β in Neutrophil Extracellular Trap Formation and Abdominal Aortic Aneurysms. *Arter. Thromb. Vasc. Biol.* **2018**, *38*, 843–853. [CrossRef] [PubMed]
445. Yan, H.; Zhou, H.-F.; Akk, A.; Hu, Y.; Springer, L.E.; Ennis, T.L.; Pham, C.T. Neutrophil Proteases Promote Experimental Abdominal Aortic Aneurysm via Extracellular Trap Release and Plasmacytoid Dendritic Cell Activation. *Arter. Thromb. Vasc. Biol.* **2016**, *36*, 1660–1669. [CrossRef]
446. Eilenberg, W.; Zagrapan, B.; Bleichert, S.; Ibrahim, N.; Knöbl, V.; Brandau, A.; Martelanz, L.; Grasl, M.-T.; Hayden, H.; Nawrozi, P.; et al. Histone citrullination as a novel biomarker and target to inhibit progression of abdominal aortic aneurysms. *Transl. Res.* **2021**, *233*, 32–46. [CrossRef] [PubMed]

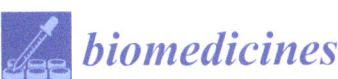

Article

The Ratio of the Size of the Abdominal Aortic Aneurysm to That of the Unchanged Aorta as a Risk Factor for Its Rupture

Maciej Jusko [1,*], Piotr Kasprzak [2], Alicja Majos [3] and Waclaw Kuczmik [1]

1. Department of General Surgery, Vascular Surgery, Angiology and Phlebology, Medical University of Silesia, 40-055 Katowice, Poland
2. Department of Vascular Surgery, University Hospital Regensburg, 93053 Regensburg, Germany
3. General and Transplant Surgery Department, Medical University of Lodz, 93-338 Lodz, Poland
* Correspondence: juskomaciej@gmail.com; Tel.: +48-793-777-193

Abstract: Background: A ruptured abdominal aortic aneurysm is a severe condition associated with high mortality. Currently, the most important criterion used to estimate the risk of its rupture is the size of the aneurysm, but due to patients' anatomical variability, many aneurysms have a high risk of rupture with a small aneurysm size. We asked ourselves whether individual differences in anatomy could be taken into account when assessing the risk of rupture. Methods: Based on the CT scan image, aneurysm and normal aorta diameters were collected from 186 individuals and compared in patients with ruptured and unruptured aneurysms. To take into account anatomical differences between patients, diameter ratios were calculated by dividing the aneurysm diameter by the diameter of the normal aorta at various heights, and then further comparisons were made. Results: It was found that the calculated ratios differ between patients with ruptured and unruptured aneurysms. This observation is also present in patients with small aneurysms, with its maximal size below the level that indicates the need for surgical treatment. For small aneurysms, the ratios help us to estimate the risk of rupture better than the maximum sac size (AUC: 0.783 vs. 0.650). Conclusions: The calculated ratios appear to be a valuable feature to indicate which of the small aneurysms have a high risk of rupture. The obtained results suggest the need for further confirmation of their usefulness in subsequent groups of patients.

Keywords: ruptured abdominal aortic aneurysm; aneurysm rupture risk factors; aneurysm rupture risk assessment

1. Introduction

A ruptured abdominal aortic aneurysm (RAAA) is a major challenge in vascular surgery. Abdominal aortic aneurysm (AAA) itself is usually asymptomatic until the moment of its rupture, when the patient's circulatory capacity suddenly collapses due to massive internal hemorrhage, and even despite the use of proper surgical treatment, serious health complications may often develop, and mortality is between 32–70% [1]. Due to such a high mortality, the effort of research teams should be focused on the most accurate estimation of which patients with AAA are most commonly predisposed to the development of aneurysm rupture and when, and therefore when they should undergo treatment in order to avoid this most serious complication [2–4]. Unfortunately, despite many years of experience in AAA treatment and numerous trials, it is difficult to predict when the aneurysm will rupture [5–8].

The rupture of the aneurysm wall is a complex process, influenced by many factors with complex relations, which to a large extent makes it difficult to fully explain the problem [7]. In recent years, in the light of new achievements, the concept of the RAAA development mechanism has changed several times. New discoveries allowed us to answer many yet-unanswered questions, but they led to many more, often much more complex ones [9–13]. Some of the considerations regarding the mechanisms by which aneurysm rupture occur are presented below.

It was originally assumed that a key role in this phenomenon was played by the pressure gradient on both sides of the vascular wall, which the aneurysm was unable to balance. The pressure exerted by the blood flowing through the aorta on its wall was calculated according to Laplace's law, which explains the way the liquid flows through cylindrical objects. Although this law describes the conditions in the physiological aorta relatively well, due to the extensive remodeling of the vessel, which unevenly affects different areas of the aorta, it cannot be used to describe the conditions in an aneurysm [14]. This prompted researchers to look for a method that could determine the local tensions of the AAA wall taking into account its often complicated shape. This was achieved thanks to the finite element method (FEM), which allowed the identification of the most vulnerable areas of the aortic wall (the so-called hot spots). FEM made it possible to better estimate which AAAs are more likely to rupture compared to Laplace's law, but in this technique the analysis is based primarily on the shape of the vessel itself. In the course of further research, it turned out that the local wall tension largely depends not only on the AAA shape and its extension, but also on the remodeling of the vascular wall [15,16]. Inside the AAA wall, a complicated inflammatory process takes place, the consequence of which is the reduction in its strength, which, to a large extent, may be the cause of its rupture. The rebuilding of the AAA wall mainly consists of smooth muscle cell atrophy, degradation of elastin fibers, increased collagen synthesis and increased neovascularization [12,13].

An additional difficulty in estimating the risk of RAAA development is the presence and size of intraluminal thrombus (ILT). According to some reports, this is a factor preventing the aneurysm from rupture, as it is a layer that isolates the AAA wall from the flowing blood [17,18]. There are also publications reporting an increased risk of RAAA development in the presence of ILT, as ILT as a condensed object is a good conductor for the stresses on the AAA wall [19]. Moreover, it has been found that the cells of the internal vascular wall are to a certain extent supplied with oxygen and nutrients by the blood flowing inside the vessel independently of the vasa vasorum. In such a case, ILT, by blocking the access of blood to the endothelium, determines the formation of an ischemic zone, which may intensify the inflammatory reaction and contribute to the weakening of aneurysm wall strength [20–22].

The combination of all the above-mentioned factors and the estimation of the risk of rupture on their basis is possible and provides valuable data; however, it causes many difficulties in assessment and is hard to perform. The reports so far that take into account most of the factors of RAAA development, i.e., aneurysm morphology, the presence of ILT and the histological structure of the vessel wall, were retrospective, and therefore cognitive. A diagnostic protocol based on the above data allowing us to modify the current indications for AAA treatment has not been developed so far and the maximum diameter of the aneurysm remains the main factor determining whether a certain patient will be treated or not [23].

The correlation between AAA diameter and the risk of its rupture is a well-known observation [5,6]. In order to measure the maximum AAA diameter, it is sufficient to analyze a single CT scan of the abdominal aorta and to perform a single measurement. The ease of making this estimation means that almost all recommendations and guidelines are mainly based on these data [23,24]. However, estimating this risk based on the diameter alone is burdened with an error resulting from not considering other factors. The same CT scan, after a more detailed analysis, may provide additional valuable data that can be used to estimate the risk of AAA rupture. Kimura et al. were comparing CT scans of patients with AAA and RAAA, and they found that the ruptured aneurysms are characterized by a smaller rounding radius (departure angle) and a smaller aspect ratio (longitudinal diameter divided by transverse) [25]. Such observations lead us to a deepening of the analysis of data that can be obtained from a CT scan, because finding the characteristic features of

RAAA other than the maximum diameter could increase the number of patients qualifying for treatment.

The initial point of this study was to question the need of sticking to the strict limits of maximum AAA diameter as the main indication for surgical treatment, which does not take into account anatomical variability between individual patients other than gender difference. Evidence of the limitations of that approach is the relatively high percentage of RAAA in patients with non-qualifying diameters identified in published studies [8,26,27]. With the current availability of healthcare services, it should be expected that some of these patients had been diagnosed with AAA and were not qualified for surgical treatment prior to aneurysm rupture.

One of the reasons for this may be the presence of different diameters of the aorta in patients with the same size of AAA. When defining an aneurysm, we base on the ratio of the diameter of a healthy artery to the dilated segment. The hypothesis of this research is potential greater risk of rupture of AAA in the case of a smaller aorta than in the case of a larger one with aneurysms of the same size. For this reason, this study analyzes the diameters of not only AAA, but also the aorta and iliac arteries at different heights. We assume that the dimensions of the unchanged vessels closest to the aneurysm will allow us to take into account individual morphological differences, and their comparison will allow for a better assessment of the risk of aneurysm rupture.

It has not been fully determined if or how profoundly the presence or absence of AAA neck segment should be regarded. The term abdominal aortic aneurysm is defined as any significantly large dilation of the aorta, from the aortic hiatus to the division into the iliac arteries. The majority of these cases are patients with an aneurysm located below the exit of the renal arteries, as in this region the histological structure determines the greater susceptibility of the vascular wall to remodeling into an aneurysm [5,10]. A rarer variant is an aneurysm present in the segment of major visceral arteries departure, and such aneurysms are often treated in clinical practice as a separate disease, not because of a different etiopathogenesis, but a different method of their treatment. However, relatively often there is an indirect variant, i.e., aneurysm, which does not cover the section where the visceral arteries depart from the aorta but begins so close to the renal arteries that there is no undilated section between them and the aneurysm sac, i.e., the neck. In this article, such aneurysms are referred to as non-neck aneurysms. Due to the same localization of aneurysms with and without the neck, in the literature referred to as infrarenal, there are no reasons to exclude non-neck aneurysms from the study group. However, all results and conclusions obtained on the basis of the measurements of the aneurysm neck section should be treated with adequate reserve, as it has not been precisely established whether and when the neck is a physiological section of the vessel or if it is already a primary lesion.

2. Materials and Methods

The study group consisted of 93 patients with infrarenal RAAA, and the control group consisted of 93 patients with infrarenal AAA operated electively on the basis of the existing criteria. The diagnoses were confirmed by angio-CT scan of the abdominal aorta. All subjects were hospitalized in the Department of General Surgery, Vascular Surgery, Angiology and Phlebology of the Upper Silesian Medical Center, Medical University of Silesia in Katowice, Poland, in 2014–2019. The control group consisted of patients treated regularly due to AAA, successively in 2018–2019.

CT scans were analyzed, and the AAA, iliac arteries and aortic diameter were measured at following levels: celiac trunk, superior mesenteric artery, renal arteries, the maximum diameter of the aneurysm sac, understood as the diameter of the AAA at the level with the highest sac circumference, the diameter of both common iliac arteries and both external iliac arteries. In addition, measurements were made of the AAA neck diameter, i.e., the diameter of the aortic section inclined at a right angle to its long axis at the level of the segment above the AAA sac and below the level of the renal arteries, provided that such segment was present at all due to AAA morphology. The diameter was measured between the outer edges of the vessel wall opposite to its center. If ILT was present inside an aneurysm sac it was also included in the measurement of maximal aneurysm diameter. The measurement was made with OsiriX DICOM Viewer program (Figure 1).

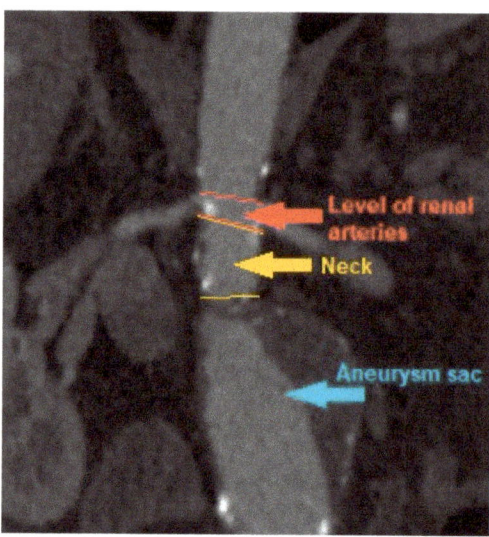

Figure 1. An example of computed tomography of patient with infrarenal abdominal aortic aneurysm with present neck segment.

The measurement of the diameter of a ruptured abdominal aortic aneurysm and its reliability remains a problematic issue, since the original diameter of the aneurysm may have changed after the rupture. For obvious clinical reasons, it is not possible to observe how the diameter of the aorta changes during an aneurysm rupture and in time after this incident, and the only test that can be referred to in order to measure a ruptured aneurysm is a CT scan performed to diagnose this incident. The possible difference in the diameter of the aneurysm just before and after rupture and its influence on the results obtained is a potential limitation of the present study.

After measuring the diameters, the aortic diameter ratios at certain levels were calculated. The ratios are the quotient of the maximum diameter of AAA and the diameter of the aorta at the level of the celiac trunk, the superior mesenteric artery, the renal arteries, the diameter of both common iliac arteries, and the diameter of both external iliac arteries. The ratios were named as the "R" and the name of the artery at the level of which the aortic diameter was measured, or the common and external iliac artery with the additional definition of the side.

In order to reveal potential differences in calculated ratios, the subjects were divided into three groups according to the maximum diameter of the aneurysm. The first group consisted of patients with AAA diameter below 5 cm, which was the size below indications for surgical intervention according to current criteria. The second was patients with a maximum diameter of AAA in the range of 5–6.5 cm, and the third was patients with AAA larger than 6.5 cm. Due to the gender disproportion in the study group (18 vs. 168), expressed even stronger after the division into subgroups, and therefore the high probability of low reliability of the results obtained in the small group, division into women and men was not used for further calculations. Patients with AAA smaller than 4 cm were not included in the analysis, because in the study group all such aneurysms had a sac-like morphology. In such a case, when AAA is not a dilation of the entire circumference of the aortic wall, but only a short segment bulge of a certain part, it seems that its rupture may be determined by other factors or of a different intensity than in the analyzed, fusiform aneurysms. To keep consistency, the study did not concern any sac-like aneurysms, regardless of their size. Additionally, subjects with iliac artery aneurysm understood as widening of the common iliac artery over 2 cm were not included in the study.

The study group and the control group were compared in terms of differences in the AAA measurement values and the calculated ratios. Next, the predictive value for the aneurysm rupture event of calculated ratios and the maximum diameter of the aneurysm was compared. The distribution of the values of the ratios in relation to the amount of RAAA subjects, which occur at a given ratio value, was analyzed. Due to the fact that the aneurysm neck segment was present only in some of the subjects, the above comparisons were made separately for the subgroups of subjects with and without the neck segment.

When comparing continuous variables, the normality was determined with the Shapiro–Wilk test. For the data that met the assumptions of the normal distribution, the groups were compared with the Student's t-test, for the data that did not meet the assumptions of the normal distribution, the Mann–Whitney U test was used. The quoted effect measures were calculated using ROC curves. The calculations were made using the Statistica 13 program.

3. Results

The group consisted of 18 women and 168 men. In the study group, the minimum diameter of RAAA was 4.4 cm, the maximum was 14.2 cm, and the median was 7.4 cm. In the control group the minimum diameter of AAA was 4.2 cm, the maximum was 9.5 cm, and the median was 5.6 cm. A total of 37 patients did not have a segment of the aorta that could be referred as an aneurysm neck; therefore, for the calculation with the use of ratio neck, the group was reduced to 149 subjects.

A problem that would not allow for all subjects to be gathered into a single cohort were the potential differences in aortic structure and aneurysm morphology between men and women, which are included in the current guidelines for the treatment of abdominal aortic aneurysms. To determine the validity of such a fusion, among groups of men and women, the separate sex subgroups were extracted, which were characterized by the same minimum and maximum diameter of the aneurysm. There were 17 women and 162 men with a minimum aneurysm diameter of 4.4 cm and a maximum diameter of 9.8 cm. The mean size was 6.4 cm for women and 6.5 cm for men, and the median was 5.8 cm for women and 6.1 cm for men. The aorta diameter above the aneurysm was compared between men and women, and for this purpose, the diameter of the aorta at the level of renal arteries was arbitrarily used for some subjects that did not have the neck segment. To simultaneously take into account the size of the aneurysm, the R Renal was compared as well. The analysis revealed no statistically significant differences both when comparing the diameter and the ratio; therefore, further measurements were made without gender division (Figure 2).

RAAA in the entire study group had a larger maximal diameter than AAA in the control group. The differences in other section sizes were not significant. The differences of all calculated ratios between the study group and the control group were statistically significant (Figure 3). There were the same results for those parameters after dividing the group into neck and non-neck subgroups (Figures 4 and 5).

As mentioned above, the test and control groups were divided into size ranges (<5; 5–6.5; >6.5 cm) and the previous calculations were made for each subgroup separately. In the group of subjects with the present aneurysm neck segment, the maximum size of the aneurysm differed significantly between the test and control groups in the size ranges of the aneurysm sac <5 cm and 5–6.5 cm. When comparing the difference in the ratios, for aneurysms smaller than 5 cm in diameter, significant differences were shown only for Ratio Neck. In the size range from 5–6.5 cm, the following ratios were significantly different: Ratio Celiac, Mesenteric, Renal, Neck, Left Iliac comm and Left iliac ext, with the difference of the latter two being less pronounced. For aneurysms larger than 6.5 cm in diameter, significant differences were shown only for the Ratio Neck (Figure 6).

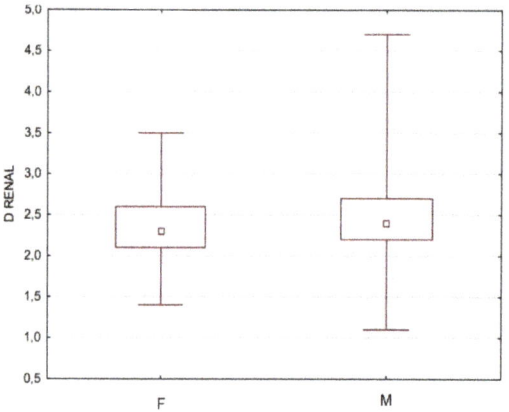 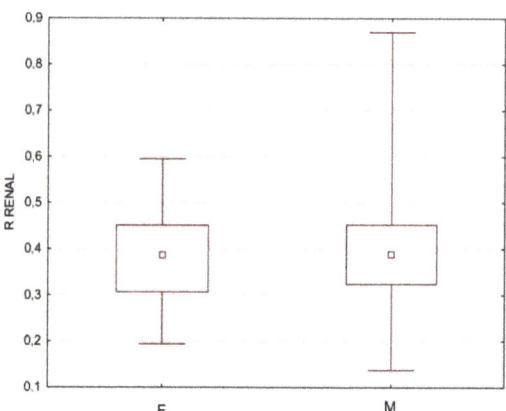

Figure 2. A comparison of aorta diameter (D RENAL) and renal ratio (R RENAL) between women (F) and men (M). D Renal for women from 1.4 to 3.5 cm with majority from 2.1 to 2.6 cm, D Renal for men from 1.1 to 4.7 cm with majority from 2.2 to 2.7 cm. R Renal for women from 0.2 to 0.6 with majority from 0.3 to 0.45, R renal for men from 0.14 to 0.88 with majority form 0.32 to 0.45. All differences insignificant $p > 0.05$.

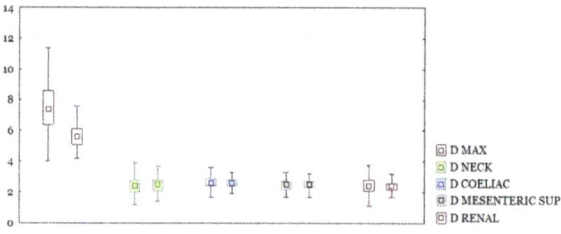 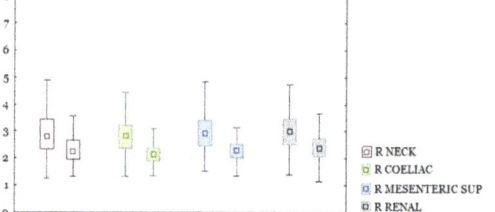

Figure 3. On the left, a comparison of diameters of the aorta at different levels and AAA diameters between ruptured and unruptured aneurysms in the whole cohort. Diameters in cm. Boxplots are shown in pairs. The left one is diameter for ruptured, the right one is diameter for unruptured aneurysms. Only D MAX difference is significant with $p < 0.05$. On the right, a comparison of ratios between ruptured and unruptured aneurysms. Boxplots are shown in pairs. The left one is ratio for ruptured, the right one is ratio for unruptured aneurysms. All differences significant at $p < 0.05$.

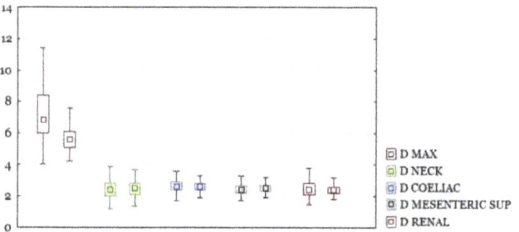 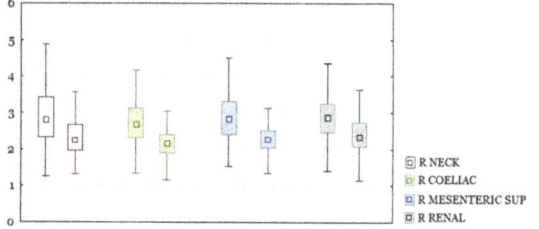

Figure 4. On the left, a comparison of diameters of the aorta between ruptured and unruptured aneurysms with the neck segment present. Diameters in cm. Boxplots are shown in pairs. The left one is diameter for ruptured, the right one is diameter for unruptured aneurysms. Only D MAX difference is significant with $p < 0.05$. On the right, a comparison of ratios between ruptured and unruptured aneurysms. Boxplots are shown in pairs. The left one is ratio for ruptured, the right one is ratio for unruptured aneurysms. All differences significant at $p < 0.05$.

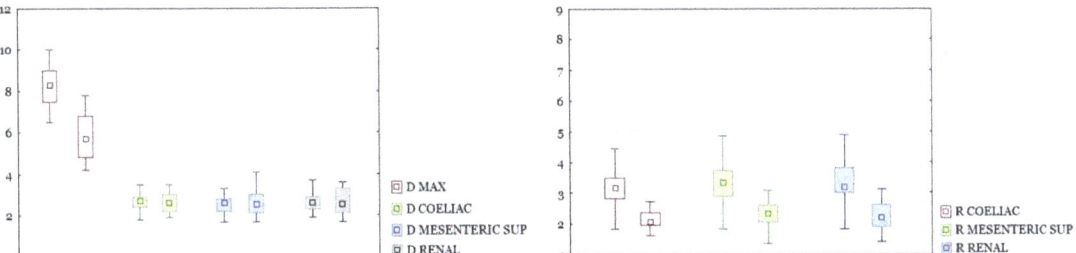

Figure 5. On the left, a comparison of diameters of the aorta between ruptured and unruptured aneurysms with the neck segment absent. Diameters in cm. Boxplots are shown in pairs. The left one is diameter for ruptured, the right one is diameter for unruptured aneurysms. Only D MAX difference is significant with $p < 0.05$. On the right, a comparison of ratios between ruptured and unruptured aneurysms. Boxplots are shown in pairs. The left one is ratio for ruptured, the right one is ratio for unruptured aneurysms. All differences significant at $p < 0.05$.

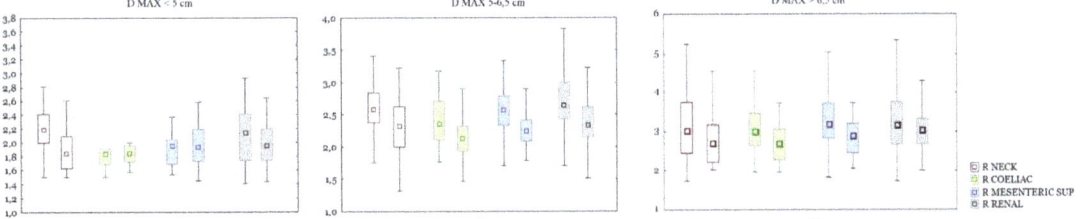

Figure 6. (**A**) A comparison of ratios of the aorta between ruptured and unruptured aneurysms with the neck segment present. Subgroup with D MAX < 5 cm. Boxplots are shown in pairs. The left one is ratio for ruptured, the right one is ratio for unruptured aneurysms. Only the R NECK difference is significant with $p < 0.05$. (**B**) A comparison of ratios of the aorta between ruptured and unruptured aneurysms with the neck segment present. Subgroup with D MAX 5–6.5 cm. Boxplots are shown in pairs. The left one is ratio for ruptured, the right one is ratio for unruptured aneurysms. All differences significant at $p < 0.05$. (**C**) A comparison of ratios of the aorta between ruptured and unruptured aneurysms with the neck segment present. Subgroup with D MAX > 6.5 cm. Boxplots are shown in pairs. The left one is ratio for ruptured, the right one is ratio for unruptured aneurysms. Only the R NECK difference is significant with $p < 0.05$.

In the group of subjects without the aneurysm neck segment, after dividing the group into size subgroups, there were too few subjects in each one of them for the results to be relied upon.

Next, the analyzed ratios were assessed for predictive value for AAA rupture. Since the only ratio showing significant differences in each of the size subgroups was the Ratio Neck, the predictive value was calculated for this parameter only and compared with the prognostic value of the maximum aneurysm sac diameter, the parameter currently used to estimate the risk of rupture. This analysis revealed that in the <5 cm subgroup, the Ratio Neck had a better prognostic value for predicting the risk of rupture than the maximum sac diameter (AUC 0.783 vs. 0.650). In the range 5–6.5 cm, the maximum diameter was a better predictor for estimating risk of rupture than the Ratio Neck (AUC 0.680 vs. 0.729), and in the >6.5 cm subgroup both parameters showed similar prognostic value for this phenomenon (AUC 0.641 vs. 0.658) (Figure 7).

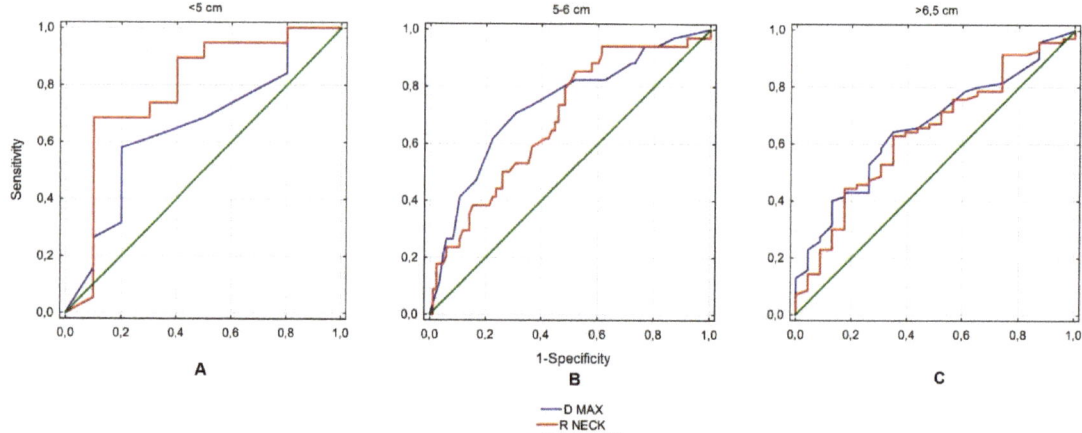

Figure 7. (**A**) ROC curves for the predictive value of R NECK compared with D MAX and the reference line in the group of aneurysms with D MAX < 5 cm. AUC for D MAX: 0.65, AUC for R NECK: 0.783. (**B**) ROC curves for the predictive value of R NECK compared with D MAX and the reference line in the group of aneurysms with D MAX 5–6.5 cm. AUC for D MAX: 0.729, AUC for R NECK: 0.68. (**C**) ROC curves for the predictive value of R NECK compared with D MAX and the reference line in the group of aneurysms with D MAX > 5 cm. AUC for D MAX: 0.658, AUC for R NECK: 0.641.

Then, the values of particular ratios in a certain percentage of patients were analyzed. To compare them between the groups, the ratio values in the 20th, 25th and 30th percentiles were analyzed. The Ratio Neck was used for the analysis, as it revealed significant differences between the study and control group in all aneurysm size subgroups. Since the Ratio Neck can only be calculated for aneurysms with a neck segment, the Ratio Renal values were additionally compared, as it would seem that it most closely describes the relation between an aneurysm sac and unchanged aorta in the patients without a neck segment. The comparison showed that in general the ratios tend to be lower for non-ruptured aneurysms. The Ratio Neck was 2.26 for 20%, 2.3 for 25% and 2.4 for 30% for ruptured aneurysms and 1.9 for 20%, 1.94 for 25% and 2.01 for 30% for non-ruptured aneurysms (Figure 8).

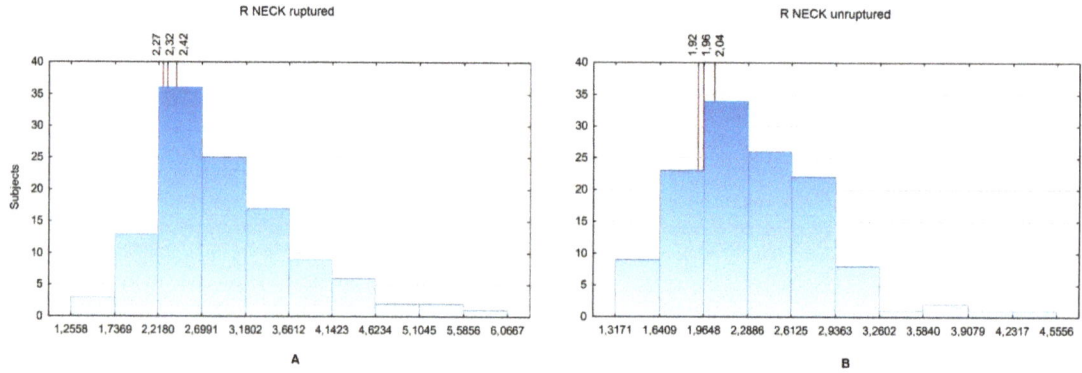

Figure 8. (**A**) R NECK values distribution in a certain number of patients with ruptured aneurysm. For the 20th percentile: 2.27, 25th percentile: 2.32, 30th percentile: 2.42. (**B**) R NECK values distribution in a certain number of patients with unruptured aneurysm. For the 20th percentile: 1.92, 25th percentile: 1.96, 30th percentile: 2.04.

The Ratio Renal analysis was performed separately for the subjects with and without the neck segment. For aneurysms with the neck segment present, the values were 2.4 for 20%, 2.41 for 25% and 2.49 for 30% for ruptured aneurysms and 2 for 20%, 2.05 for 25% and 2.18 for 30% for non-ruptured aneurysms (Figure 9).

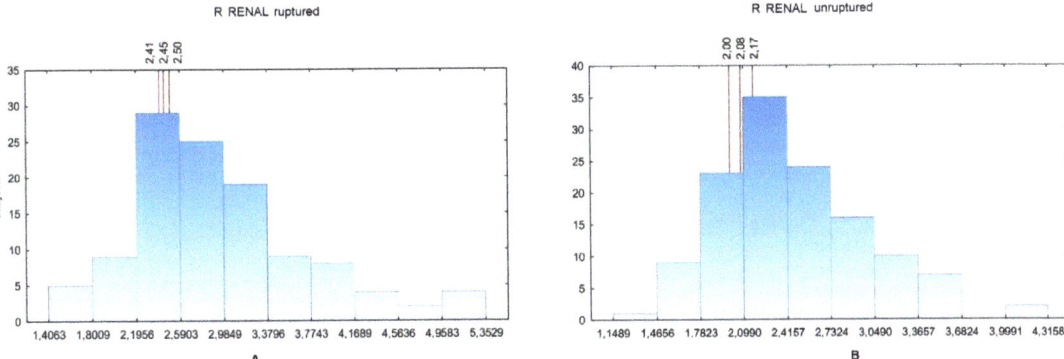

Figure 9. (**A**) R RENAL values distribution in a certain number of patients with ruptured aneurysm with neck segment present. For the 20th percentile: 2.41, 25th percentile: 2.45, 30th percentile: 2.5. (**B**) R RENAL values distribution in a certain number of patients with unruptured aneurysm with neck segment present. For the 20th percentile: 2, 25th percentile: 2.08, 30th percentile: 2.17.

For aneurysms without necks, the values were 2.78 for 20%, 3 for 25% and 3 for 30% for ruptured aneurysms and 1.8 for 20%, 1.91 for 25% and 2 for 30% for non-ruptured aneurysms (Figure 10).

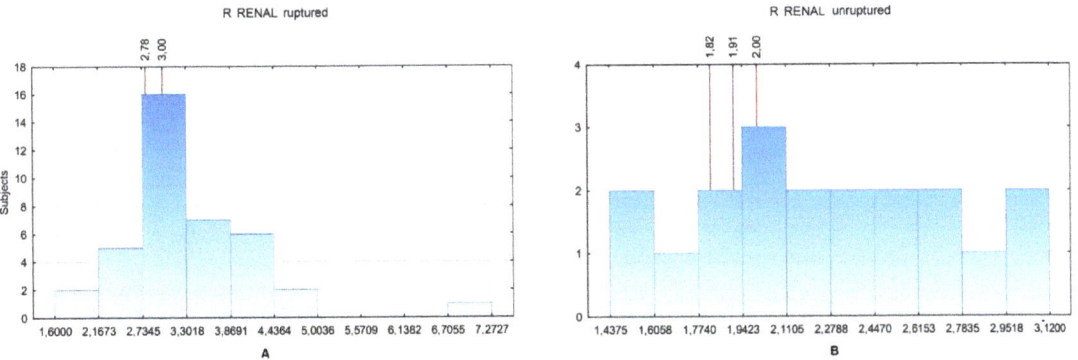

Figure 10. (**A**) R RENAL values distribution in a certain number of patients with ruptured aneurysm with neck segment absent. For the 20th percentile: 2.78, 25th percentile: 3, 30th percentile: 3. (**B**) R RENAL values distribution in a certain number of patients with unruptured aneurysm with neck segment absent. For the 20th percentile: 1.82, 25th percentile: 1.91, 30th percentile: 2.

4. Discussion

AAA is a pathological lesion with a very heterogeneous structure and shape when compared between individual patients. The differences in AAA morphology, the length and characteristics of the aortic section it covers, as well as the histological structure of the vascular wall make it reasonable to look for individual factors that would allow the patient to be provided with surgical treatment. There may be factors other than the maximum size of the aneurysm, which, according to the variables mentioned above, could in some cases lower the diameter importance [7,10,25]. In the current guidelines, the only manifestations of taking into account the individual characteristics of a certain patient are lowering the AAA size range due to the female gender and qualifying patients for surgical treatment with AAA, which increases its maximum size relatively quickly [23,24]. The latter factor, although important in clinical practice, turns out to be difficult to assess, as it requires at least two computed tomography (CT) scans per year in a specific patient. Given the widespread use of ultrasound diagnostics used in vascular outpatient clinics, providing a fairly good, but incomplete, picture of the disease, this is rarely practiced. Ultrasound measurements are subject to some error from the lack of standardization of this method, which may result in the delivery of many false positive and false negative results of a rapid increase in the maximum diameter of AAA [28]. Moreover, intravenous administration of a contrast agent, which, with frequent examinations, may cause or lead to an exacerbation of the present renal failure is not without significance [29]. Due to the above-mentioned difficulties, a group of patients may be mistakenly classified as low-risk RAAA patients, and they are not qualified for surgical treatment as they should be.

The starting point of this study is the assumption that even a single CT scan can provide more data indicating an increased risk of AAA rupture in a certain patient than the maximal aneurysm size alone. A study by Kimura et al. took into account, for example, the fillet radius and the aspect ratio, the parameters whose values, obtained through a single CT scan, distinguished RAAA from AAA [25]. In our study, emphasis was placed on taking into account the size of the unchanged aorta and iliac arteries and comparing them to the size of aneurysm sac. It was assumed that even in the case of a relatively small aneurysm, when there is also a small size of healthy vessels, the peak wall stress (PWS) may be significant. The normal abdominal aorta has a very similar diameter throughout its entire length down to the division into the iliac arteries. However, abdominal aneurysms commonly have diverse morphologies and may be accompanied by dilations in other parts of the aorta that are not sufficiently large to be classified as aneurysms. We therefore determined the dimensions of the aorta at several separate sites. Similarly, the calculations concerning the diameter of iliac arteries were enrolled.

The study assumes that the degree of enlargement of the aneurysm sac in relation to the initial size of the aorta is a significant risk factor for AAA rupture. Unfortunately, verifying the validity of this statement in each RAAA patient turns out to be difficult to enroll. The mean diameter of ruptured abdominal aneurysms encountered in clinical practice is larger than the threshold at which an aneurysm becomes eligible for surgical treatment Since no one undermines the benefits of surgical treatment in patients with large AAA, aneurysms of a size on the threshold of current indications for surgery and smaller have become the object of special interest in this study. Because of that, we divided our group into the subgroups based on the aneurysm size. Thanks to this division, it was possible to visualize the differences between patients with similar aneurysms but different aorta sizes, which was reflected in the calculated ratios. If no differences in the values of the ratios were observed, this would mean that the comparison of the size of the unchanged aorta to the size of the aneurysm is irrelevant and the only anatomical factor determining the rupture is the maximum size of the aneurysm sac. An interesting observation is the presence of numerous significant differences in the 5–6.5 cm subgroup, with only single ones in the remaining subgroups. In large aneurysms (>6.5) this may be due to the variety of sizes of the aneurysm sacs, still present in this subgroup even after division. This diversity does not allow us to prove the potential value of the ratios; however, in these subjects the mere fact of the presence of a large aneurysm indicates a risk of rupture high enough for the patient to be qualified for surgical treatment. The lack of differences in the values of the ratios in the group of small aneurysms (<5 cm) with only single exception indicates that there are no particular anatomical differences between ruptured and unruptured aneurysms of such size, so their rupture is rather induced by non-anatomical risk factors.

Another interesting observation is the comparison of the predictive value of the calculated ratios and the maximum AAA size for the estimation of the risk of rupture. It is noteworthy that in the studied group, in the size range <5 cm, the predictive value of maximum diameter of the aneurysm sac is characterized by the AUC for the ROC curve at the level of 0.655, which means that it has a slightly better predictive value for predicting AAA rupture than a coin toss (0.500) and does not meet the significance for a good aneurysm rupture risk predictor. The remaining parameter, R Neck, fares better in this respect with AUC 0.787, which in our opinion proves the predictive value is high enough to analyze this parameter in other study groups, as it could potentially become a new indication for surgical treatment of small aneurysms. In the remaining analyzed subgroups, the Ratio Neck size presented a prognostic value similar to or worse than the maximum AAA sac size, which limits its potential use.

In order to complete this analysis, it is necessary to look at what values each ratio has and what these values indicate. It was assumed that the value of a certain ratio in the appropriate percentile of its distribution reflects the percentage risk of rupture in the study group. The values of the ratios that had significant differences between groups were arbitrarily selected for the 20th, 25th and 30th percentiles as it was decided that the information about such a risk would be most clinically useful if the role of the ratios were to be more widely recognized. On the basis of the obtained results, it can be noticed that in most of the analyzed cases the ratios tended to be greater than or equal to 2 in the case of ruptured aneurysms, while in the case of non-ruptured aneurysms, the ratio exceeds this value only in sporadic cases. In other words, a 20% or greater risk of aneurysm rupture in this study group is when the aneurysm is at least twice the diameter of the unchanged aorta.

In our opinion, the obtained results constitute an interesting and helpful aspect for predicting the risk of AAA rupture and identifying patients particularly at risk of this incident. The role of the ratios calculated in this way should be verified in other research groups and taking into account additional risk factors. The use of additional techniques such as FEM for the assessment of PWS within individual AAA and RAAA could be particularly helpful in verifying the usefulness of the ratios [30]. For example, Urrutia et al. observed that PWS, calculated using FEM, apart from the maximum size of the aneurysm, is equally well correlated with other parameters such as: T (tortuosity), DDr (maximum diameter to neck diameter ratio), S (wall surface area), K-median (median of the Gaussian surface curvature), C-max (maximum lumen compactness), and M-mode (mode of the mean surface curvature) [31]. Zelaya et al. proposed estimating the PWS using a so-called linear model. The authors compared the vascular wall tension between patient-specific AAA models with the results obtained using conventional approaches and a hypothetical AAA reference model. It has been shown that such a linear model allows for a simple and effective estimation of PWS on the basis of a single CT scan, without referring to complicated analytical methods [32].

In recent years, there were some other attempts to assess the risk of AAA rupture based on aneurysm morphology. Netio-Palomo et al. were performing complex and detailed statistical analysis of individual aneurysm risk of rupture based on its size, shape and wall stress [33]. The authors made some very interesting observations linking the increased risk of aneurysm rupture with parameters other than the maximum diameter, such as the length of the aneurysm, its symmetry coefficient or the way blood flows through the aorta. The analysis is based on the creation of an accurate three-dimensional graphic model of a given aneurysm and it allows for much more precise measurements than in the case of the ratios calculated by us, but the difficulty of its implementation and the precise criteria that a given aneurysm had to meet in order to be analyzed determined the small size of the study group. For the same reason, ruptured aneurysms were not included in the study, so it is not possible to make any comparisons using the technique presented by the authors in this field.

An approach to the analyzed problem similar to ours was presented by Vande Geest et al. In their work, the authors calculated the rupture potential index (RPI), which is the ratio containing the relation of wall stress to wall strength and they compared it between patients with ruptured and non-ruptured AAA [33]. On the basis of the calculations performed, no differences were found between the groups, but their small number makes one ask whether the studied individuals were group-representative enough to abandon this direction of research.

In our work, we emphasized the simplicity of calculations, which, although limiting their accuracy, allowed us to create a larger group than in many of the cited studies [33–35]. We hoped that observing a given feature in a larger population would emphasize its significance and we believe that further development of the study group, especially with patients from other centers, would confirm the significance of the ratios we calculated. We realize that taking into account the individually variable dimensions of the aorta when estimating the risk of aneurysm rupture is only one of many elements of the individual characteristics of the patient that could be included in the calculations. Apart from increasing the size of the study group, the use of basic biometric data could be extremely valuable in this aspect. In our study, we showed that for two patients with the same size of AAA, the one with a smaller aorta has a higher risk of rupture, which confirms the significance of individual differences between patients. The most obvious physical difference between people is, of course, their height and weight. Incorporating these data in correlation with aortic and aneurysm sizes could significantly affect the reliability of the data, and this is a direction that should be followed in future analyses. Unfortunately, although these data appear to be easy to obtain, in some severe and unstable cases of RAAA, it is not possible to precisely measure height and weight or obtain them from the patient.

The results obtained by our team and other authors seems to be promising enough to consider the gathering of missing data and complexing the calculations with more advanced three-dimensional models. If that had been achieved, we would have had truly individual abdominal aortic aneurysm rupture risk assessment.

5. Conclusions

The ratio of aneurysm size to the size of the unchanged aorta visibly differs between ruptured and unruptured aneurysms, which results from the larger maximum size of ruptured aneurysms. In the study group, while maintaining the same size of the aneurysm, the aorta was smaller in ruptured aneurysms than in non-ruptured aneurysms. In the case of small aneurysms, their maximum size does not determine the risk of rupture high enough to predict this incident. The ratio of the aneurysm diameter to the iliac arteries is not applicable in assessing the risk of rupture. The ratio of the aneurysm sac to aorta diameter is a better prognostic factor for rupture, but only in small aneurysms with a present neck segment. In the study group, the aneurysm size enlarging twice as compared to the unchanged aorta determined at least a 20% risk of aneurysm rupture. In order to confirm the usefulness of calculated ratios for the assessment of the risk of rupture, further studies on other groups of patients are necessary.

Author Contributions: Conceptualization, P.K. and M.J.; methodology, P.K. and M.J.; software, A.M.; validation, P.K., W.K. and M.J.; formal analysis, M.J.; investigation, M.J.; resources, M.J.; data curation, A.M.; writing—original draft preparation, M.J.; writing—review and editing, P.K. and W.K.; visualization, A.M.; supervision, P.K. and W.K.; project administration, M.J.; funding acquisition, W.K. All authors have read and agreed to the published version of the manuscript.

Funding: This research received no external funding.

Institutional Review Board Statement: Ethical review and approval were waived for this study due to the study material concerned only CT-scan measurement data without patients' personal records and without biological material sampling the Bioethical Commission of Medical University of Silesia in Katowice at the meeting on 8 February 2022 declared that our study does not need the commission approval.

Informed Consent Statement: Not applicable.

Data Availability Statement: Data available on request from corresponding author.

Conflicts of Interest: The authors declare no conflict of interest.

References

1. Noel, A.A.; Gloviczki, P.; Cherry, K.J., Jr.; Bower, T.C.; Panneton, J.M.; Mozes, G.I.; Harmsen, W.S.; Jenkins, G.D.; Hallett, J.W. Ruptured abdominal aortic aneurysms: The excessive mortality rate of conventional repair. *J. Vasc. Surg.* **2001**, *34*, 41–46. [CrossRef] [PubMed]
2. Raux, M.; Marzelle, J.; Kobeiter, H.; Dhonneur, G.; Allaire, E.; Cochennec, F.; Becquemin, J.-P.; Desgranges, P. Endovascular balloon occlusion is associated with reduced intraoperative mortality of unstable patients with ruptured abdominal aortic aneurysm but fails to improve other outcomes. *J. Vasc. Surg.* **2015**, *61*, 304–308. [CrossRef] [PubMed]
3. van Beek, S.; Vahl, A.; Wisselink, W.; Reekers, J.; Legemate, D.; Balm, R. Midterm Re-interventions and Survival After Endovascular Versus Open Repair for Ruptured Abdominal Aortic Aneurysm. *Eur. J. Vasc. Endovasc. Surg.* **2015**, *49*, 661–668. [CrossRef]
4. Luebke, T.; Brunkwall, J. Risk-Adjusted Meta-analysis of 30-Day Mortality of Endovascular Versus Open Repair for Ruptured Abdominal Aortic Aneurysms. *Ann. Vasc. Surg.* **2015**, *29*, 845–863. [CrossRef]
5. Limet, R.; Sakalihassan, N.; Albert, A. Determination of the Expansion Rate and Incidence of Rupture of Abdominal Aortic Aneurysms. *J. Vasc. Surg.* **1991**, *14*, 540–548. [CrossRef]
6. Cronenwett, J.L. Variables That Affect the Expansion Rate and Rupture of Abdominal Aortic Aneurysms. *Ann. N. Y. Acad. Sci.* **1996**, *800*, 56–67. [CrossRef]
7. Choke, E.; Cockerill, G.; Wilson, W.; Sayed, S.; Dawson, J.; Loftus, I.; Thompson, M. A Review of Biological Factors Implicated in Abdominal Aortic Aneurysm Rupture. *Eur. J. Vasc. Endovasc. Surg.* **2005**, *30*, 227–244. [CrossRef]
8. Galyfos, G.; Sigala, F.; Mpananis, K.; Vouros, D.; Kimpizi, D.; Theodoropoulos, C.; Zografos, G.; Filis, K. Small Abdominal Aortic Aneurysms: Has Anything Changed So Far? *Trends Cardiovasc. Med.* **2020**, *30*, 500–504. [CrossRef]
9. Venkatasubramaniam, A.K.; Fagan, M.J.; Mehta, T.; Mylankal, K.J.; Ray, B.; Kuhan, G.; Chetter, I.C.; McCollum, P.T. A Comparative Study of Aortic Wall Stress Using Finite Element Analysis for Ruptured and Non-ruptured Abdominal Aortic Aneurysms. *Eur. J. Vasc. Endovasc. Surg.* **2004**, *28*, 168–176.
10. Vallabhaneni, S.R.; Gilling-Smith, G.L.; How, T.V. Heterogeneity of Tensile Strength and Matrix Metalloproteinase Activity in the Wall of Abdominal Aortic Aneurysms. *J. Endovasc. Ther.* **2004**, *11*, 494–502. [CrossRef]
11. Maguire, E.M.; Pearce, S.W.A.; Xiao, R.; Oo, A.Y.; Xiao, Q. Matrix Metalloproteinase in Abdominal Aortic Aneurysm and Aortic Dissection. *Pharmaceuticals* **2019**, *12*, 118. [CrossRef] [PubMed]
12. Tang, W.; Yao, L.; Hoogeveen, R.; Alonso, A.; Couper, D.; Lutsey, P.L.; Steenson, C.C.; Guan, W.; Hunter, D.W.; Lederle, F.A.; et al. The Association of Biomarkers of Inflammation and Extracellular Matrix Degradation with the Risk of Abdominal Aortic Aneurysm: The ARIC Study. *Angiology* **2019**, *70*, 130–140. [CrossRef] [PubMed]
13. MA3RS Study Investigators. Aortic Wall Inflammation Predicts Abdominal Aortic Aneurysm Expansion, Rupture, and Need for Surgical Repair. *Circulation* **2017**, *136*, 787–797. [CrossRef] [PubMed]
14. Stringfellow, M.M.; Lawrence, P.F.; Stringfellow, R.G. The influence of aorta-aneurysm geometry upon stress in the aneurysm wall. *J. Surg Res.* **1987**, *42*, 425–433. [CrossRef]
15. Mower, W.E.; Baraff, L.J.; Sneyd, J. Stress Distributions in Vascular Aneurysms: Factors Affecting Risk of Aneurysm Rupture. *J. Surg. Res.* **1993**, *55*, 155–161. [CrossRef] [PubMed]
16. Elger, D.F.; Blackketter, D.M.; Budwig, R.S.; Johansen, K.H. The Influence of Shape on the Stresses in Model Abdominal Aortic Aneurysms. *J. Biomech. Eng.* **1996**, *118*, 326–332. [CrossRef]
17. Di Martino, E.; Mantero, S.; Inzoli, F.; Melissano, G.; Astore, D.; Chiesa, R.; Fumero, R. Biomechanics of abdominal aortic aneurysm in the presence of endoluminal thrombus: Experimental characterisation and structural static computational analysis. *Eur. J. Vasc. Endovasc. Surg.* **1998**, *15*, 290–299. [CrossRef]
18. Domonkos, A.; Staffa, R.; Kubíček, L. Effect of Intraluminal Thrombus on Growth Rate of Abdominal Aortic Aneurysms. *Int. Angiol.* **2019**, *38*, 39–45. [CrossRef]
19. Schurink, G.W.H.; van Baalen, J.M.; Visser, M.J.T.; van Bockel, J.H. Thrombus within an aortic aneurysm does not reduce pressure on the aneurysmal wall. *J. Vasc. Surg.* **2000**, *31*, 501–506. [CrossRef]
20. Vorp, D.A.; Wang, D.H.J.; Webster, M.W.; Federspiel, W.J. Effect of Intraluminal Thrombus Thickness and Bulge Diameter on the Oxygen Diffusion in Abdominal Aortic Aneurysm. *J. Biomech. Eng.* **1998**, *120*, 579–583. [CrossRef]
21. Vorp, D.A.; Lee, P.C.; Wang, D.H.; Makaroun, M.S.; Nemoto, E.M.; Ogawa, S.; Webster, M.W. Association of intraluminal thrombus in abdominal aortic aneurysm with local hypoxia and wall weakening. *J. Vasc. Surg.* **2001**, *34*, 291–299. [CrossRef] [PubMed]
22. Fontaine, V.; Jacob, M.-P.; Houard, X.; Rossignol, P.; Plissonnier, D.; Angles-Cano, E.; Michel, J.-B. Involvement of the Mural Thrombus as a Site of Protease Release and Activation in Human Aortic Aneurysms. *Am. J. Path.* **2002**, *161*, 1701–1710. [CrossRef]
23. Chaikof, E.L.; Dalman, R.L.; Eskandari, M.K.; Jackson, B.M.; Lee, W.A.; Mansour, M.A.; Mastracci, T.M.; Mell, M.; Murad, M.H.; Nguyen, L.L.; et al. The Society for Vascular Surgery Practice Guidelines on the Care of Patients with an Abdominal Aortic Aneurysm. *J. Vasc. Surg.* **2018**, *67*, 2–77.e2. [CrossRef] [PubMed]

24. Moll, F.L.; Powell, J.T.; Fraedrich, G.; Verzini, F.; Haulon, S.; Waltham, M.; van Herwaarden, J.A.; Holt, P.J.E.; van Keulen, J.W.; Rantner, B.; et al. Management of Abdominal Aortic Aneurysms Clinical Practice Guidelines of the European Society for Vascular Surgery. *Eur. J. Vasc. Endovasc Surg.* **2011**, *41* (Suppl. S1), S1–S58. [CrossRef]
25. Kimura, M.; Hoshina, K.; Miyahara, K.; Nitta, J.; Kobayashi, M.; Yamamoto, S.; Ohshima, M. Geometric analysis of ruptured and nonruptured abdominal aortic aneurysms. *J. Vasc. Surg.* **2019**, *69*, 86–91. [CrossRef]
26. Cronenwett, J.L.; Murphy, T.F.; Zelenock, G.B.; Whitehouse, W.M., Jr.; Lindenauer, S.M.; Graham, L.M.; Quint, L.E.; Silver, T.M.; Stanley, J.C. Actuarial analysis of variables associated with rupture of small abdominal aortic aneurysms. *Surgery* **1985**, *98*, 472–483.
27. Lederle, F.A.; Wilson, S.E.; Johnson, G.R.; Reinke, D.B.; Littooy, F.N.; Acher, C.W.; Ballard, D.J.; Messina, L.M.; Gordon, I.L.; Chute, E.P.; et al. Immediate Repair Compared with Surveillance of Small Abdominal Aortic Aneurysms. *N. Engl. J. Med.* **2002**, *346*, 1437–1444. [CrossRef]
28. Concannon, E.; McHugh, S.; Healy, D.A.; Kavanagh, E.; Burke, P.; Moloney, M.C.; Walsh, S.R. Diagnostic accuracy of non-radiologist performed ultrasound for abdominal aortic aneurysm: Systematic review and meta-analysis. *Int. J. Clin. Pract.* **2014**, *68*, 1122–1129. [CrossRef]
29. Rundback, J.H.; Nahl, D.; Yoo, V. Contrast-induced nephropathy. *J. Vasc. Surg.* **2011**, *54*, 575–579. [CrossRef]
30. Soto, B.; Vila, L.; Dilmé, J.F.; Escudero, J.R.; Bellmunt, S.; Camacho, M. Increased Peak Wall Stress, but Not Maximum Diameter, Is Associated with Symptomatic Abdominal Aortic Aneurysm. *Eur. J. Vasc. Endovasc. Surg.* **2017**, *54*, 706–711. [CrossRef]
31. Urrutia, J.; Roy, A.; Raut, S.; Antón, R.; Muluk, S.C.; Finol, E.A. Geometric surrogates of abdominal aortic aneurysm wall mechanics. *Med. Eng. Phys.* **2018**, *59*, 43–49. [CrossRef]
32. Zelaya, J.E.; Goenezen, S.; Dargon, P.T.; Azarbal, A.-F.; Rugonyi, S. Improving the efficiency of abdominal aortic aneurysm wall stress computations. *PLoS ONE* **2014**, *9*, e101353. [CrossRef] [PubMed]
33. Nieto-Palomo, F.; Pérez-Rueda, M.; Lipsa, L.-M.; Vaquero-Puerta, C.; Vilalta-Alonso, J.-A.; Vilalta-Alonso, G.; Soudah-Prieto, E. Statistical techniques for predicting rupture risk in abdominal aortic aneurysms: A contribution based on bootstrap. *Sci. Prog.* **2021**, *104*, 1–21. [CrossRef] [PubMed]
34. Georgakarakos, E.; Ioannou, C.; Kamarianakis, Y.; Papaharilaou, Y.; Kostas, T.; Manousaki, E.; Katsamouris, A. The Role of Geometric Parameters in the Prediction of Abdominal Aortic Aneurysm Wall Stress. *Eur. J. Vasc Surg.* **2010**, *39*, 42–48. [CrossRef] [PubMed]
35. Geest, J.P.V.; DI Martino, E.S.; Bohra, A.; Makaroun, M.S.; Vorp, D.A. A biomechanics-based rupture potential index for abdominal aortic aneurysm risk assessment: Demonstrative application. *Ann. N. Y. Acad. Sci.* **2006**, *1085*, 11–21. [CrossRef]

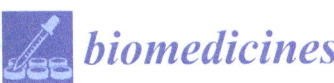

Article

Use of MALDI Mass Spectrometry Imaging to Identify Proteomic Signatures in Aortic Aneurysms after Endovascular Repair

Matthias Buerger [1,†], Oliver Klein [2,†], Sebastian Kapahnke [1], Verena Mueller [1], Jan Paul Frese [1], Safwan Omran [1], Andreas Greiner [1], Manuela Sommerfeld [3], Elena Kaschina [3], Anett Jannasch [4], Claudia Dittfeld [4], Adrian Mahlmann [5] and Irene Hinterseher [1,6,*]

1. Berlin Institute of Health, Vascular Surgery Clinic, Charité—Universitätsmedizin Berlin, Freie Universität Berlin and Humboldt-Universität zu Berlin, Hindenburgdamm 30, 12203 Berlin, Germany; matthias.buerger@charite.de (M.B.); sebastian.kapahnke@charite.de (S.K.); verena.mueller@charite.de (V.M.); jan-paul-bernhard.frese@charite.de (J.P.F.); safwan.omran@charite.de (S.O.); andreas.greiner@charite.de (A.G.)
2. BIH Center for Regenerative Therapies BCRT, Berlin Institute of Health at Charité—Universitätsmedizin Berlin, Augustenburger Platz 1, 13353 Berlin, Germany; oliver.klein@charite.de
3. Center for Cardiovascular Research (CCR), Institute of Pharmacology, Charité—Universitätsmedizin Berlin, Freie Universität Berlin and Humboldt-Universität zu Berlin, Hessische Str. 3-4, 10115 Berlin, Germany; manuela.sommerfeld@charite.de (M.S.); elena.kaschina@charite.de (E.K.)
4. Department of Cardiac Surgery, Herzzentrum Dresden, Medical Faculty Carl Gustav Carus Dresden, Technische Universität Dresden, 01307 Dresden, Germany; anett.jannasch@tu.dresden.de (A.J.); claudia.dittfeld@tu-dresden.de (C.D.)
5. University Center for Vascular Medicine, Department of Medicine—Section Angiology, University Hospital Carl Gustav Carus, Technische Universität, 01307 Dresden, Germany; adrian.mahlmann@uniklinikum-dresden.de
6. Medizinische Hochschule Brandenburg Theordor Fontane, 16816 Neuruppin, Germany
* Correspondence: irene.hinterseher@charite.de; Tel.: +49-30-450-522725
† Contributed equally to this work.

Abstract: Endovascular repair (EVAR) has become the standard procedure in treating thoracic (TAA) or abdominal aortic aneurysms (AAA). Not entirely free of complications, a persisting perfusion of the aneurysm after EVAR, called Endoleak (EL), leads to reintervention and risk of secondary rupture. How the aortic wall responds to the implantation of a stentgraft and EL is mostly uncertain. We present a pilot study to identify peptide signatures and gain new insights in pathophysiological alterations of the aortic wall after EVAR using matrix-assisted laser desorption or ionization mass spectrometry imaging (MALDI-MSI). In course of or accompanying an open aortic repair, tissue sections from 15 patients (TAA = 5, AAA = 5, EVAR = 5) were collected. Regions of interest (tunica media and tunica adventitia) were defined and univariate (receiver operating characteristic analysis) statistical analysis for subgroup comparison was used. This proof-of-concept study demonstrates that MALDI-MSI is feasible to identify discriminatory peptide signatures separating TAA, AAA and EVAR. Decreased intensity distributions for actin, tropomyosin, and troponin after EVAR suggest impaired contractility in vascular smooth muscle cells. Furthermore, inability to provide energy caused by impaired respiratory chain function and continuous degradation of extracellular matrix components (collagen) might support aortic wall destabilization. In case of EL after EVAR, this mechanism may result in a weakened aortic wall with lacking ability to react on reinstating pulsatile blood flow.

Keywords: aortic aneurysm; EVAR; endoleak; proteomic signature; MALDI-MSI

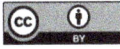

1. Introduction

Defined as a dilatation of the aortic wall by 1.5 times of the physiological diameter, aortic aneurysm is a common disease with an age-dependent prevalence of 8% and is a leading cause of death in men >65 years old. If left untreated, the risk of further dilatation and rupture increases. With a mortality of up to 80%, aortic rupture is an acutely life-threatening event [1].

The aortic wall consists of a three-layered structure. On the luminal site, a single layer of endothelial cells is forming the tunica intima. The tunica media is formed by adjacent vascular smooth muscle cells (VSMC) and structural proteins, such as elastin and collagen. The outermost tunica adventitia is composed of mostly fibroblasts and collagen fibers [2]. The formation of an aortic aneurysm is considered a multifactorial process caused by genetic and epigenetic alterations supported by behavioral risk factors such as smoking and atherosclerotic degradation. However, the exact pathophysiology remains to be elucidated. Histologically, aortic aneurysms are characterized by inflammation, VSMC apoptosis, extracellular matrix (ECM) degradation and oxidative stress [3,4]. This results in a weakened and instable aortic wall which is no longer able to withstand luminal blood pressure.

To prevent aortic rupture, aortic aneurysm repair should be considered from a threshold diameter of 60 mm or 55 mm in thoracic (TAA) and abdominal aortic aneurysm (AAA), respectively (depending on localization, configuration, and patient gender). Furthermore, rapid aneurysm growth is an additional risk factor for aortic rupture requiring aortic repair. Endovascular stent grafts became state of the art in the treatment of TAA and AAA [5]. Several studies have shown an early survival benefit of patients treated with EVAR compared to conventional open aortic repair for elective surgery in infrarenal AAA in short-term follow-ups [6–8]. Nevertheless, the emergence of late complications after EVAR leads to a loss of the initial survival benefit during long-term observations [9,10]. The most common complication leading to secondary intervention is persisting perfusion of the aneurysm sac, a so-called endoleak (EL) [11,12]. As a result of persisting EL, the risk of aortic rupture is increased [13].

The underlying pathophysiological changes in the aortic wall leading to EL and rupture after EVAR are unclear. Findings of structural atrophy due to a significant thinning of the aneurysm wall layers accompanied by cell deficiency suggest a weakened aneurysm wall after EVAR. Cell-depletion supported by alterations of extracellular matrix (ECM) components, such as collagen, may result in a status of instability [14]. Furthermore, new insights into the role of VSMC as the predominant existing cell type in aortic walls underline their importance for aortic wall integrity. The exact sequential pathophysiology of AAA formation remains uncertain, but VSMC contractile and synthetic phenotypes are considered to have an impact on aneurysm formation [15]. While the synthetic phenotype provides manufacturing of ECM, the contractile properties of VSMC encompass mechanical force distribution by regulating their linkage to ECM components [16,17]. It has been shown that mutations in genes, encoding for contractile proteins of VSMC, such as smooth muscle actin (ACTA2) and smooth muscle myosin heavy chain (MYH11), predispose for hereditary TAA and aortic dissections [17,18]. Recently, evaluations of VSCM contractility suggest both an impaired contractile function in AAA patients and patients formerly treated by EVAR [19]. Therefore, pathophysiological changes of ECM components accompanied by alterations of VSCM properties are of particular interest to understand mechanisms leading to complications after EVAR.

The unraveling of molecular changes often remains hidden due to tissue heterogeneity. Proteomic methods have been successfully used to characterize pathophysiological processes in various diseases [20,21]. In current studies, fluid-based proteomic approaches such as liquid chromatography are combined with mass spectrometry after tissue microdissection to discover new disease-related markers in muscle tissue [22–24]. However, obtaining a sufficient amount of material is labor-intensive and provides little insight into the actual spatial distribution of pathophysiological regions.

Recently, matrix-assisted laser desorption or ionization mass spectrometry imaging (MALDI-MSI), a tissue-based technology for analyzing human specimens, entered the field of diagnostics for a variety of diseases [25,26]. Several studies have demonstrated the advantages of high resolution MSI data in microdissected tissue sections while preserving spatial specificity with accurate protein assignment [27–29]. Due to long processing time for both microdissection and mass spectrometry and the higher costs, these promising techniques are not well suited for large scale studies. In contrast, spatially distinct peptide signatures obtained from MALDI tissue imaging data can be acquired in a shorter time frame, a larger sample cohort, and at a lower cost [30–32]. Combining a mass spectrometric technique with conventional histological evaluation on a single tissue section allows the analysis of a variety of molecules. Furthermore, by preserving the spatial coordinates in the analyzed tissue sections, it generates a unique molecular intensity map and thus allows conclusions about location-related alterations in specific regions of interest. Referring to aortic diseases, Mohamed et al. emphasized the potential of the MALDI technique in a proof-of-concept study to provide useful information for underlying pathogenesis in aneurysms of the thoracic ascending aorta [26].

The aim of this pilot study was to investigate the feasibility and potential of using MALDI-MSI combined with univariate statistical analysis to differentiate between TAA, AAA, and EVAR and to discriminate remodeling processes in aortic wall specimens after EVAR. Alterations in proteomic signatures after EVAR might be used to gain insights into the underlying pathophysiological remodeling leading to complications such as EL or aortic rupture.

2. Experimental Section

The study was approved by the institutional ethic review board at the Charité Universitätsmedizin Berlin on 7 July 2020 (project identification code EA4/108/20) and written consent was obtained from all patients.

2.1. Patient and Sample Cohort

Human aortic tissue samples were obtained during elective open aortic surgeries for TAA, AAA, or EL, and aneurysm sac enlargement after EVAR, respectively. Specimens were removed intraoperatively from the area of largest diameter of the aneurysmal formation in the thoracic or abdominal aorta. Subsequently, aneurysmal aortic tissue sections from TAA (n = 5), AAA (n = 5), and EVAR (n = 5) were transported to the laboratory for further processing and preparation of formalin-fixed paraffin-embedded (FFPE) tissue sections.

2.2. MALDI-MSI

FFPE tissue samples were prepared for MALDI-IMS analysis as previously reported [33]. Briefly, all FFPE tissue sections were 6 µm thick, cut by microtome (HM325, Thermo Fisher, Bremen, Germany) and mounted onto conductive glass slides coated in indium tin oxide (Bruker Daltonik GmbH, Bremen, Germany). Sections were preheated to 80 °C for 15 min before deparaffinization. Paraffin was removed in xylene, and tissue sections were processed through 100% isopropanol and successive hydration steps of 100% ethanol followed by 96%, 70%, and 50% ethanol, each for 5 min. Sections were fully rehydrated in Milli-Q-purified water (MilliQ-water). Heat-induced antigen retrieval was performed in MilliQ-water for 20 min in a steamer. After drying slides for 10 min, tryptic digestion was performed. An automated spraying device (HTX TM-Sprayer, HTX Technologies LLC, ERC GmbH Riemerling, Germany) was used to deliver onto each section, 16 layers of tryptic solution (20µg Promega® Sequencing Grade Modified Porcine Trypsin in 800 µL digestion buffer; 20 mM ammonium bicarbonate with 0.01% glycerol) at 30 °C. Tissue sections were incubated for 2 h at 50 °C in a humidity chamber saturated with potassium sulfate solution, then the HTX TM Sprayer applied 4 layers of the matrix solution (7 g/L a-cyano-4-hydroxycinnamic acid in 70% acetonitrile and 1% trifluoroacetic acid) at 75 °C. MALDI imaging was conducted on the rapifleX® MALDI Tissuetyper® (Bruker Daltonik GmbH, Bremen, Germany) in reflector mode with the detection range of 600–3200 m/z, 500 laser shots per spot, a 1.25 GS/s sampling rate, and raster width of 50 µm. FlexImaging 5.1 and flexControl 3.0 software (Bruker Daltonik GmbH, Bremen, Germany) coordinated the MALDI imaging run. External calibration was performed using a peptide calibration standard (Bruker Daltonik GmbH, Bremen, Germany). The matrix was removed from tissue sections with 70% ethanol after MALDI imaging, and sections were stained with hematoxylin and eosin for histology. Subsequently, aortic wall layers were annotated in QuPath software [34] and transferred into SCiLS Lab software (Version 2019c Pro, Bruker Daltonik GmbH, Bremen, Germany). In general, we stuck to the previously published standard operation procedure by Ly et al. [35].

2.3. Protein Identification by Electrospray Ionization Tandem Mass Spectrometry

Protein identification for peptide values was performed on adjacent tissue sections using a bottom-up nano-liquid chromatography electrospray ionization tandem mass spectrometry approach as previously described [33]. Similar to their preparation for MALDI-MSI, sections were preheated to 80 °C for 15 min before deparaffinization. Paraffin removal, antigen retrieval, and tryptic digestion were carried out as for MALDI-MSI. After incubation at 50 °C in a humidity chamber saturated with potassium sulfate solution for 2 h, peptides were extracted separately from each tissue section into 40 µL of 0.1% trifluoroacetic acid and incubated 15 min at room temperature. Digests were filtered using a ZipTip® C18 following the manufacturer's instructions, and the eluates were vacuum concentrated (Eppendorf® Concentrator 5301, Eppendorf AG, Hamburg, Germany,) and reconstituted separately in 20 µL 0.1% trifluoroacetic acid, from which 2 µL were injected into a NanoHPLC (Dionex UltiMate 3000, Thermo Fisher Scientific, Bremen, Germany) coupled to an ESI-QTOF ultrahigh-resolution mass spectrometer (Impact II™, Bruker Daltonic GmbH, Bremen, Germany). The peptide mixture was loaded onto an Acclaim PepMap™ 100 C18 trap column (100 µm × 2 cm, PN 164564, Thermo Fisher Scientific, Bremen, Germanyand calibrated with 10 mM sodium hypofluorite (flowrate 20 µL/h) before separation in an Acclaim PepMap™ RSLC C18 column (75 µm × 50 cm, PN 164564, Thermo Fisher Scientific, Bremen, Germany) with an increasing acetonitrile gradient of 2–35% in 0.1% formic acid (400 nL/min flow rate, 10–800 bar pressure range) for 90 min while the column was kept at 60 °C. Released charged peptides were detected by a tandem mass spectrometer using a full-mass scan (150–2200 m/z) at a resolution of 50,000 FWHM. The autoMS/MS InsantExpertise was used to select peaks for fragmentation by collision-induced dissociation. Acquired raw MS/MS spectra were converted into mascot generic files (.mgf) for amino acid sequences using ProteoWizard software [36], and used to search the human UniProt database using the Mascot search engine (version 2.4, MatrixScience Inc., London, UK) with the significance threshold of $p < 0.05$ and the settings for trypsin as the proteolytic enzyme; a maximum of 1 missed cleavage; 10 ppm peptide tolerance; peptide charges of 2+, 3+, or 4+; oxidation allowed as variable modification; 0.8 Da MS/MS tolerance and a MOWSE score > 13 to identify the corresponding protein. Mascot results were exported as .csv files. To match aligned m/z values from MALDI-MSI (Supplementary Table S1) with the peptides identified by nanoLC-MS/MS (Supplementary Table S2), we developed an excel macro in-house. The macro was applied with settings accommodating previously described parameters [37]. Briefly, the comparison of MALDI-MSI and LC−MS/MS m/z values required the identification of >1 peptide (mass differences < 0.9 Da). The peptides with highest MOWSE peptide score, smallest mass differences between MALDI-MSI and LC-MS/MS data and a correlation coefficient >0.1 or <0.1 were accepted as correctly identified.

2.4. MALDI-MSI Data Processing for Statistical Analyses

MALDI-MSI raw data were imported into the SCiLS Lab software version 2019c Pro (Bruker Daltonik GmbH) using settings preserving total ion count without baseline removal and converted into the SCiLS base data .sbd file and .slx file. An attribute table was built for the sample number and the different aortic wall layers tunica media and tunica adventitia. Attributes were used to divide the data set into independent data sets from different spatial spectral regions in tissue sections. Peak finding and alignment were conducted across a data set (interval width = 0.3 Da) using a standard segmentation pipeline (SciLS Lab software) in maximal interval processing mode with TIC normalization, medium noise reduction and no smoothing (Sigma: 0.75) [38,39].

2.5. Statistical Data Analysis

The top-down segmentation using bisecting k-means clustering analysis was performed on the partitioned data sets from tissue sections, as previously described [40], to defined proteomic signatures. Both analyses used settings for 0.3 Da interval width, include all individual spectra, and medium noise reduction and correlation distance. Discriminative MALDI-MSI m/z values were identified using supervised ROC analysis on the partitioned data sets from different tissue regions such as tunica media and tunica adventitia. The area under the ROC curve (AUC) varies between 0 and 1, where values close to 0 and 1 indicate peptides to be discriminatory and 0.5 indicates no discriminatory value. Since the number of m/z values from comparison groups must be similar for analysis, 35,000 m/z values were randomly selected per group. For those peptides with an AUC > 0.6 or <0.4, a univariate hypothesis test (Wilcoxon rank sum test) was used to test the statistical significance of m/z values. Peptides with p-value < 0.001 and a peak correlation ratio > 0.5 were selected as candidate markers.

3. Results

3.1. Clinical Characterization

General patient characteristics are shown in Table 1. All patients were non-diabetic men. The mean overall age was 67 ± 10 years. No significant difference in subgroup comparison was observed for age (TAA = 59 ± 10 years vs. AAA = 73 ± 6 years vs. EVAR = 70 ± 7 years, p = 0.077). The mean aortic diameter was 69 ± 16 mm. Patients with AAA (AAA = 80 ± 19 mm vs. TAA = 54 ± 5 mm, p = 0.01) or EVAR (EVAR = 72 ± 12 mm vs. TAA = 54 ± 5 mm, p = 0.02) had a significantly larger aortic diameter compared to those with TAA.

Indications for open aortic repair included rapid aneurysm growth (>5 mm in six months or >10 mm in one year, n = 2) or exceeded a threshold diameter of 55 mm (n = 8) for TAA and AAA patients. Patients formerly treated by EVAR developed several types of EL requiring open surgery for EL type Ia (n = 1), EL type II (n = 2), EL type III (n = 1), and EL type V (n = 1).

3.2. MALDI-MSI Data

Primary proteomic screenings were performed simultaneously for TAA, AAA, and EVAR tissue sections. Subsequently, mass spectra for the annotated regions of interest (ROI, tunica media, and tunica adventitia) were obtained and statistically analyzed using SCiLS Lab software (Bruker, Bremen, Germany). Analysis of the whole tissue sections revealed 46.446, 75.128 and 126.259 spectra for TAA, AAA, and EVAR specimens, respectively. Annotated ROIs in TAA, AAA, and EVAR revealed 10.014, 11.988, and 27.112 spectra for tunica adventitia and 22.661, 8932, and 16.588 spectra for tunica media, respectively. Average exemplary spectra are shown for TAA, AAA, and EVAR subregions in Figure 1. The peptide signatures extracted from the analyzed tissue samples yielded 476 aligned peptide values (Supplementary Table S1) in a mass range for tryptic peptides (m/z value range: 600–3200).

Table 1. Indications and patient characteristics.

Subgroup	Gender	Age	Maximum Aneurysm Diameter (mm)	Comorbidities
TAA_1	M	62	58	CAD, HI
TAA_2	M	67	59	HI
TAA_3	M	54	52	HI
TAA_4	M	43	57	HI
TAA_5	M	68	46	CAD, HI, AHT, HLP, COPD, CRF
AAA_1	M	78	60	CAD, AHT, HLP
AAA_2	M	72	81	CRF, AHT
AAA_3	M	78	80	CAD, HLP
AAA_4	M	63	110	AHT
AAA_5	M	76	68	CAD, HI, AHT
EVAR_1	M	67	75	CAD, PAD, AHT
EVAR_2	M	64	90	CAD, AHT, HLP
EVAR_3	M	80	65	AF, PAD
EVAR_4	M	73	59	CAD, CRF
EVAR_5	M	65	69	AHT, PAD

CAD = coronary artery disease, HI = heart insufficiency, AHT = arterial hypertension, HLP = hyperlipidemia, COPD = chronic obstructive pulmonary disease, CRF = chronic renal failure, PAD = peripheral artery disease, AF = atrial fibrillation.

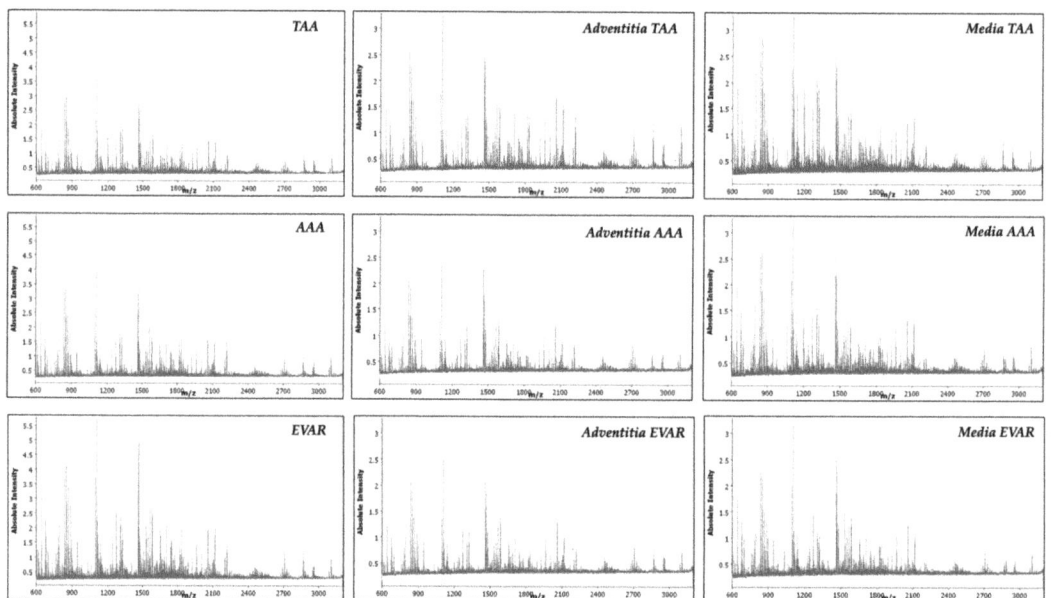

Figure 1. MALDI-MSI average spectra from the whole tissue sections and annotated regions of interest of tunica adventitia and tunica media in TAA, AAA, and EVAR tissue samples.

3.3. Discriminative Proteins from TAA, AAA, and EVAR Tissue Sections Based on MALDI-MSI Data

To provide a better understanding of the pathophysiological differences in aortic wall layers, specific localized peptide values were explored in TAA, AAA, and EVAR tissue sections. Based on the typical wall structure of the aorta, sections of tunica media, and tunica adventitia were defined for analysis.

The identification of peptide values might provide insights into aneurysm formation and alterations of aortic wall structure after EVAR. To identify the corresponding proteins to the discriminatory tryptic peptide fragments, we performed a bottom-up LC-MS/MS approach in adjacent tissue sections. In total, 476 peptide values were detected via MALDI-MSI in annotated ROIs. Of those, 284 peptide values could be assigned to peptide values derived from LC-MS/MS (mass differences < 1 Da) corresponding to 91 proteins (Supplementary Table S2). After comparison of MALDI-MSI and LC−MS/MS (Supplementary Table S3) peptide values (requiring identification of >1 peptide to one protein), 84 peptide values revealed 28 corresponding proteins. ROC analysis was used on the total 284 aligned peptide peaks from annotated tunica adventitia (Supplementary Table S4) and tunica media (Supplementary Table S5) in AAA, TAA, and EVAR tissue sections. Overall, analysis for tunica adventitia revealed 82 and 62 discriminative peptide values for comparison of AAA and TAA and for EVAR and TAA, respectively. For tunica media, 63, 52, and 257 discriminative peptide values have been identified for subgroup comparison (AAA vs. EVAR, AAA vs. TAA, and EVAR vs. TAA). As the formation of an aortic aneurysm is largely caused by changes within the tunica media, we focus our interpretation of the results only on the peptide alterations observed in this area.

Corresponding proteins to peptide values are correctly identified when the validating approach identifies at least two peptide values (detected in MALDI-MSI) from the same protein (AUC < 0.4, >0.6, p < 0.001) [36]. This revealed 47 peptide values with 17 corresponding proteins (ACTA, CAD13, CO1A1, CO1A2, CO6A3, KCRM, DESM, ETFB, H13, H4, MYH6, PGAM2, TPM1, TNNI3, TNNT2, TBB5, VME). In comparison to EVAR, nine peptide values with their corresponding four proteins (ACTA, ETFB, TPM1, TBB5) were increased in AAA tissue sections. Moreover, 46 m/z values from 17 corresponding proteins (ACTA, CAD13, CO1A1, CO1A2, CO6A3, KCRM, DESM, ETFB, H13, H4, MYH6, PGAM2, TPM1, TNNI3, TNNT2, TBB5, VME) are decreased in EVAR specimens compared to TAA tissue sections. The peptide values corresponding to ACTA were decreased in AAA specimens compared to TAA specimens (Table 2). As an example, we show intensity distributions in separate tissue sections for ETFB in Figure 2 and Supplementary Figure S1. Moreover, illustrative intensity distributions for actin, tropomyosin, and troponin are shown in Figure 3. The remaining peptides and their corresponding protein intensity distributions are shown in Supplementary Figure S2.

Table 2. Differential peptides (MALDI-MSI) and their corresponding proteins from the tunica media in TAA, AAA, and EVAR tissue sections.

MALDI-MSI m/z Value [Da]	ROC [AUC] Media AAA vs. EVAR	ROC [AUC] Media AAA vs. TAA	ROC [AUC] Media EVAR vs. TAA	LC-MS [MH + Calc.]	Scores	Sequence	Gene Symbol	Protein
976.43	0.62	0.35	0.22	976.4468194	88.56	AGFAGDDAPR		
1198.65	0.66	0.29	0.10	1198.51941	57.19	DSYVGDEAQSK		
1198.65	0.66	0.29	0.10	1198.703002	41.77	AVFPSIVGRPR	ACTA2	Actin, aortic smooth muscle
1580.684	0.56	0.45	0.39	1580.800411	43.04	MQKEITALAPSTMK		
1790.904	0.57	0.36	0.27	1790.891339	28.06	SYELPDGQVITIGNER		
1564.883	0.59	0.42	0.33	1564.905355	31.49	SIVVSPILIPENQR	CDH13	Cadherin-13
1835.908	0.58	0.44	0.34	1836.842546	32.84	MTAFDADDPATDNALLR		

Table 2. Cont.

MALDI-MSI m/z Value [Da]	ROC [AUC] Media AAA vs. EVAR	ROC [AUC] Media AAA vs. TAA	ROC [AUC] Media EVAR vs. TAA	LC-MS [MH + Calc.]	Scores	Sequence	Gene Symbol	Protein
836.417	0.59	0.42	0.31	836.4361428	49.08	GPAGPQGPR	COL1A1	Collagen alpha-1(I) chain
852.418	0.61	0.40	0.28	851.4249814	43.88	GFSGLDGAK		
868.42	0.59	0.42	0.31	868.4253882	34.63	GEAGPQGPR		
886.421	0.56	0.43	0.36	886.4359955	47.39	GSEGPQGVR		
784.412	0.58	0.45	0.37	785.3889089	48.12	GDQGPVGR	COL1A2	Collagen alpha-2(I) chain
1561.883	0.60	0.48	0.37	1562.79067	87.57	GETGPSGPVGPAGAVGPR		
1237.653	0.57	0.43	0.37	1238.651334	47.18	VAVFFSNTPTR	COL6A3	Collagen alpha-3(VI) chain
1459.673	0.61	0.43	0.32	1459.860756	25.39	IGDLHPQIVNLLK		
1462.674	0.55	0.44	0.39	1462.763096	27.26	QINVGNALEYVSR		
1508.678	0.60	0.40	0.32	1507.799786	83.26	LSVEALNSLTGEFK	CKM	Creatine kinase M-type Desmin
1508.678	0.60	0.40	0.32	1507.699725	58.36	GGDDLDPNYVLSSR		
1767.902	0.57	0.47	0.39	1768.83488	32.75	DGEVVSEATQQQHEVL		
2088.931	0.56	0.45	0.39	2088.091512	51.57	TFGGAPGFPLGSPLSSPVFPR		
853.418	0.61	0.40	0.27	853.5233919	55.31	LGPLQVAR	ETFB	Electron transfer flavoprotein subunit beta
1340.663	0.60	0.44	0.34	1339.720602	51.07	LSVISVEDPPQR		
974.429	0.56	0.43	0.38	973.6021152	45.36	SGVSLAALKK	H1-3	Histone H1.3
1106.641	0.58	0.42	0.32	1107.565851	47.87	ALAAAGYDVEK		
1198.65	0.66	0.29	0.10	1198.666651	64.14	ASGPPVSELITK		
1325.661	0.59	0.44	0.36	1325.752447	45.61	DNIQGITKPAIR	H4C1	Histone H4
1466.674	0.60	0.42	0.32	1466.801839	61.03	TVTAMDVVYALKR		
1533.68	0.58	0.44	0.34	1533.775171	82.04	VVDSLQTSLDAETR	MYO6	Myosin-6
1850.909	0.59	0.44	0.34	1851.041427	48.84	VQLLHSQNTSLINQKK		
2088.931	0.56	0.45	0.39	2088.123001	33.09	YRILNPVAIPEGQFIDSR		
2199.941	0.57	0.46	0.39	2200.123705	49.68	GTLEDQIIQANPALEAFGNAK		
976.43	0.62	0.35	0.22	975.4887038	36.63	AMEAVAAQGK	PGAM2	Phosphoglycerate mutase 2
1150.645	0.56	0.43	0.38	1150.666958	45.55	VLIAAHGNSLR		
875.42	0.57	0.44	0.37	875.4465169	30.27	SLEAQAEK	TPM1	Tropomyosin alpha-1 chain
1460.674	0.62	0.43	0.31	1460.731208	39.4	KATDAEADVASLNR		
1516.679	0.61	0.43	0.32	1516.819568	27.34	SKQLEDELVSLQK		
1305.659	0.58	0.41	0.34	1306.638768	44.38	KNIDALSGMEGR	TNNI3	Troponin I, cardiac muscle
1479.675	0.54	0.43	0.40	1479.727686	42.27	ISADAMMQALLGAR		
1889.913	0.57	0.46	0.38	1890.031221	44.46	NITEIADLTQKIFDLR		
758.41	0.55	0.45	0.40	757.4673223	35.39	ILAERR	TNNT2	Troponin T, cardiac muscle
906.423	0.55	0.43	0.37	906.5021046	26.65	YEINVLR		
1797.904	0.57	0.46	0.40	1796.934971	29.11	SFMPNLVPPKIPDGER		
1143.445	0.60	0.42	0.31	1143.632775	28.94	LAVNMVPFPR	TUBB	Tubulin beta chain
1320.661	0.64	0.38	0.24	1319.701066	49.82	IMNTFSVVPSPK		
1269.656	0.56	0.43	0.37	1270.559399	37.29	LGDLYEEEMR	VIM	Vimentin
1428.671	0.55	0.33	0.28	1428.710851	40.41	SLYASSPGGVYATR		
2498.168	0.55	0.49	0.44	2497.256473	42.86	LLQDSVDFSLADAINTEFKNTR		

The relative peptide expression (color bar) is shown for MALDI m/z ion peaks with the highest significant area under the curve (AUC) values (>0.6, $p < 0.001$, on top) in receiver operator characteristic (ROC) analysis and the lowest AUC values (<0.4, $p < 0.001$, bottom MALDI images). Red lines represent tunica media. Hematoxylin and eosin (H&E) staining in sections is shown for orientation.

Relative peptide expression (color bar) is shown for MALDI m/z ion peaks with the highest significant area under the curve (AUC) values (>0.6, $p < 0.001$, left) in receiver operator characteristic (ROC) analysis and the lowest AUC values (<0.4, $p < 0.001$, right MALDI images). Red lines represent tunica media and green lines represent tunica adventitia. Hematoxylin and eosin (H&E) staining in sections is shown for orientation.

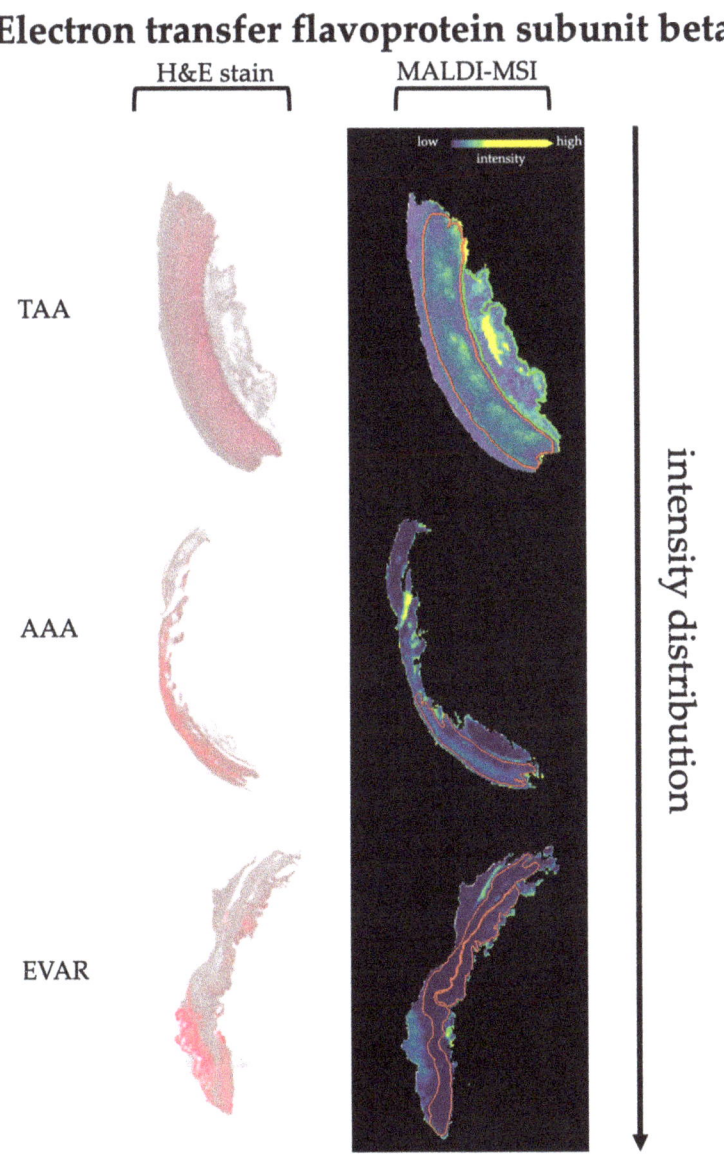

Figure 2. Differential intensity distributions of electron transfer flavoprotein subunit beta between TAA, AAA, and EVAR specimens.

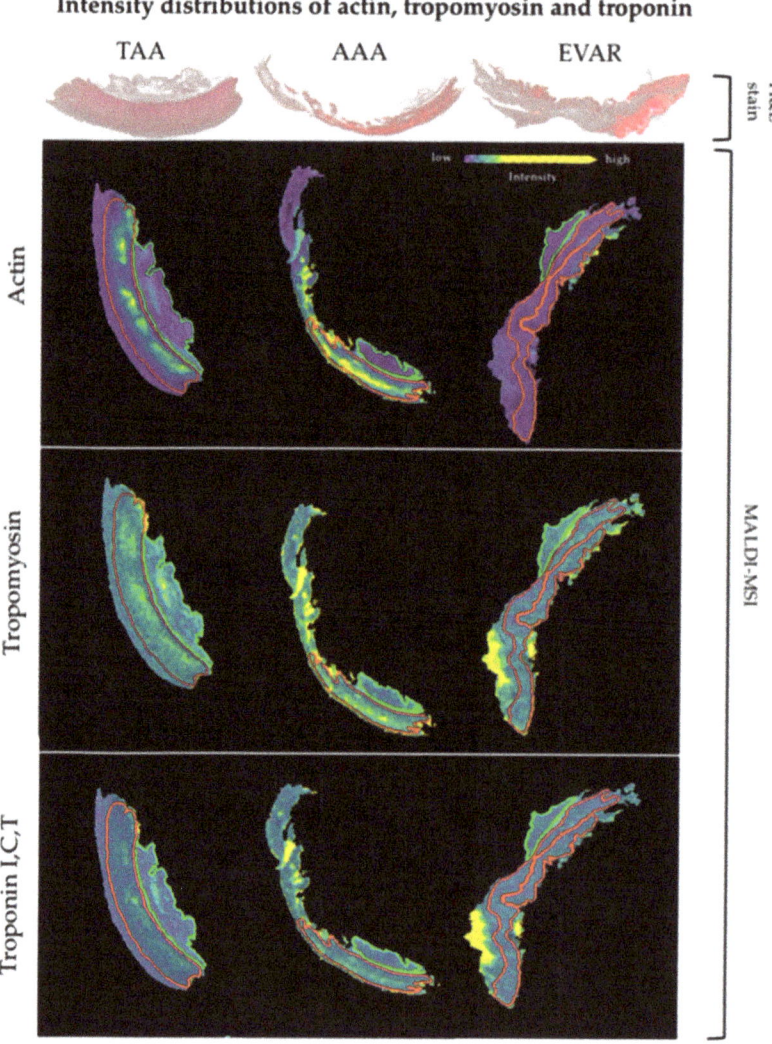

Figure 3. Differential intensity distributions of actin, tropomyosin, and troponin between TAA, AAA, and EVAR specimens.

4. Discussion

4.1. Summary

As a unique mass spectrometric technique which combines spatial molecular analysis and histological assessment, MALDI-MSI identified proteomic signatures in aortic walls in TAA, AAA, and after, EVAR. Since little is known about pathophysiological changes after EVAR, the advantage of MALDI-MSI is seen in the absence of requirements for labelling or knowledge of molecular targets to analyze the distribution of hundreds of peptides. Furthermore, preservation of the spatial coordinates allows the linkage of alterations in protein distributions to specific regions inside the aortic wall layers. Thus, MALDI-MSI as a new technique seems to be an optimal tool to gain new insights on underlying changes inside the aortic wall.

Acquired spatial proteomic signatures revealed 17 proteins with altered distributions among the tissue sections in EVAR and TAA or AAA, respectively. Actin, tropomyosin, and troponin, associated with the contractile unit in VSMC, showed decreased intensity distribution after EVAR. Furthermore, a decrease in extracellular matrix (collagen) or cytoskeletal proteins (desmin, tubulin) and electron carrier protein (electron transferring flavoprotein) could be observed in aortic wall specimens after EVAR. Based on these results, three spatial alterations could contribute to impaired wall stability after EVAR: (1) loss of function of the contractile unit in VSMC, (2) continuous degradation of extracellular matrix (ECM) proteins, and (3) reduced capacity to provide energy.

4.2. Impaired Vascular Smooth Muscle Cell Contractility after EVAR

Although the exact pathophysiological mechanism in aortic aneurysm formation remains unclear, VSCM are considered to play a central role depending on their phenotype [15]. Degradation of ECM induced by increased production of elastolytic enzymes, such as matrix metalloproteinases (MMP) by synthetic VSMC, is assumed to be one of the main reasons for aneurysm growth and rupture [3,4]. However, most VSMC in the aortic wall display a contractile phenotype responsible for regulating vascular tone.

To maintain contractile function, VSMCs express α-smooth muscle actin (aSMA), which forms the thin filament of the contractile unit with tropomyosin (Tm), calmodulin, and caldesmon [41]. Although it has been demonstrated that mutations affecting the contractile unit, such as ACTA2 and MYH11-gene mutations [17,18], contribute to the formation of thoracic aneurysms or dissections, still, little is known about the loss of VSMC contractile function in the pathogenesis of aortic aneurysm.

Recently, Bogunovic et al. [19] reported about the contractility in VSMC isolated from controls and sporadic AAA in human specimens by using electric cell-substrate impedance sensing (ECIS). No significant overall difference between AAA-patients and the control group in mean and maximum contraction was observed. Therefore, patients were subsequently divided into low and high contracting groups (defined as lower or higher than two standard deviations of results in the control group). Nevertheless, based on the findings that 28% (6/21) and 23% (5/21) of AAA patients showed lower contractility and low maximum contraction, respectively, the authors hypothesized that an impaired contractile function in VSMC in AAA patients might play a pathophysiological role in aneurysm formation. Furthermore, four patients formerly treated by EVAR were analyzed. Interestingly, VSMC obtained from those patients demonstrated a nearly significant ($p = 0.05$) trend of lower maximum contraction compared to the control group. Our data showed a lower intensity distribution of aSMA in the EVAR tissue sections compared to AAA and TAA specimens, respectively. In particular, this might explain the trend of impaired VSMC contraction in EVAR patients already observed by Bogunovic et al.

However, the functionality of the contractile unit is complemented by other modulating proteins such as Tm and troponin. Although, Tm had neither been reported in AAA formation nor in EVAR complications, its importance to maintain contractile function as a calcium sensor is well established [41]. Historical assumptions that Tn proteins are not expressed in VSCM have been shown to be incorrect [42,43]. The exact role of Tn during the process of contraction in smooth muscle cells, particularly in VSMC, remains unclear. Kajioka et al. [43] not only provided evidence of the presence of all subunits of Tn in smooth muscle cells outside of cardiac muscle (e.g., aortic VSMC, trachea, urinary bladder) but also demonstrated its role in smooth muscle cell contraction. Their results suggest that particularly the complex of tropomyosin and TnT make a substantial contribution to smooth muscle contraction. With the detection of TnT and TnI, we confirm the expression of Tn outside the cardiac muscle. Furthermore, we see a significantly lower level of Tm, TnT, and TnI within the aortic wall after EVAR supporting the thesis of reduced VSMC contractility after stentgraft implantation.

In conclusion and based on our results of only a small-sample-sized patient cohort, the interaction of aSMA, myosin, Tm, and Tn assumably plays a central role in smooth muscle cell contraction. Our data provide evidence that, particularly after EVAR, a significant reduction of proteins elementarily important for VSMC contraction (aSMA, Tm, Tn) can be observed. If the aneurysm sac is successfully eliminated after EVAR, there is no risk of secondary rupture due to decreased contractility of the VSMC. However, if an EL occurs, the loss of the ability to respond to pulsatile blood flow by contraction may possibly promote rupture of the aortic wall.

4.3. Increased ECM Degradation after EVAR

In addition to the VSMCs, ECM is essential to maintain this physiological function. Within the three-layered structure of the aortic walls, a variety of ECM proteins compose a three-dimensional organization [16].

Collagen and elastic fibers comprise approximately 50% of the dry weight of larger arteries and function as the main proteins providing tensile strength and expandability [44]. Additionally, they play a key role in modulating the adhesion, proliferation, and migration of VSMC by interacting with various integrins and proteins [45]. ECM degradation in tunica media and tunica adventitia has proven to be involved in aneurysm formation [3,4].

Collagen, as the main structural protein in the aortic wall, mainly consists of fibrillar collagens type I and III, accounting for 80–90% of the total collagen. Both increased collagen I/III levels enhancing arterial stiffness and decreased collagen I/III levels weakening the aortic wall have been proven to favor aortic aneurysm and dissection [46,47]. Augmented expression of MMPs is well documented in human and mouse aortic aneurysm [48] leading to degradation of aortic ECM and collagen cleavage in particular. In contrast, Menges et al. [14] revealed an altered collagen composition in AAA and EVAR patients compared to healthy aorta with a high abundance of collagen I and decreased expression of collagen III, respectively. Underlining the importance of collagen integrity, Lee et al. [49] associated the use of fluoroquinolones to collagen degradation and higher risk of aortic aneurysm formation aortic dissection. Particularly with a significant decrease in collagen types I and III seen after EVAR, our data might provide further evidence that collagen is continued to be cleaved and degraded after stentgraft implantation. Based on this assumption, this may result in progression of aneurysm formation and lowers the tensile strength of the remaining aortic wall in case of reinstating pulsatile blood flow in case of EL.

As previously mentioned, depending on the phenotype, the increased expression of elastolytic enzymes by synthetic VSMC results in ECM degradation. The shift of the VSMC phenotype from actin- and desmin-expressing contractile phenotype to synthetic phenotype weakens the aortic wall [50,51]. Desmin, actin, and tubulin [52] can be used to define contractile phenotype in VSMC. In comparison to non-AAA samples, AAA samples contain significantly less actin and desmin, suggesting higher levels of synthetic VSMC in AAA patients [47].

Bogunovic et al. [19] examined if the observed decreased contractility might depend on the phenotype defect of VSMC. Therefore, changes in VSMC-specific marker genes (ACTA2, CNN1, TAGLN) and protein expression (aSMA, Calponin, SM22) of VSMC marker proteins were studied using quantitative PCR and Western blot, respectively. Again, the heterogeneous results in the small-sized comparison groups prevented a significant result. We observed a lower expression of desmin and tubulin after EVAR, which could be a potential sign of a lower level of contractile VSMCs. Aforementioned, we already assume to provide evidence for reduced VSMC contractility due to decreased expression of proteins necessary for contractile function. In addition, the lower expression of desmin and tubulin might support the idea that not only reduced expression of contractile proteins but also a lower proportion of contractile VSMCs in the aortic wall after EVAR might be able to reduce resistance of the aortic wall in case of pulsatile blood flow. Thus, ECM degradation and reduced VSMC contractility might benefit the risk of rupture due to aortic wall destabilization.

4.4. Alteration of the Energy Supply after EVAR

The transport of electrons to the membrane-bound respiratory chain also involves electron transferring falvoproteins (ETFs) [53]. ETFs are soluble heterodimeric FAD-containing proteins [54] and function as electron carriers between various flavoprotein-containing dehydrogenases. At least nine mitochondrial matrix flavoprotein dehydrogenases (acyl-CoA dehydrogenase, isovaleryl-CoA dehydrogenase, 2-methyl branched-chain acyl-CoA dehydrogenase, glutaryl-CoA dehydrogenase, dimethyl-glycine and sarcosine dehydrogenases) donor electrons to ETFs. Thus, ETFs are indirectly involved in several energetic pathways (fatty acid β-oxidation, amino acid oxidation, choline metabolism [55,56]. Electrons are transported by ETFB to the membrane-bound ETF-ubiquinone oxidoreductase [57], which results in a reduction of ubiquinone to ubiquinol.

No studies are available regarding impaired mitochondrial function or respiratory chain disorders in TAA and/or AAA formation. Nevertheless, our data might provide evidence for a reduced or nearly eliminated capacity of the ETF in AAA and EVAR patients. Particularly after implantation of an endovascular stentgraft, restricted nutrition might be the reason for reduced energy production. Under normal conditions, cells of the aortic wall are largely dependent on intimal diffusion [58]. Not only ending endoluminal diffusion, the endovascular implantation of the stentgraft may restrict the collateral supply of nutrition brought by the vasa vasorum. However, the significantly lower concentration of ETF in AAA than in TAA may additionally suggest a relevant role in the formation of AAA through reduced energy supply. Since ATP as a universally usable energy carrier is indispensable for triggering a muscle contraction and thus also the contraction of the VSMCs; additionally, the circle might be closed to the assumption of a limited functional capacity of the contractile unit.

5. Conclusions

In summary, our data successfully demonstrate the feasibility of using MALDI-MSI to discriminate aortic wall specimens in patients with aneurysm disease and after the implantation of an endovascular stentgraft. Not only by detecting various alterations of protein distributions in general but also by directly assigning them to specific wall layers, MALDI-MSI is ideally suited for detecting ongoing remodeling processes after EVAR. The advantage of preserving the spatial coordinates could be used to link remodeling alterations to specific regions, even to regions inside the single aortic layers, and might allow conclusions about location-related changes in specific regions of interest.

The collected data might support the hypothesis of impaired contractility of VSMCs in the aortic wall after EVAR due to reduced synthesis of aSMA, Tm, and Tn, proteins that are elementally important for contraction. In addition, a reduced supply of the energy carrier ATP could promote decreased contractility through reduced electron transport to the respiratory chain. In combination with a continuous degradation of ECM proteins, this might result in a weakened aortic wall not able to react on reinstating pulsatile blood flow in case of EL after EVAR.

Nevertheless, the findings should only be interpreted in the context of a small sample size. Additionally, comparison to non-AAA samples and further analysis with methods such as immunohistochemistry could validate the results and might help to support the hypothesis. However, if the results can be confirmed in further studies, MALDI-MSI appears to be an excellent method to detect initial remodeling processes leading to complications after EVAR and could be an important tool for initiating subsequent preventive therapy concepts.

Supplementary Materials: The following are available online at https://www.mdpi.com/article/10.3390/biomedicines9091088/s1, Figure S1: Differential intensity distributions of electron transfer flavoprotein subunit beta in all specimens Relative peptide expression (color bar) is shown for MALDI m/z ion peaks. Red lines represents tunica media. Figure S2: Differential intensity distributions of vimentin, tubulin, collagen alpha-1 (I) chain and desmin in TAA, AAA and EVAR specimens Relative peptide expression (color bar) is shown for MALDI m/z ion peaks. Red lines represents tunica media and green lines represent tunica adventitia. Hematoxylin and eosin (H&E) staining in sections is shown for orientation. Table S1: Overall differential intensity distributions of m/z values in TAA, AAA and EVAR specimens. Table S2: Peptides identified by nanoLC-MS/MS. Table S3: Differential intensity distributions of all peptides (MALDI-MSI) and their corresponding proteins from the tunica adventitia in TAA, AAA and EVAR tissue sections. Table S4: Differential intensity distributions of all peptides (MALDI-MSI) and their corresponding proteins from the tunica media in TAA, AAA and EVAR tissue sections. Table S5: Differential intensity distributions of all peptides (MALDI-MSI) and their corresponding proteins from the tunica media in TAA, AAA and EVAR tissue sections.

Author Contributions: Conceptualization, M.B. and I.H.; methodology, M.B., I.H., E.K. and O.K.; software, O.K.; validation, I.H., O.K. and E.K., formal analysis, O.K.; investigation, M.B. and O.K.; resources, M.B., I.H., V.M., J.P.F., S.O., A.G., M.S., E.K., A.M., A.J. and C.D.; data curation, O.K.; writing—original draft preparation, M.B.; writing—review and editing, I.H., S.K., V.M., J.P.F., M.S., E.K., A.J., C.D., A.M., S.O., A.G. and O.K.; visualization, M.B. and O.K.; supervision, I.H., A.G. and E.K.; project administration, I.H.; All authors have read and agreed to the published version of the manuscript.

Funding: This research received no external funding.

Institutional Review Board Statement: Ethical approval for use of residual tissue samples in this research was awarded by the local ethics committee of the Charité—Universitätsmedizin Berlin (protocol code, EA4/108/20; 7 July 2020).

Informed Consent Statement: Written informed consent was given by patients or legal guardians of the patients treated according to the study protocol for use of aortic samples in research. No individual patients can be identified from data presented in this paper.

Data Availability Statement: Data are contained within the article or supplementary material. The MALDI-MSI data presented in this study are available on request from the corresponding author.

Conflicts of Interest: The authors declare no conflict of interest.

References

1. Nordon, I.M.; Hinchliffe, R.J.; Loftus, I.M.; Thompson, M.M. Pathophysiology and epidemiology of abdominal aortic aneurysms. *Nat. Rev. Cardiol.* **2011**, *8*, 92–102. [CrossRef]
2. Ruddy, J.M.; Jones, J.A.; Spinale, F.G.; Ikonomidis, J.S. Regional heterogeneity within the aorta: Relevance to aneurysm disease. *J. Thorac. Cardiovasc. Surg.* **2008**, *136*, 1123–1130. [CrossRef]
3. Boddy, A.M.; Lenk, G.M.; Lillvis, J.H.; Nischan, J.; Kyo, Y.; Kuivaniemi, H. Basic research studies to understand aneurysm disease. *Drug News Perspect.* **2008**, *21*, 142–148.
4. Wassef, M.; Baxter, B.T.; Chisholm, R.L.; Dalman, R.L.; Fillinger, M.F.; Heinecke, J.; Humphrey, J.D.; Kuivaniemi, H.; Parks, W.C.; Pearce, W.H.; et al. Pathogenesis of abdominal aortic aneurysms: A multidisciplinary research program supported by the National Heart, Lung, and Blood Institute. *J. Vasc. Surg.* **2001**, *34*, 730–738. [CrossRef]
5. Parodi, J.C.; Palmaz, J.C.; Barone, H.D. Transfemoral Intraluminal Graft Implantation for Abdominal Aortic Aneurysms. *Ann. Vasc. Surg.* **1991**, *5*, 491–499. [CrossRef] [PubMed]
6. Greenhalgh, R.M.; Brown, L.C.; Kwong, G.P.; Powell, J.T.; Thompson, S.G. Comparison of endovascular aneurysm repair with open repair in patients with abdominal aortic aneurysm (EVAR trial 1), 30-day operative mortality results: Randomised controlled trial. *Lancet* **2004**, *364*, 843–848. [CrossRef]
7. Prinssen, M.; Verhoeven, E.L.; Buth, J.D.; Cuypers, P.W.; Van Sambeek, M.R.; Balm, R.; Buskens, E.; Grobbee, D.E.; Blankensteijn, J. A Randomized Trial Comparing Conventional and Endovascular Repair of Abdominal Aortic Aneurysms. *N. Engl. J. Med.* **2004**, *351*, 1607–1618. [CrossRef] [PubMed]
8. Lederle, F.A.; Freischlag, J.A.; Kyriakides, T.C.; Padberg, F.T., Jr.; Matsumura, J.S.; Kohler, T.R.; Lin, P.H.; Jean-Claude, J.M.; Cikrit, D.F.; Swanson, K.M.; et al. Outcomes Following Endovascular vs Open Repair of Abdominal Aortic AneurysmA Randomized Trial. *JAMA* **2009**, *302*, 1535–1542. [CrossRef]
9. Greenhalgh, R.M.; Brown, L.C.; Powussell, J.T.; Thompson, S.G.; Epstein, D.; Sculpher, M.J. Endovascular versus Open Repair of Abdominal Aortic Aneurysm. *N. Engl. J. Med.* **2010**, *362*, 1863–1871. [CrossRef]
10. Lederle, F.A.; Kyriakides, T.C.; Stroupe, K.T.; Freischlag, J.A.; Padberg, F.T., Jr.; Matsumura, J.S.; Huo, Z.; Johnson, G.R. Open versus Endovascular Repair of Abdominal Aortic Aneurysm. *N. Engl. J. Med.* **2019**, *380*, 2126–2135. [CrossRef] [PubMed]
11. Lal, B.K.; Zhou, W.; Li, Z.; Kyriakides, T.; Matsumura, J.; Lederle, F.A.; Freischlag, J. Predictors and outcomes of endoleaks in the Veterans Affairs Open Versus Endovascular Repair (OVER) Trial of Abdominal Aortic Aneurysms. *J. Vasc. Surg.* **2015**, *62*, 1394–1404. [CrossRef]

12. Mehta, M.; Sternbach, Y.; Taggert, J.B.; Kreienberg, P.B.; Roddy, S.P.; Paty, P.S.; Ozsvath, K.J.; Darling, R.C., 3rd. Long-term outcomes of secondary procedures after endovascular aneurysm repair. *J. Vasc. Surg.* **2010**, *52*, 1442–1449. [CrossRef]
13. Patel, R.; Sweeting, M.J.; Powell, J.T.; Greenhalgh, R.M. Endovascular versus open repair of abdominal aortic aneurysm in 15-years' follow-up of the UK endovascular aneurysm repair trial 1 (EVAR trial 1): A randomised controlled trial. *Lancet* **2016**, *388*, 2366–2374. [CrossRef]
14. Menges, A.-L.; Busch, A.; Reutersberg, B.; Trenner, M.; Kath, P.; Chernogubova, E.; Maegdefessel, L.; Eckstein, H.-H.; Zimmermann, A. The structural atrophy of the aneurysm wall in secondary expanding aortic aneurysms with endoleak type II. *J. Vasc. Surg.* **2019**, *70*, 1318–1326.e1315. [CrossRef]
15. Petsophonsakul, P.; Furmanik, M.; Forsythe, R.; Dweck, M.; Schurink, G.W.; Natour, E.; Reutelingsperger, C.; Jacobs, M.; Mees, B.; Schurgers, L. Role of Vascular Smooth Muscle Cell Phenotypic Switching and Calcification in Aortic Aneurysm Formation. *Arterioscler. Thromb. Vasc. Biol.* **2019**, *39*, 1351–1368. [CrossRef]
16. Jana, S.; Hu, M.; Shen, M.; Kassiri, Z. Extracellular matrix, regional heterogeneity of the aorta, and aortic aneurysm. *Exp. Mol. Med.* **2019**, *51*, 1–15. [CrossRef]
17. Milewicz, D.M.; Trybus, K.M.; Guo, D.-C.; Sweeney, H.L.; Regalado, E.; Kamm, K.; Stull, J.T. Altered Smooth Muscle Cell Force Generation as a Driver of Thoracic Aortic Aneurysms and Dissections. *Arterioscler. Thromb. Vasc. Biol.* **2017**, *37*, 26–34. [CrossRef] [PubMed]
18. Milewicz, D.M.; Guo, D.-C.; Tran-Fadulu, V.; Lafont, A.L.; Papke, C.L.; Inamoto, S.; Kwartler, C.S.; Pannu, H. Genetic Basis of Thoracic Aortic Aneurysms and Dissections: Focus on Smooth Muscle Cell Contractile Dysfunction. *Annu. Rev. Genom. Hum. Genet.* **2008**, *9*, 283–302. [CrossRef] [PubMed]
19. Bogunovic, N.; Meekel, J.P.; Micha, D.; Blankensteijn, J.D.; Hordijk, P.L.; Yeung, K.K. Impaired smooth muscle cell contractility as a novel concept of abdominal aortic aneurysm pathophysiology. *Sci. Rep.* **2019**, *9*, 6837. [CrossRef] [PubMed]
20. Ohlendieck, K. Skeletal muscle proteomics: Current approaches, technical challenges and emerging techniques. *Skelet. Muscle* **2011**, *1*, 6. [CrossRef] [PubMed]
21. Lewis, C.; Carberry, S.; Ohlendieck, K. Proteomic profiling of x-linked muscular dystrophy. *J. Muscle Res. Cell Motil.* **2009**, *30*, 267–269. [CrossRef]
22. Cox, J.; Mann, M. Quantitative, High-Resolution Proteomics for Data-Driven Systems Biology. *Annu. Rev. Biochem.* **2011**, *80*, 273–299. [CrossRef]
23. Anderson, N.L.; Anderson, N.G. The Human Plasma Proteome: History, character, and diagnostic prospects. *Mol. Cell. Proteom.* **2002**, *1*, 845–867. [CrossRef] [PubMed]
24. Maerkens, A.; Kley, R.A.; Olivé, M.; Theis, V.; van der Ven, P.F.; Reimann, J.; Milting, H.; Schreiner, A.; Uszkoreit, J.; Eisenacher, M.; et al. Differential proteomic analysis of abnormal intramyoplasmic aggregates in desminopathy. *J. Proteom.* **2013**, *90*, 14–27. [CrossRef] [PubMed]
25. Aichler, M.; Walch, A. MALDI Imaging mass spectrometry: Current frontiers and perspectives in pathology research and practice. *Lab. Investig.* **2015**, *95*, 422–431. [CrossRef] [PubMed]
26. Mohamed, S.A.; Taube, E.T.; Thiele, H.; Noack, F.; Nebrich, G.; Mohamady, K.; Hanke, T.; Klein, O. Evaluation of the Aortopathy in the Ascending Aorta: The Novelty of Using Matrix-Assisted Laser Desorption/Ionization Imaging. *Proteom. Clin. Appl.* **2020**, *15*, e2000047. [CrossRef] [PubMed]
27. Dilillo, M.; Ait-Belkacem, R.; Esteve, C.; Pellegrini, D.; Nicolardi, S.; Costa, M.; Vannini, E.; Graaf, E.L.; Caleo, M.; McDonnell, L.A. Ultra-High Mass Resolution MALDI Imaging Mass Spectrometry of Proteins and Metabolites in a Mouse Model of Glioblastoma. *Sci. Rep.* **2017**, *7*, 603. [CrossRef]
28. Mezger, S.T.P.; Mingels, A.M.A.; Bekers, O.; Heeren, R.M.A.; Cillero-Pastor, B. Mass Spectrometry Spatial-Omics on a Single Conductive Slide. *Anal. Chem.* **2021**, *93*, 2527–2533. [CrossRef]
29. Spraggins, J.M.; Rizzo, D.G.; Moore, J.L.; Noto, M.J.; Skaar, E.P.; Caprioli, R.M. Next-generation technologies for spatial proteomics: Integrating ultra-high speed MALDI-TOF and high mass resolution MALDI FTICR imaging mass spectrometry for protein analysis. *Proteomics* **2016**, *16*, 1678–1689. [CrossRef]
30. Klein, O.; Kanter, F.; Kulbe, H.; Jank, P.; Denkert, C.; Nebrich, G.; Schmitt, W.D.; Wu, Z.; Kunze, C.A.; Sehouli, J.; et al. MALDI-Imaging for Classification of Epithelial Ovarian Cancer Histotypes from a Tissue Microarray Using Machine Learning Methods. *Proteom. Clin. Appl.* **2019**, *13*, e1700181. [CrossRef] [PubMed]
31. Mascini, N.E.; Teunissen, J.; Noorlag, R.; Willems, S.M.; Heeren, R.M. Tumor classification with MALDI-MSI data of tissue microarrays: A case study. *Methods* **2018**, *151*, 21–27. [CrossRef] [PubMed]
32. Klein, O.; Fogt, F.; Hollerbach, S.; Nebrich, G.; Boskamp, T.; Wellmann, A. Classification of Inflammatory Bowel Disease from Formalin-Fixed, Paraffin-Embedded Tissue Biopsies via Imaging Mass Spectrometry. *Proteom. Clin. Appl.* **2020**, *14*, 1900131. [CrossRef]
33. Klein, O.; Strohschein, K.; Nebrich, G.; Oetjen, J.; Trede, D.; Thiele, H.; Alexandrov, T.; Giavalisco, P.; Duda, G.N.; Von Roth, P.; et al. MALDI imaging mass spectrometry: Discrimination of pathophysiological regions in traumatized skeletal muscle by characteristic peptide signatures. *Proteomics* **2014**, *14*, 2249–2260. [CrossRef] [PubMed]
34. Bankhead, P.; Loughrey, M.B.; Fernández, J.A.; Dombrowski, Y.; McArt, D.G.; Dunne, P.D.; McQuaid, S.; Gray, R.T.; Murray, L.J.; Coleman, H.G.; et al. QuPath: Open source software for digital pathology image analysis. *Sci. Rep.* **2017**, *7*, 16878. [CrossRef] [PubMed]

35. Ly, A.; Longuespée, R.; Casadonte, R.; Wandernoth, P.; Schwamborn, K.; Bollwein, C.; Marsching, C.; Kriegsmann, K.; Hopf, C.; Weichert, W.; et al. Site-to-Site Reproducibility and Spatial Resolution in MALDI–MSI of Peptides from Formalin-Fixed Paraffin-Embedded Samples. *Proteom. Clin. Appl.* **2019**, *13*, e1800029. [CrossRef]
36. Chambers, M.C.; Maclean, B.; Burke, R.; Amodei, D.; Ruderman, D.L.; Neumann, S.; Gatto, L.; Fischer, B.; Pratt, B.; Egertson, J.; et al. A cross-platform toolkit for mass spectrometry and proteomics. *Nat. Biotechnol.* **2012**, *30*, 918–920. [CrossRef] [PubMed]
37. Cillero-Pastor, B.; Heeren, R.M. Matrix-Assisted Laser Desorption Ionization Mass Spectrometry Imaging for Peptide and Protein Analyses: A Critical Review of On-Tissue Digestion. *J. Proteome Res.* **2014**, *13*, 325–335. [CrossRef]
38. Alexandrov, T.; Becker, M.; Deininger, S.O.; Ernst, G.; Wehder, L.; Grasmair, M.; von Eggeling, F.; Thiele, H.; Maass, P. Spatial Segmentation of Imaging Mass Spectrometry Data with Edge-Preserving Image Denoising and Clustering. *J. Proteome Res.* **2010**, *9*, 6535–6546. [CrossRef]
39. Alexandrov, T.; Becker, M.; Guntinas-Lichius, O.; Ernst, G.; von Eggeling, F. MALDI-imaging segmentation is a powerful tool for spatial functional proteomic analysis of human larynx carcinoma. *J. Cancer Res. Clin. Oncol.* **2012**, *139*, 85–95. [CrossRef]
40. Trede, D.; Schiffler, S.; Becker, M.; Wirtz, S.; Steinhorst, K.; Strehlow, J.; Aichler, M.; Kobarg, J.H.; Oetjen, J.; Dyatlov, A.; et al. Exploring Three-Dimensional Matrix-Assisted Laser Desorption/Ionization Imaging Mass Spectrometry Data: Three-Dimensional Spatial Segmentation of Mouse Kidney. *Anal. Chem.* **2012**, *84*, 6079–6087. [CrossRef]
41. Marston, S.; El-Mezgueldi, M. Role of tropomyosin in the regulation of contraction in smooth muscle. *Adv. Exp. Med. Biol.* **2008**, *644*, 110–123. [CrossRef] [PubMed]
42. Moran, C.M.; Garriock, R.J.; Miller, M.K.; Heimark, R.L.; Gregorio, C.C.; Krieg, P.A. Expression of the fast twitch troponin complex, fTnT, fTnI and fTnC, in vascular smooth muscle. *Cell Motil. Cytoskelet.* **2008**, *65*, 652–661. [CrossRef]
43. Kajioka, S.; Takahashi-Yanaga, F.; Shahab, N.; Onimaru, M.; Matsuda, M.; Takahashi, R.; Asano, H.; Morita, H.; Morimoto, S.; Yonemitsu, Y.; et al. Endogenous Cardiac Troponin T Modulates (Ca2+)—Mediated Smooth Muscle Contraction. *Sci. Rep.* **2012**, *2*, 979. [CrossRef] [PubMed]
44. Wagenseil, J.E.; Mecham, R.P. Vascular Extracellular Matrix and Arterial Mechanics. *Physiol. Rev.* **2009**, *89*, 957–989. [CrossRef]
45. Clyman, R.I.; McDonald, K.A.; Kramer, R.H. Integrin receptors on aortic smooth muscle cells mediate adhesion to fibronectin, laminin, and collagen. *Circ. Res.* **1990**, *67*, 175–186. [CrossRef] [PubMed]
46. Carmo, M.; Colombo, L.; Bruno, A.; Corsi, F.R.; Roncoroni, L.; Cuttin, M.S.; Radice, F.; Mussini, E.; Settembrini, P.G. Alteration of Elastin, Collagen and their Cross-links in Abdominal Aortic Aneurysms. *Eur. J. Vasc. Endovasc. Surg.* **2002**, *23*, 543–549. [CrossRef] [PubMed]
47. Blassova, T.; Tonar, Z.; Tomasek, P.; Hosek, P.; Hollan, I.; Treska, V.; Molacek, J. Inflammatory cell infiltrates, hypoxia, vascularization, pentraxin 3 and osteoprotegerin in abdominal aortic aneurysms—A quantitative histological study. *PLoS ONE* **2019**, *14*, e0224818. [CrossRef]
48. Keeling, W.B.; Armstrong, P.A.; Stone, P.A.; Bandyk, D.F.; Shames, M.L. An Overview of Matrix Metalloproteinases in the Pathogenesis and Treatment of Abdominal Aortic Aneurysms. *Vasc. Endovasc. Surg.* **2005**, *39*, 457–464. [CrossRef]
49. Lee, C.-C.; Lee, M.-T.G.; Chen, Y.-S.; Lee, S.-H.; Chen, Y.-S.; Chen, S.-C.; Chang, S.-C. Risk of Aortic Dissection and Aortic Aneurysm in Patients Taking Oral Fluoroquinolone. *JAMA Intern. Med.* **2015**, *175*, 1839–1847. [CrossRef]
50. Ailawadi, G.; Moehle, C.W.; Pei, H.; Walton, S.P.; Yang, Z.; Kron, I.L.; Lau, C.L.; Owens, G.K. Smooth muscle phenotypic modulation is an early event in aortic aneurysms. *J. Thorac. Cardiovasc. Surg.* **2009**, *138*, 1392–1399. [CrossRef]
51. López-Candales, A.; Holmes, D.R.; Liao, S.; Scott, M.J.; Wickline, S.A.; Thompson, R.W. Decreased vascular smooth muscle cell density in medial degeneration of human abdominal aortic aneurysms. *Am. J. Pathol.* **1997**, *150*, 993–1007.
52. Jiao, L.; Xu, Z.; Xu, F.; Zhang, S.; Wu, K. Vascular smooth muscle cell remodelling in elastase-induced aortic aneurysm. *Acta Cardiol.* **2010**, *65*, 499–506. [CrossRef] [PubMed]
53. Toogood, H.S.; Leys, D.; Scrutton, N.S. Dynamics driving function – new insights from electron transferring flavoproteins and partner complexes. *FEBS J.* **2007**, *274*, 5481–5504. [CrossRef] [PubMed]
54. Roberts, D.L.; Frerman, F.E.; Kim, J.J. Three-dimensional structure of human electron transfer flavoprotein to 2.1—A resolution. *Proc. Natl. Acad. Sci. USA* **1996**, *93*, 14355–14360. [CrossRef] [PubMed]
55. Chohan, K.K.; Jones, M.; Grossmann, J.G.; Frerman, F.E.; Scrutton, N.S.; Sutcliffe, M.J. Protein Dynamics Enhance Electronic Coupling in Electron Transfer Complexes. *J. Biol. Chem.* **2001**, *276*, 34142–34147. [CrossRef] [PubMed]
56. Frerman, F.E. Acyl-CoA dehydrogenases, electron transfer flavoprotein and electron transfer flavoprotein dehydrogenase. *Biochem. Soc. Trans.* **1988**, *16*, 416–418. [CrossRef] [PubMed]
57. Beckmann, J.D.; Frerman, F.E. Electron transfer flavoprotein-ubiquinone oxidoreductase from pig liver: Purification and molecular, redox, and catalytic properties. *Biochemistry* **1985**, *24*, 3913–3921. [CrossRef]
58. Wolinsky, H.; Glagov, S. Comparison of Abdominal and Thoracic Aortic Medial Structure in Mammals. Deviation of man from the usual pattern. *Circ. Res.* **1969**, *25*, 677–686. [CrossRef]

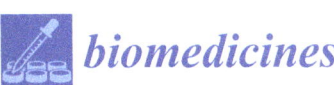

Article

Identification of the Key Genes and Potential Therapeutic Compounds for Abdominal Aortic Aneurysm Based on a Weighted Correlation Network Analysis

Lin Li [1,2], Kejia Kan [1,2], Prama Pallavi [1,2] and Michael Keese [1,2,*]

1 Department of Vascular Surgery, Medical Faculty Mannheim, Heidelberg University, 68167 Mannheim, Germany; lin.li@medma.uni-heidelberg.de (L.L.); kejia.kan@medma.uni-heidelberg.de (K.K.); prama.pallavi@medma.uni-heidelberg.de (P.P.)
2 European Center for Angioscience ECAS, Medical Faculty Mannheim, Heidelberg University, 68167 Mannheim, Germany
* Correspondence: michael.keese@umm.de; Tel.: +49-621-383-1501; Fax: +49-621-383-2166

Abstract: Background: There is still an unmet need for therapeutic drugs for patients with an abdominal aortic aneurysm (AAA), especially for candidates unsuitable for surgical or interventional repair. Therefore, the purpose of this in silico study is to identify significant genes and regulatory mechanisms in AAA patients to predicate the potential therapeutic compounds for significant genes. Methods: The GSE57691 dataset was obtained from Gene Expression Omnibus (GEO) and used to identify the differentially expressed genes (DEGs) and weighted correlation network analysis (WGCNA). The biological function of DEGs was determined using gene ontology (GO) and the Kyoto Encyclopedia of Genes and Genomes (KEGG). AAA-related genes were obtained from the Comparative Toxicogenomics Database (CTD) using the keywords: aortic aneurysm and abdominal. The hub genes in AAA were obtained by overlapping DEGs, WGCNA-based hub genes, and CTD-based genes. The diagnostic values of hub genes were determined using ROC curve analysis. Hereby, a TF-miRNA-hub gene network was constructed based on the miRnet database. Using these data, potential therapeutic compounds for the therapy of AAA were predicted based on the Drug Gene Interaction Database (DGIdb). Results: A total of 218 DEGs (17 upregulated and 201 downregulated) and their biological function were explored; 4093 AAA-related genes were derived by text mining. Three hub modules and 144 hub genes were identified by WGCNA. asparagine synthetase (ASNS), axin-related protein 2 (AXIN2), melanoma cell adhesion molecule (MCAM), and the testis-specific Y-encoded-like protein 1 (TSPYL1) were obtained as intersecting hub genes and the diagnostic values were confirmed with ROC curves. As potential compounds targeting the hub genes, asparaginase was identified as the target compound for ASNS. Prednisolone and abiraterone were identified as compounds targeting TSPYL1. For MCAM and TSPYL1, no potential therapeutic compound could be predicted. Conclusion: Using WGCNA analysis and text mining, pre-existing gene expression data were used to provide novel insight into potential AAA-related protein targets. For two of these targets, compounds could be predicted.

Keywords: AAA; WGCNA; CTD

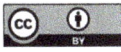

1. Introduction

Abdominal aortic aneurysm (AAA) is a common and potentially life-threatening disease that leads to more than 150,000 global deaths yearly [1–5]. While there is conclusive data on the role of environmental factors in the development of AAA in patients, there are also distinct genetic factors that have been found to play an important role in AAA progression [6]. These large dataset-based RNA-seq and microarrays datasets include differentially expressed single genes (for example, H19, BRG1-associated factor 60A (BAF60a), Kruppel-like factor 5 (Klf5), and thyroid receptor-interacting protein 13 (TRIP13)) [7–9], single nucleotide polymorphism (SNP) of genes such as the matrix metalloproteinase (MMP) family, transforming growth factor-beta (TGFBR2), and sortilin (SORT1) [10], or gene families such as the MMP family.

MicroRNAs (miRNAs) are a class of non-coding RNAs that regulate target gene expression by region binding to the 3′ UTR of target mRNA and regulation of many bioprocesses to silence and activate the target gene expression at the transcriptional and post-transcriptional level [11–13]. These oligonucleotides have also been associated with the development of AAA [14]. Interestingly, a large number of miRNAs have been shown to be associated with the regulation of key gene expression during the pathophysiology of AAA. One example of these is miRNA-21 (miR-21). Overexpression of miR-21 can inhibit the viability of vascular smooth muscle cells (VSMCs) and stabilize the aortic wall in animal models of AAA by downregulating the expression of phosphatase and tensin homolog (PTEN) [15].

MiRNAs may also interact with other key players for the development of AAA: transcription factors (TFs). By interacting with miRNAs, TFs act as master regulators of several genes at once by constituting transcriptional complexes. Identifying miRNAs and their respective TFs from co-expressed genes can thus provide important insights into the regulatory mechanism affecting vascular disorders such as AAA [14,16]. During AAA progression, miRNAs have been shown to regulate the extracellular matrix (ECM) turnover, the matrix metalloproteinase (MMP) family, different inflammatory components, and VSMCs by forming TF–miRNA network networks [17].

Based on the public dataset and bioinformatic analysis, multiple studies have been conducted to explore the regulatory mechanism of AAA at the genetic level [18–21]. Public datasets for further analysis are still scarce. In our study, we combined the GEO dataset with the Comparative Toxicogenomics Database (CTD) dataset to identify differential genes and reveal potential TF–miRNA-hub gene regulatory networks related to AAA.

2. Materials and Methods

2.1. Data Download and Processing

Microarray data of the GSE57691 dataset, which includes 49 AAA samples (20 patients with small AAA (≤55 mm), 29 patients with large AAA (>55 mm)), and 10 normal control full-thickness aortic wall biopsies and corresponding clinical data were downloaded from gene expression omnibus (GEO, https://www.ncbi.nlm.nih.gov/geo/, 23 August 2021) [22]. The expression data were generated by Illumina HumanHT-12 V4.0 expression bead chips [22]. In the present study, the normalized data were downloaded and used for subsequent analyses. Figure 1 displays the flow chart of the data analysis.

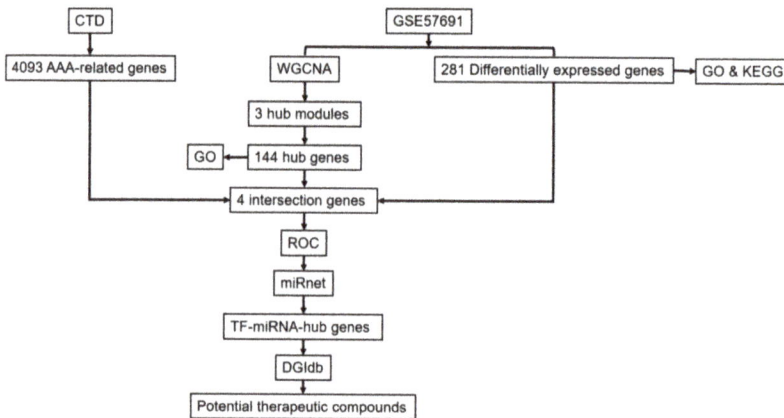

Figure 1. Flowchart of the data analysis.

2.2. AAA-Related Genes Obtained from Comparative Toxicogenomics Database (CTD)

The Comparative Toxicogenomics Database (CTD: http://ctdbase.org, 23 August 2021) is a public database that contains a wide spectrum of information on chemicals, genes, phenotypes, diseases, and exposures to advance the understanding of human health [11,18]. A total of 21,684 AAA-related genes were obtained from CTD using the keywords aortic aneurysm and abdominal and 4093 AAA-related genes were found according to previous studies (Table S5) [19,20].

2.3. Identification of the Differentially Expressed Genes (DEGs) in AAA and Normal Tissues

The DEGs between AAA and normal tissues were screened by the Limma R 3.46.0 package [22] with cutoff values of $|\log2 \text{(fold change, FC)}| > 1$ and p-value < 0.05. All results were visualized by the ggplot2 R 3.3.3 package [22].

2.4. Gene Ontology (GO) Annotation and Kyoto Encyclopedia of Genes and Genomes (KEGG) Analysis

Gene ontology (GO) annotation and Kyoto Encyclopedia of Genes and Genomes (KEGG) pathway enrichment analysis, GO annotation including biological process (BP), cellular component (CC), molecular function (MF), and KEGG pathway enrichment analyses were performed by the cluster profile R 3.14.3 package [23] with false discovery rate (FDR) < 0.05 and the analyses were visualized by the ggplot2 R 3.3.3 package.

2.5. Weighted Gene Co-Expression Network Analysis (WGCNA)

The transcripts and samples from the GSE57691 dataset were analyzed by the WGCNA R 1.70-3 package [22]. All samples were clustered according to Pearson's correlation analysis and the outliers were removed. The community dissimilarity was speculated according to the similarity. Afterward, the adjacency matrix was transformed into a topological overlap matrix (TOM). Genes were assigned to different gene modules according to the TOM-related dissimilarity measure and the soft-thresholding setting. The numbers of gene modules were obtained according to the dissimilarity and the criterion of dynamic tree cutting with a minimal module size of 30 genes. The modules that correlated the most with the clinical traits were identified as AAA-related modules in this study. All biological functions of the hub genes with gene significance (GS) > 0.2 and module membership (MM) > 0.8 were analyzed by GO enrichment.

2.6. Identification of the Hub Genes in AAA Based on Receiver Operating Characteristic (ROC) Curve Analysis

Two-hundred and eighteen DEGs between AAA and normal tissues, 4093 AAA-related genes from CTD, and 144 hub genes from WGCNA were overlapped to identify the intersection genes in AAA. The diagnostic values of four intersection genes for AAA were detected by ROC curve analysis and the area under the ROC curve (AUC) using the pROC R 1.17.0.1 package [24].

2.7. Construction of the Transcription Factor (TF)-miRNA-Hub Gene Network

MiRNAs and TFs related to four hub genes were screened out based on the miRNet2/0 online database (https://www.mirnet.ca, 23 August 2021) [18]. Nine TFs and 290 miRN0As related to four hub genes were identified and constructed in the network using Cytoscape (San Diego, CA, USA) [24].

2.8. Screening the Potential Therapeutic Compounds for AAA in Drug-Gene Interaction Database (DGIdb)

DGIdb (https://www.dgidb.org, 23 August 2021) was used as a drug–gene interaction database to supply the drug–gene interactions and gene–drug ability information from papers, databases, and web resources [24]. In the present study, the target therapeutic compounds for four hub genes were identified based on the DGIdb.

3. Results

3.1. Identification of the DEGs and Analysis of Their Function in AAA

A total of 218 DEGs, including 17 upregulated and 201 downregulated DEGs, were identified from the GSE57691 dataset using the Limma R package [22–24] with the thresholds | log2 (FC) | > 1 and p-value < 0.05 (Figure 2A and Table S1). The biological function of these genes was explored by GO and KEGG enrichment analyses with FDR < 0.05. The most significant BP terms included establishment of protein localization to endoplasmic reticulum, signal recognition particle (SRP)-dependent co-translational protein targeting to membrane, detoxification, cellular response to cadmium ion, and co-translational protein targeting to membrane (Figure 2B and Table S2). The significant CC terms included I band, cytosolic ribosome, contractile fiber, sarcomere, and cytosolic large ribosomal subunit. The significant MF terms included haptoglobin binding, oxygen carrier activity, structural constituent of ribosome, cytochrome-c oxidase activity, and heme-copper terminal oxidase activity. Several genes were also significantly associated with several degenerative disease-related pathways and others, such as ribosome, cardiac muscle contraction, oxidative phosphorylation, fatty acid degradation, pyruvate metabolism, and diabetic cardiomyopathy based on KEGG (Figure 2C and Table S3).

3.2. Identification of the Hub Modules and Genes by WGCNA

A total of 17,784 genes were derived from the 49 samples from the GSE57691 dataset. These genes were used to construct the co-expression network. The results of the cluster analysis of the samples are shown in Figures 3 and 4A,B. All outliers, including GSM1386795, GSM1386831, and GSM1386798 were removed and the remaining 46 samples were used for subsequent analysis (Figure 3A,B). Because the scale-free topology fit index (signed R^2) was less than 0.85 (Figure 4A), a soft-setting of threshold power was achieved according to the criterion with samples > 40 (Figure 3A). When the soft-threshold power was set as 12 and 13, modules could be identified with a minimal module size of 30 genes (Figure 4B).

To correlate the modules with sample information, we analyzed the data according to the heatmap of module–clinical trait correlations. Hereby, we correlated data for the clinical traits. Hereby, red, green, and pink modules were identified as the most correlated with clinical traits (Figure 4C). The red and green ones, which were identified as the hub modules associated with clinical traits, were used to deeply explore the correlation between module membership (MM) and gene significance (GS) to identify the hub genes in AAA. In the results demonstrated in Figure 4D–F and Table S4, 47, 60, and 37 hub genes were respectively identified from red, green, and pink modules with the MM > 0.8 and GS > 0.2. Furthermore, the biological function of the hub genes from three modules was analyzed by GO analysis with FDR < 0.05. The results revealed that the hub genes of the red module are mostly enriched in tissue homeostasis, bone resorption, disaccharide metabolic process, monosaccharide metabolic process, mononuclear cell migration, anatomical structure homeostasis, lymphocyte migration, and hexose metabolic process. All genes are associated with GTPase activator activity (Figure 4G). The hub genes of the green module significantly correlated with mitochondrial matrix (Figure 4H). The hub genes of the pink module are enriched in ribosome biogenesis, rRNA processing, rRNA metabolism process, ncRNA processing, ncRNA metabolism processing, and ribonucleoprotein complex biogenesis. The CC terms included organellar, large ribosomal subunit, mitochondrial large ribosomal subunit, ribosome, large ribosome subunit, organellar ribosome, mitochondrial ribosome, mitochondrial protein-containing complex, and mitochondrial inner membrane (Figure 4I).

3.3. Identification and Validation of AAA-Related Hub Genes

Based on CTD (search keywords: aortic aneurysm and abdominal), a total of 21,684 AAA-related genes were obtained. Moreover, 4093 AAA-related genes included genes with more than 4 references (Table S2). By overlapping the AAA-related 218 DEGs, the 144 WGCNA-based hub genes, and the 4093 CTD-based genes, 4 AAA-related genes were obtained (Figure 5A). Then, the diagnostic values of four genes for AAA were confirmed by ROC curve analysis and the AUC value. As shown in Figure 5B, the AUC values of ASNS, AXIN2, MCAM, and TSPYL1 were shown to be of prognostic power in AAA with 0.8612, 0.9276, 0.9082, 0.8745, respectively.

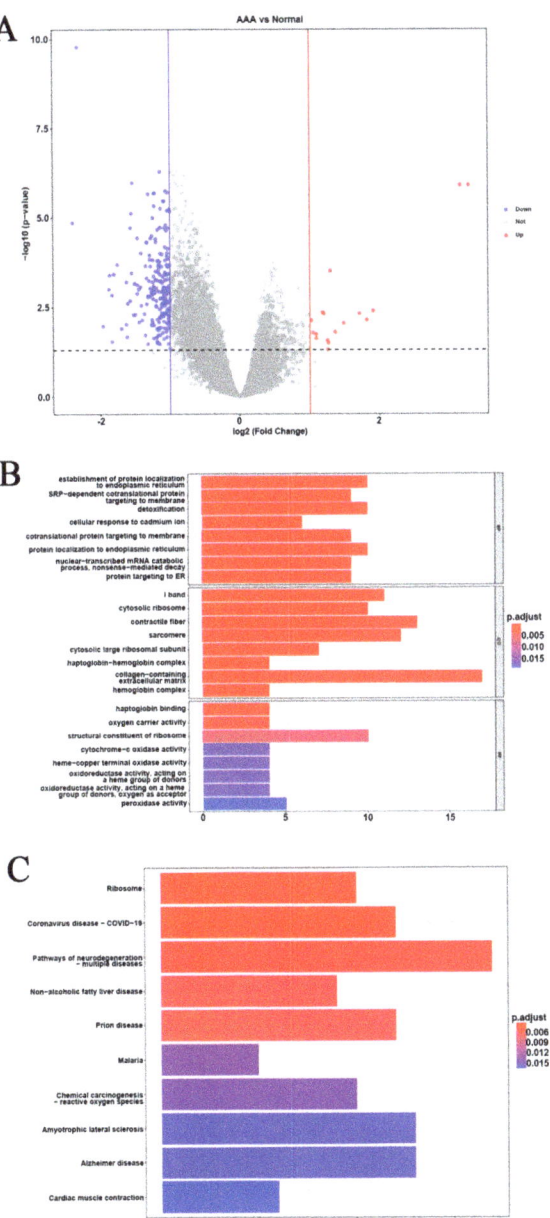

Figure 2. Identification of DEGs and analysis of their function in AAA. (**A**) Volcano plot of DEGs with cutoff value |log2 (FC)| > 1 and *p*-values < 0.05. (**B**) Bar charts of the GO analysis with FDR > 0.05, including BP, CC, and MF terms. (**C**) Bar charts of the KEGG pathway enrichment analysis with FDR > 0.05.

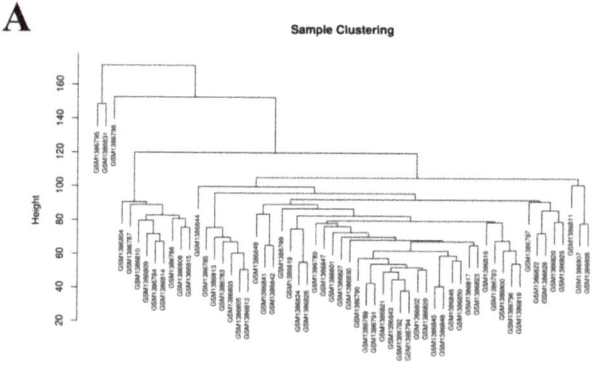
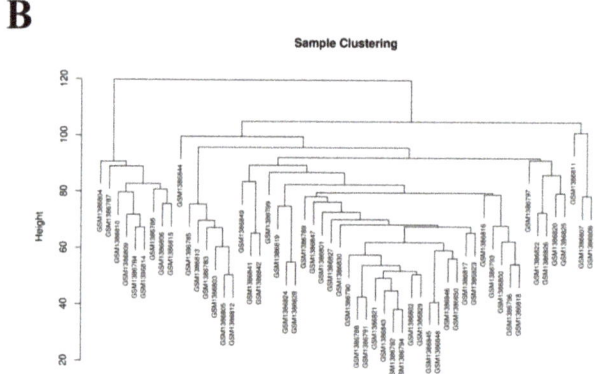
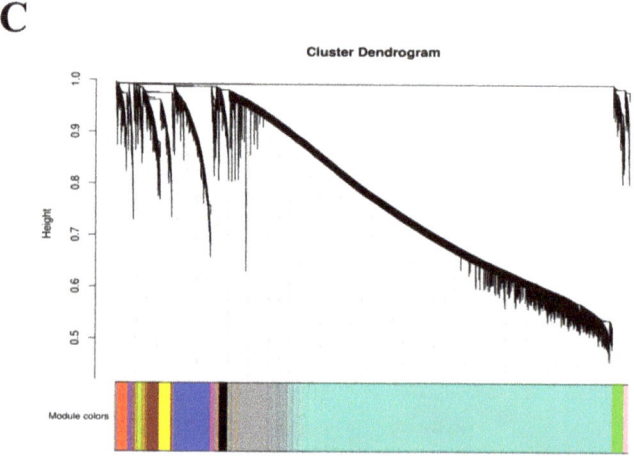

Figure 3. Soft-setting of threshold power. (**A**,**B**) GSM1386795, GSM1386831, and GSM1386798 were excluded as outliers. (**C**) The minimum number of genes per module was set to 30 according to the criteria of the dynamic tree-cutting algorithm. Thirteen modules were generated. Genes are grouped into modules by hierarchical clustering, with different colors representing different modules, where the grey default is for genes that cannot be grouped into any module.

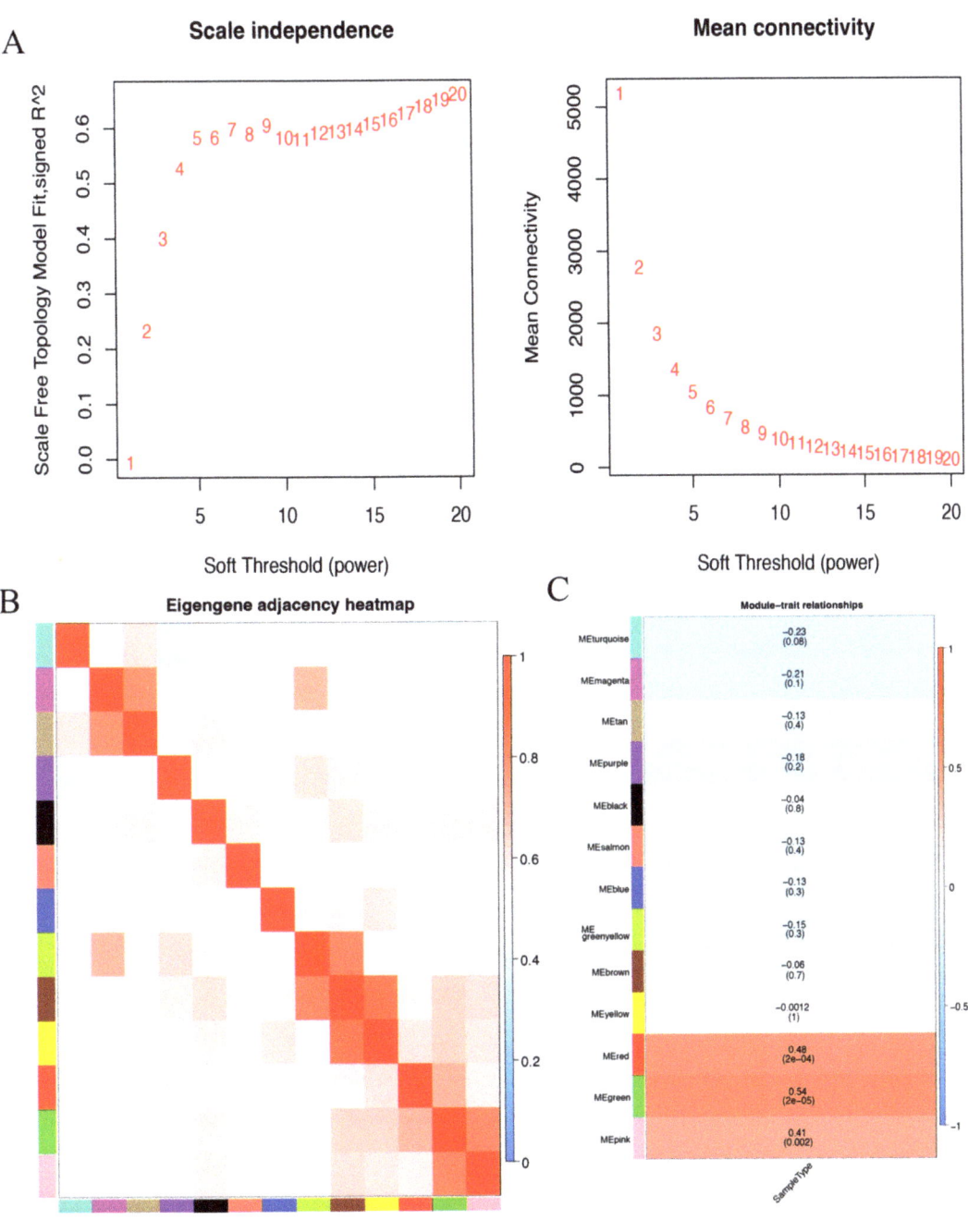

Figure 4. *Cont.*

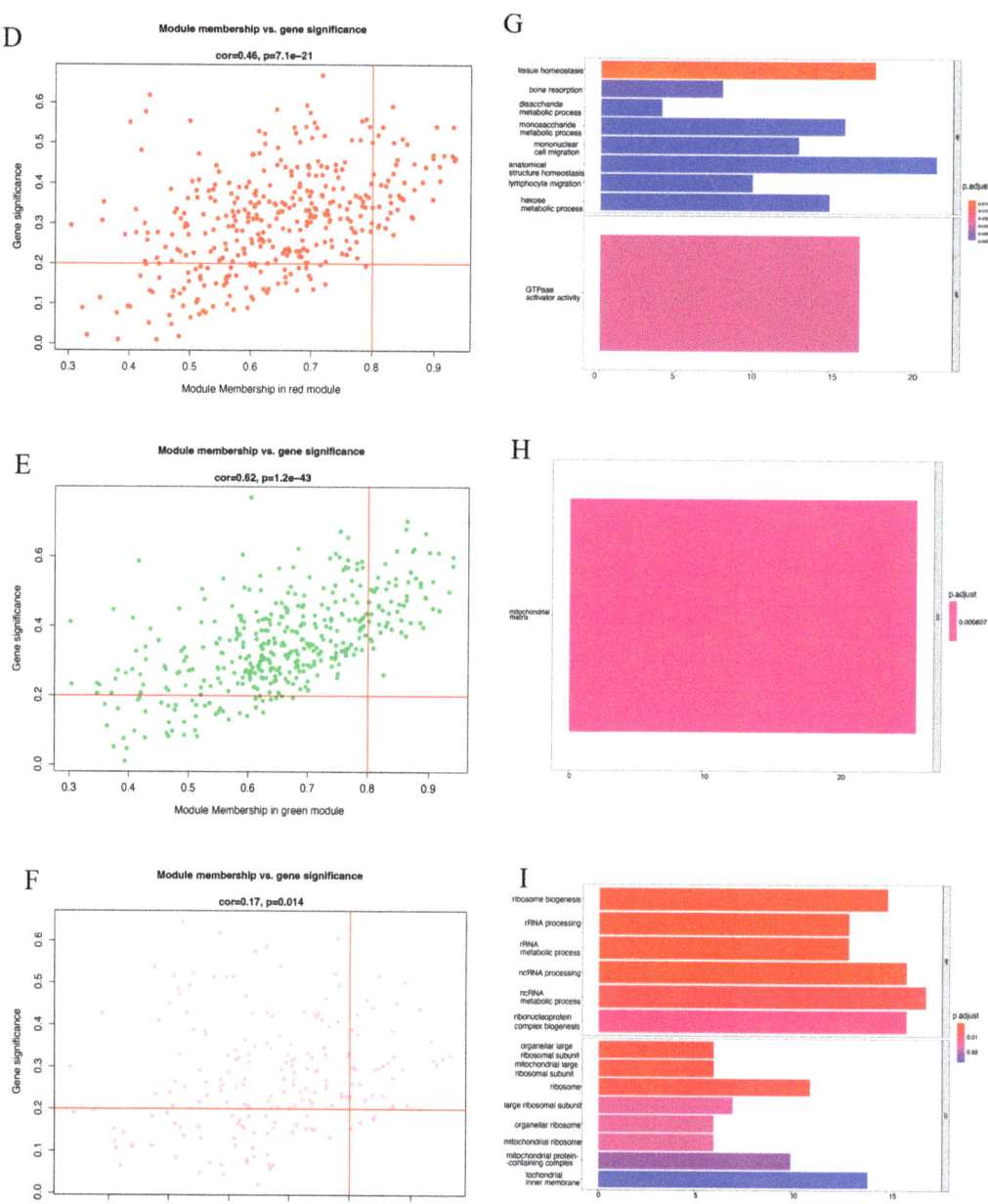

Figure 4. Identification of the hub modules and genes by WGCNA. (**A**) The soft-threshold power selecting processes included the scale-free fit index (left) and the mean connectivity (right) analysis. (**B**) Eigengene adjacency heatmap of correlation between the modules. (**C**) Heatmap of the correlation between module eigengenes and clinical traits of AAA. (**D–F**) Scatter plots of the correlation between MM and GS of red, green, and pink modules, respectively. (**G–I**) Bar charts of the GO analysis of genes from red, green, and pink modules, respectively.

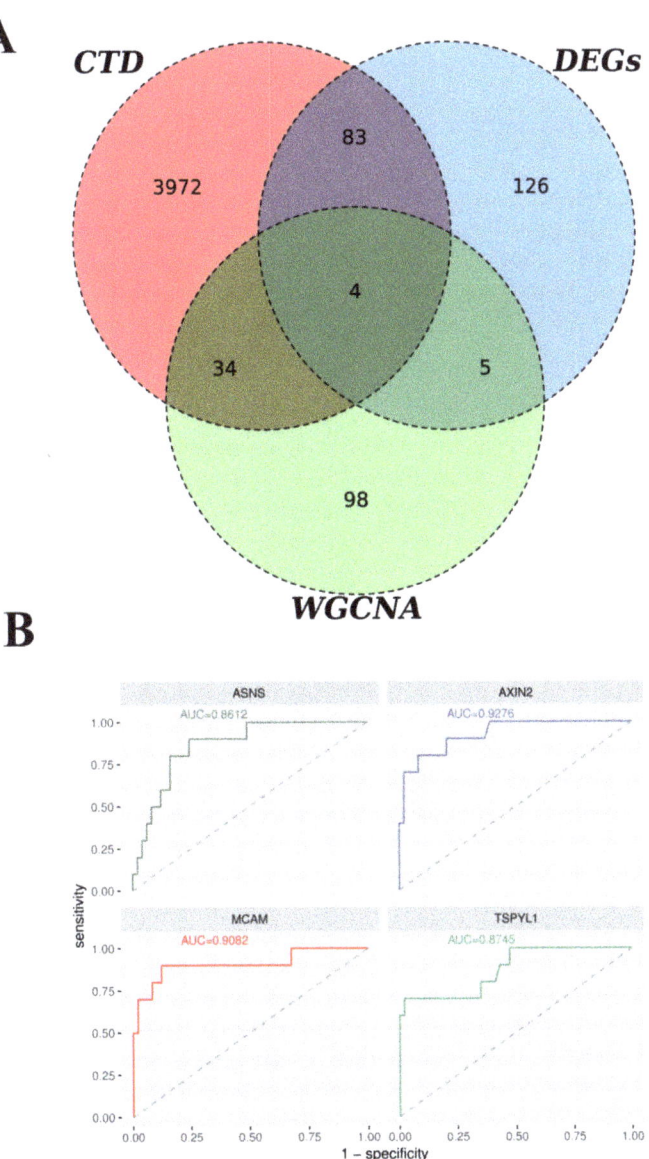

Figure 5. Identification and validation of the AAA-related hub genes. (**A**) Venn plots of intersection genes among the AAA-related 218 DEGs, 144 WGCNA-based hub genes, and 4093 CTD-based genes. (**B**) ROC curves and AUC values of the ASNS, AXIN2, MCAM, and TSPYL1. x-axis indicates specificity; y-axis indicates sensitivity.

3.4. Construction of the TF-miRNA-Hub Gene Network in AAA

We further investigated the regulatory mechanism of these four genes in AAA. The target miRNAs and TFs of four genes were identified and then the TF–miRNA-hub gene network was constructed based on miRnet. Finally, a TF–miRNA-hub gene network, which included 4 genes, 9 TFs, and 290 miRNAs, was constructed with 347 edges (Figure 6).

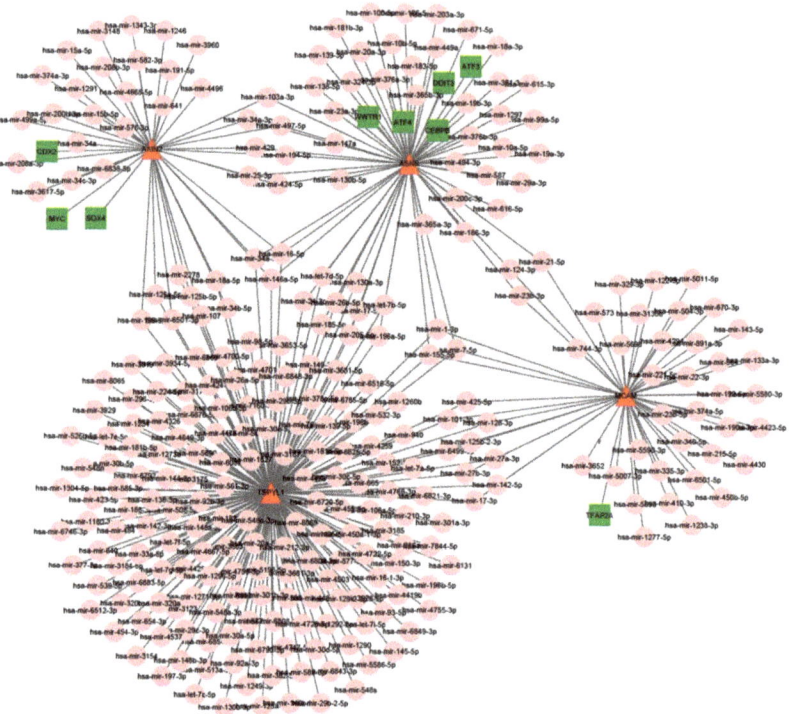

Figure 6. Construction of the TF–miRNA-hub gene network in AAA based on miRnet. Red triangle indicates 4 hub genes (ASNS, AXIN2, MCAM, TSPYL1), pink circles display miRNAs, and green squares show TFs.

3.5. Identification of the Potential Therapeutic Compounds for AAA

In the search for common potential therapeutic compounds for the four hub genes, DGIdb was used (Table 1). Asparaginase has been identified as the target compound of ASNS; prednisolone and abiraterone were found as the target compounds of TSPYL1. For the other two genes, no drug compound could be identified.

Table 1. The potential compounds of two genes were identified using DGIdb.

Gene	Drug	Interaction Type	Sources	PMIDs
ASNS	ASPARAGINASE	NASE	NCI, CIViC, PharmGKB	28069604, 24268318, 11556848
TSPYL1	PREDNISOLONE	LONE	PharmGKB	
TSPYL1	ABIRATERONE	ONE	PharmGKB	

4. Discussion

To date, several druggable molecules have been described to play roles in AAA development, progression, and rupture, such as the matrix metalloproteinase (MMP) family, transforming growth factor beta receptor 2 (TGFBR2), and sortilin 1 (SORT1) [10]. However, not only single protein-expressing genes may be involved but also whole pathway networks may be deregulated, such as the Wnt/β-catenin pathway and TGF beta/SMAD pathway. This may be mediated by miRNAs. MiRNAs have been studied to be associated with the pathophysiological process of many diseases [11]. Various studies have reported that miRNAs are involved in the occurrence and development of AAA [12]. Especially, it is important to construct TF–miRNA-hub gene networks for miRNAs as they may regulate several pathways. These networks may help to find novel therapeutic compounds for significant genes.

Here, we built an in silico approach TF–miRNA-hub gene network depending on the shared dataset and published literature. Unlike our previous study which only focused on WCGNA to mine key genes of mouse AAA progression [21], we here applied text mining and WCGNA. Hereby, four hub genes (ASNS, AXIN2, MCAM, TSPYL1) were obtained. These four hub genes are all reported to be associated with the function of vascular cells, but no study has so far studied the connection between these four hub genes and the pathophysiology of AAA [23,24].

Asparagine synthetase (ASNS) is associated with asparaginase therapy in acute lymphoblastic leukemia [25]. ASNS is also reported to be essential for endothelial cell growth and angiogenesis [26]. Interestingly, the proliferation of fibroblasts is impaired under conditions of asparagine deprivation which may be the potential link connecting ASNS and AAA pathogenesis [26].

Testis-specific protein, Y-encoded-like 1 (TSPYL1) is a member of the TSPYL protein family which exerts its regulatory effects on vascular cells and promotes endothelial cell proliferation, migration, and neoangiogenesis [27]. AXIN2, a scaffold protein involved in the degradation of β-catenin, plays a vital role in the Wnt/β-catenin pathway and its gene expression is suggested to be associated with endothelial cell proliferation and function [28]. AXIN2 mutations have been studied in different cancer entities including digestive tract tumors and melanoma [29]. MCAM is highly expressed in many tumors and endothelial cells. It plays an important role in the regulation of vascular permeability, cell–cell cohesion, leukocyte transmigration, and angiogenesis [30].

MiRNAs may be a potential tie between TSPYL5, AXIN2, and MCAM and AAA formation. MiRNAs have been shown to regulate the ECM turnover, MMP family, different inflammatory components, and VSMCs by forming TF–miRNA network networks [17].

We here identified nine TFs and 290 miRNAs as the master regulators of the resulting gene regulatory network, as they have the largest connectivity with the co-expressed four genes associated with AAA. The diagnostic values of the four genes for AAA were confirmed using ROC curves. These data confirmed that ASNS, AXIN2, MCAM, and TSPYL1 showed significant prognostic values in AAA.

The compound search was based on the analysis of a TF–miRNA-hub gene network. Increasing evidence has indicated that TF-related networks exert key roles in cancer. A prominent example is the SOX4–Axin2 network and the CDX2–Axin2 network, both of which are reported to inhibit the proliferation and tumor formation of cancer cells by suppressing Wnt/β-catenin signaling [31]. The WWTR1–ASNS network, ATF4–ASNS network, and DDIT3–ASNS network are reported to inhibit the proliferation and tumor formation of cancer cells [32]. The CEBPB–ASNS network and ATF3–ASNS network can activate the placental mammalian amino acid response pathway [33]. Furthermore, the TFAP2A–MCAM network is reported to be associated with melanoma metastasis [34]. All TF–miRNA networks have been previously associated with the development of AAA.

With the help of DGIdb, the target therapeutic compounds for two of the hub genes were identified. Asparaginase has been identified as the target compound of ASNS, while prednisolone and abiraterone were identified as target compounds of TSPYL1. Since all four hub genes were firstly connected to AAA in the present study, there is so far no experimental evidence for the drug compounds. This will also be an issue for further experimental studies.

In summary, our study has firstly demonstrated a novel TF–miRNA-hub network linked to AAA based on text mining and WCGNA analysis. While this is a novel approach with novel findings, our work also has some limitations. Our work has focused on potential regulators of the most significantly overexpressed genes, TFs, and miRNAs of AAA, without ruling out the possibility that other regulatory mechanisms, which may not only depend on gene overexpression, may still be important in the development and progression of AAA. Therefore, our in silico findings will have to be confirmed by in vitro and in vivo AAA models.

Moreover, the number of datasets available is still limited. We here used the GSE57691 dataset as the most complete available dataset to combine hits with the AAA-related genes that we obtained from CTD to identify the DEGs.

Supplementary Materials: The following supporting information can be downloaded at: https://www.mdpi.com/article/10.3390/biomedicines10051052/s1, Table S1: Differentially expressed gene; Table S2: GO analysis; Table S3: KEGG analysis; Table S4: hub genes of hub modules; Table S5: AAA-related genes from CTD.

Author Contributions: Conceptualization, Methodology and formal analysis: L.L. and K.K.; writing and formal analysis: M.K. and P.P. All authors have read and agreed to the published version of the manuscript.

Funding: K.K. was supported by the China Scholarship Council (CSC), No. 201706230257.

Institutional Review Board Statement: Not applicable.

Informed Consent Statement: Not applicable.

Data Availability Statement: All datasets of this study are available in the GEO database (https://www.ncbi.nlm.nih.gov/geo/, accessed on 23 August 2021).

Acknowledgments: We thank "Zhilong Su" for sharing the knowledge of bioinformatics analysis.

Conflicts of Interest: The authors declare no conflict of interest.

References

1. Golledge, J.; Muller, J.; Daugherty, A.; Norman, P. Abdominal aortic aneurysm: Pathogenesis and implications for management. *Arterioscler. Thromb. Vasc. Biol.* **2006**, *26*, 2605–2613. [CrossRef]
2. Ullery, B.W.; Hallett, R.L.; Fleischmann, D. Epidemiology and contemporary management of abdominal aortic aneurysms. *Abdom. Radiol.* **2018**, *43*, 1032–1043. [CrossRef]
3. GBD 2013 Mortality and Causes of Death Collaborators. Global, regional, and national age-sex specific all-cause and cause-specific mortality for 240 causes of death, 1990–2013: A systematic analysis for the Global Burden of Disease Study 2013. *Lancet* **2015**, *385*, 117–171. [CrossRef]
4. Sampson, U.K.; Norman, P.E.; Fowkes, F.G.; Aboyans, V.; Yanna, S.; Harrell, F.E.; Forouzanfar, M.H.; Naghavi, M.; Denenberg, J.O.; McDermott, M.M.; et al. Global and regional burden of aortic dissection and aneurysms: Mortality trends in 21 world regions, 1990 to 2010. *Glob. Heart.* **2014**, *9*, 171–180.e10. [CrossRef]
5. Sakalihasan, N.; Limet, R.; Defawe, O.D. Abdominal aortic aneurysm. *Lancet* **2005**, *365*, 1577–1589. [CrossRef]
6. Golledge, J. Abdominal aortic aneurysm: Update on pathogenesis and medical treatments. *Nat. Rev. Cardiol.* **2019**, *16*, 225–242. [CrossRef] [PubMed]
7. Li, D.Y.; Busch, A.; Jin, H.; Chernogubova, E.; Pelisek, J.; Karlsson, J.; Sennblad, B.; Liu, S.; Lao, S.; Hofmann, P.; et al. H19 induces abdominal aortic aneurysm development and progression. *Circulation* **2018**, *138*, 1551–1568. [CrossRef] [PubMed]
8. He, X.; Wang, S.; Li, M.; Zhong, L.; Zheng, H.; Sun, Y.; Lai, Y.; Chen, X.; Wei, G.; Si, X.; et al. Long noncoding RNA GAS5 induces abdominal aortic aneurysm formation by promoting smooth muscle apoptosis. *Theranostics* **2019**, *9*, 5558–5576. [CrossRef]
9. Tsai, S.H.; Hsu, L.A.; Tsai, H.Y.; Yeh, Y.H.; Lu, C.Y.; Chen, P.C.; Wang, J.C.; Chiu, Y.L.; Lin, C.Y.; Hsu, Y.J. Aldehyde dehydrogenase 2 protects against abdominal aortic aneurysm formation by reducing reactive oxygen species, vascular inflammation, and apoptosis of vascular smooth muscle cells. *FASEB J.* **2020**, *34*, 9498–9511. [CrossRef] [PubMed]
10. Davis, F.M.; Rateri, D.L.; Daugherty, A. Abdominal aortic aneurysm: Novel mechanisms and therapies. *Curr. Opin. Cardiol.* **2015**, *30*, 566–573. [CrossRef]
11. Giraud, A.; Zeboudj, L.; Vandestienne, M.; Joffre, J.; Esposito, B.; Potteaux, S.; Vilar, J.; Cabuzu, D.; Kluwe, J.; Seguier, S.; et al. Gingival fibroblasts protect against experimental abdominal aortic aneurysm development and rupture through tissue inhibitor of metalloproteinase-1 production. *Cardiovasc. Res.* **2017**, *113*, 1364–1375. [CrossRef] [PubMed]
12. Bogunovic, N.; Meekel, J.P.; Micha, D.; Blankensteijn, J.D.; Hordijk, P.L.; Yeung, K.K. Impaired smooth muscle cell contractility as a novel concept of abdominal aortic aneurysm pathophysiology. *Sci. Rep.* **2019**, *9*, 6837. [CrossRef] [PubMed]
13. Raffort, J.; Lareyre, F.; Clement, M.; Mallat, Z. Micro-RNAs in abdominal aortic aneurysms: Insights from animal models and relevance to human disease. *Cardiovasc. Res.* **2016**, *110*, 165–177. [CrossRef]
14. Goodall, G.J.; Wickramasinghe, V.O. RNA in cancer. Nature reviews. *Cancer* **2021**, *21*, 22–36.
15. Kumar, S.; Boon, R.A.; Maegdefessel, L.; Dimmeler, S.; Jo, H. Role of noncoding RNAs in the pathogenesis of abdominal aortic aneurysm: Possible therapeutic targets? *Circ. Res.* **2019**, *124*, 619–630. [CrossRef]

16. Rupaimoole, R.; Slack, F.J. MicroRNA therapeutics: Towards a new era for the management of cancer and other diseases. Nature reviews. *Drug Discov.* **2017**, *16*, 203–222. [CrossRef]
17. Pu, M.; Chen, J.; Tao, Z.; Miao, L.; Qi, X.; Wang, Y.; Ren, J. Regulatory network of miRNA on its target: Coordination between transcriptional and post-transcriptional regulation of gene expression. *Cell Mol. Life Sci.* **2019**, *76*, 441–451. [CrossRef] [PubMed]
18. Davis, A.P.; Grondin, C.J.; Johnson, R.J.; Sciaky, D.; Wiegers, J.; Wiegers, T.C.; Mattingly, C.J. Comparative Toxicogenomics Database (CTD): Update 2021. *Nucleic Acids Res.* **2021**, *49*, D1138–D1143. [CrossRef]
19. Nordon, I.M.; Hinchliffe, R.J.; Loftus, I.M.; Thompson, M.M. Pathophysiology and epidemiology of abdominal aortic aneurysms. *Nat. Rev. Cardiol.* **2011**, *8*, 92–102. [CrossRef]
20. Navas-Madroñal, M.; Rodriguez, C.; Kassan, M.; Fité, J.; Escudero, J.R.; Cañes, L.; Martínez-González, J.; Camacho, M.; Galán, M. Enhanced endoplasmic reticulum and mitochondrial stress in abdominal aortic aneurysm. *Clin. Sci.* **2019**, *133*, 1421–1438. [CrossRef]
21. Kan, K.J.; Guo, F.; Zhu, L.; Pallavi, P.; Sigl, M.; Keese, M. Weighted gene co-expression network analysis reveals key genes and potential drugs in abdominal aortic aneurysm. *Biomedicines* **2021**, *9*, 546. [CrossRef] [PubMed]
22. Langfelder, P.; Horvath, S. WGCNA: An R package for weighted correlation network analysis. *BMC Bioinform.* **2008**, *9*, 559. [CrossRef] [PubMed]
23. Chang, L.; Zhou, G.; Soufan, O.; Xia, J. miRNet 2.0: Network-based visual analytics for miRNA functional analysis and systems biology. *Nucleic Acids Res.* **2020**, *48*, W244–W251. [CrossRef] [PubMed]
24. Cotto, K.C.; Wagner, A.H.; Feng, Y.Y.; Kiwala, S.; Coffman, A.C.; Spies, G.; Wollam, A.; Spies, N.C.; Griffith, O.L.; Griffith, M. DGIdb 3.0: A redesign and expansion of the drug-gene interaction database. *Nucleic Acids Res.* **2018**, *46*, D1068–D1073. [CrossRef]
25. Lomelino, C.L.; Andring, J.T.; McKenna, R.; Kilberg, M.S. Asparagine synthetase: Function, structure, and role in disease. *J. Biol. Chem.* **2017**, *292*, 19952–19958. [CrossRef]
26. Häberle, J.; Görg, B.; Rutsch, F.; Schmidt, E.; Toutain, A.; Benoist, J.F.; Gelot, A.; Suc, A.L.; Höhne, W.; Schliess, F.; et al. Congenital glutamine deficiency with glutamine synthetase mutations. *N. Engl. J. Med.* **2005**, *353*, 1926–1933. [CrossRef]
27. Na, H.J.; Yeum, C.E.; Kim, H.S.; Lee, J.; Kim, J.Y.; Cho, Y.S. TSPYL5-mediated inhibition of p53 promotes human endothelial cell function. *Angiogenesis* **2019**, *22*, 281–293. [CrossRef]
28. Zhang, Y.; Chidiac, R.; Delisle, C.; Gratton, J.P. Endothelial NO Synthase-Dependent S-Nitrosylation of β-Catenin Prevents Its Association with TCF4 and Inhibits Proliferation of Endothelial Cells Stimulated by Wnt3a. *Mol. Cell Biol.* **2017**, *37*, e00089-17. [CrossRef]
29. Rivera, B.; Perea, J.; Sánchez, E.; Villapún, M.; Sánchez-Tomé, E.; Mercadillo, F.; Robledo, M.; Benítez, J.; Urioste, M. A novel AXIN2 germline variant associated with attenuated FAP without signs of oligondontia or ectodermal dysplasia. *Eur. J. Hum. Genet.* **2014**, *22*, 423–426. [CrossRef]
30. Wang, Z.; Xu, Q.; Zhang, N.; Du, X.; Xu, G.; Yan, X. CD146, from a melanoma cell adhesion molecule to a signaling receptor. *Signal Transduct. Target Ther.* **2020**, *5*, 148. [CrossRef]
31. Yu, J.; Liu, D.; Sun, X.; Yang, K.; Yao, J.; Cheng, C.; Wang, C.; Zheng, J. CDX2 inhibits the proliferation and tumor formation of colon cancer cells by suppressing Wnt/β-catenin signaling via transactivation of GSK-3β and Axin2 expression. *Cell Death Dis.* **2019**, *10*, 26. [CrossRef] [PubMed]
32. Lancho, O.; Herranz, D. The MYC Enhancer-ome: Long-range transcriptional regulation of MYC in cancer. *Trends Cancer* **2018**, *4*, 810–822. [CrossRef] [PubMed]
33. Strakovsky, R.S.; Zhou, D.; Pan, Y.X. A low-protein diet during gestation in rats activates the placental mammalian amino acid response pathway and programs the growth capacity of offspring. *J. Nutr.* **2010**, *140*, 2116–2120. [CrossRef] [PubMed]
34. Mobley, A.K.; Braeuer, R.R.; Kamiya, T.; Shoshan, E.; Bar-Eli, M. Driving transcriptional regulators in melanoma metastasis. *Cancer Metastasis Rev.* **2012**, *31*, 621–632. [CrossRef] [PubMed]

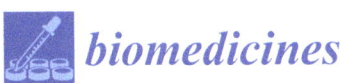

Article

Weighted Gene Co-Expression Network Analysis Reveals Key Genes and Potential Drugs in Abdominal Aortic Aneurysm

Ke-Jia Kan [1,2,†], Feng Guo [1,2,†], Lei Zhu [1,3], Prama Pallavi [1,2], Martin Sigl [4] and Michael Keese [1,2,*]

1 Department of Surgery, Medical Faculty Mannheim, Heidelberg University, 68167 Mannheim, Germany; Kejia.Kan@medma.uni-heidelberg.de (K.-J.K.); Feng.Guo@medma.uni-heidelberg.de (F.G.); Lei.Zhu@medma.uni-heidelberg.de (L.Z.); Prama.Pallavi@medma.uni-heidelberg.de (P.P.)
2 European Center of Angioscience (ECAS), Medical Faculty Mannheim, Heidelberg University, 68167 Mannheim, Germany
3 German Cancer Research Center (DKFZ), Junior Clinical Cooperation Unit Translational Surgical Oncology (A430), 69120 Heidelberg, Germany
4 First Department of Medicine, Medical Faculty Mannheim, Heidelberg University, 68167 Mannheim, Germany; martin.sigl@umm.de
* Correspondence: michael.keese@umm.de; Tel.: +49-621-383-1501
† These authors contributed equally.

Abstract: Abdominal aortic aneurysm (AAA) is a prevalent aortic disease that causes high mortality due to asymptomatic gradual expansion and sudden rupture. The underlying molecular mechanisms and effective pharmaceutical therapy for preventing AAA progression have not been fully identified. In this study, we identified the key modules and hub genes involved in AAA growth from the GSE17901 dataset in the Gene Expression Omnibus (GEO) database through the weighted gene co-expression network analysis (WGCNA). Key genes were further selected and validated in the mouse dataset (GSE12591) and human datasets (GSE7084, GSE47472, and GSE57691). Finally, we predicted drug candidates targeting key genes using the Drug–Gene Interaction database. Overall, we identified key modules enriched in the mitotic cell cycle, GTPase activity, and several metabolic processes. Seven key genes (CCR5, ADCY5, ADCY3, ACACB, LPIN1, ACSL1, UCP3) related to AAA progression were identified. A total of 35 drugs/compounds targeting the key genes were predicted, which may have the potential to prevent AAA progression.

Keywords: abdominal aortic aneurysm; weighted gene co-expression network; key module; hub gene; functional enrichment; drug–gene prediction

1. Introduction

Abdominal aortic aneurysm (AAA) is a localized dilation or bulging of the abdominal aorta, commonly occurring in the infrarenal region [1]. Most patients with AAA remain asymptomatic for years or even decades. It is estimated that around 200,000 AAA rupture cases are diagnosed worldwide annually, and the mortality after rupture remains around 80% [2–4].

Currently, AAA requiring intervention, e.g., large aneurysms with a diameter more than 5.5 cm, aneurysms that expand rapidly in a short period, or aneurysms that compromise the perfusion to distant organs are indicated for open surgical or endovascular aortic repair. However, the outcomes from these measures are not so satisfactory [5,6]. For patients with small AAAs or those who are not eligible for AAA repair, close aneurysm surveillance and adjuvant therapy are recommended [5]. So far, no effective pharmacological treatments have been developed to prevent AAA growth or rupture [7,8]. Hence, there is a need to elucidate the possible mechanisms of AAA progression and explore corresponding pharmaceutical treatments.

A number of preclinical mouse AAA models have been developed to understand the pathogenesis of AAA [9,10]. Among these models, angiotensin II-infused ApoE$^{-/-}$ mice

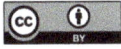

are the commonly used [11–15]. Although the inherent pathology of aneurysm is different between mice and humans, it shares some of the important properties of human AAA, like pronounced inflammatory responses and aortic rupture [11–15]. Based on the findings from mouse models and human samples, AAA is currently accepted as an inflammation-driven disease, as many related processes (such as infiltration of macrophages, neutrophils, B cells and T cells, and activation of inflammatory pathways) were found both in humans and mice [16–19]. Overactivation of the inflammatory response leads to the destruction of aortic media through the release of proteolytic enzymes and the death of vascular smooth muscle cells, which further promote AAA development [20].

Several studies based on the high-throughput microarray profiling further confirmed the involvement of the above biological processes in AAA, including the immune response, chronic inflammation, and reactive oxygen species [21–23]. Dozens of genes related to AAA development were identified through gene expression profiles [24–26]. However, these studies exclusively focused on the differentially expressed genes (DEGs) between AAA and control groups, which ignored some key genes that are highly correlated to specific sample traits of AAA. Weighted gene co-expression network analysis (WGCNA) is a bioinformatics algorithm developed by Horvath et al. [27]. By constructing a scale-free weighted network, WGCNA can investigate biologically meaningful gene sets connected to sample features and explore inner module hub genes that are highly associated inside the co-expression module. WGCNA has been successfully used to identify key modules and hub genes related to cardiovascular diseases, such as atherosclerosis, heart failure, and acute myocardial infarction [28–30]. So far, data collected at different time points of AAA progression have not been subjected to WGCNA analysis to identify the critical modules and hub genes.

In this study, WGCNA analysis was performed using the explore dataset GSE17901 in the Gene Expression Omnibus (GEO) database. Key modules of AAA development and hub genes in each module were identified. Gene functional enrichment analysis of key modules was applied to show their potential biological activities. Hub genes were screened in the STRING database and further selected in the Cytoscape software (San Diego, CA, USA). Key genes from hub genes were validated using mouse AAA model GSE12591 dataset and human AAA sample GSE7084, GSE47472, and GSE57691 datasets. Candidate drugs for AAA treatment were screened in the Drug Gene Interaction Database (DGIdb) based on the above-identified key genes.

2. Materials and Methods

2.1. Data Sources and Preprocessing

The workflow of this study is shown in Figure 1. Datasets related to AAA—GSE17901, GSE12591, GSE7084, GSE47472 and GSE57691 (Table 1) were downloaded from the GEO database (accessed on 1 April 2020 from https://www.ncbi.nlm.nih.gov/geo/). In the explore dataset GSE17901 [26], aortic samples were taken on day 7, day 14, and day 28 from ApoE$^{-/-}$ mice treated by angiotensin II or saline. The diameters of the treated aortas increased throughout the 28-day course, which we defined as the progression of AAA, so samples with AAA ($n = 18$) were selected for weighted gene co-expression network (WGCNA) analysis. Mouse dataset (GSE12591) and human datasets (GSE7084, GSE47472, and GSE57691) were used to validate the hub genes. The GSE12591 dataset included 18 mouse aortas exposed to saline ($n = 6$) or angiotensin II ($n = 12$) infusion [25]. The GSE7084 included control samples ($n = 10$) and AAA samples from patients ($n = 9$) [24]. The GSE47472 contained AAA neck specimen ($n = 14$) and normal aortic tissue from organ donors ($n = 8$). The GSE57691 included AAA samples ($n = 49$) and normal aortic specimens of organ donors ($n = 10$) [31]. Each dataset was processed by background correction, including removal of batch effect using the sva R package (version 3.12) and quantile normalization with the limma R package (version 3.38.3) [32] for further analysis.

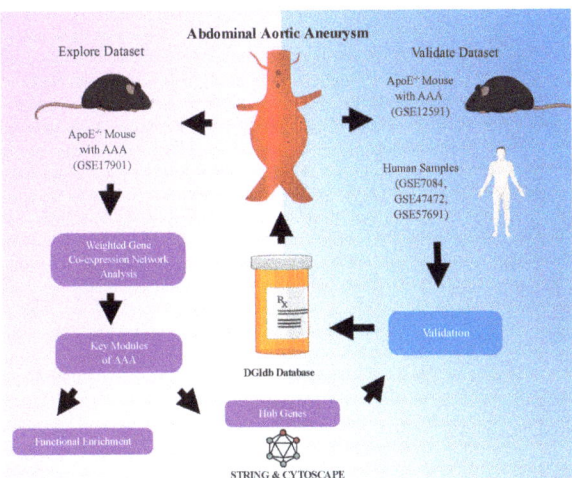

Figure 1. Flowchart of analysis in the study. GSE17901 was a mouse dataset containing AAA samples collected on day 7, day 14 and day 28, which was used for exploring the key modules and hub genes related to AAA progression. Hub genes were identified through the STRING database and Cytoscape software (San Diego, CA, USA). Key genes were further selected from the hub genes and validated in the mouse (GSE12591) and human (GSE7084, GSE47472 and GSE57691) AAA datasets. Finally, potential drugs or compounds targeting these key genes were screened in the DGIdb database. AAA: abdominal aortic aneurysm. The flowchart was created with BioRender.com (accessed on 11 April 2021).

Table 1. GSE datasets included in the study.

Catalog.	GSE Dataset	Organism	Sample Number *	PMID
Explore dataset	GSE17901	Mouse	AAA day7: 7, AAA day14: 5, AAA day28: 6	21712436
Validate dataset	GSE12591	Mouse	Control: 6, AAA: 5	19580648
	GSE7084	Human	Donor: 10, AAA: 9	17634102
	GSE47472	Human	Donor: 8, AAA: 14	NA
	GSE57691	Human	Donor: 10, AAA: 49	NA

*: Number of samples (control or AAA) used in this study; NA: not applicable.

2.2. Construction of WGCNA

The WGCNA R package (version 1.69) was used to perform the weighted co-expression network analysis. Genes with the top 25% variance from the explore dataset GSE17901 were selected for the following analysis step. Using the pick Soft Threshold function, the soft-thresholding power was determined and used to construct a scale-free network. Thereafter, gene co-expression modules were identified using the one-step network construction method and labeled with different colors. The reassign threshold was set at 0.25, and the minimum number of genes in each module was 30.

2.3. Selection of Key Modules Corresponding to Sample Traits

To explore the key modules that are significantly associated with sample traits of AAA, we calculated the relevancy between module eigengene (ME), which summarizes each module's expression profiles. The correlation results were shown using the ggcorrplot R package (version 0.1.3) [33]. Furthermore, Gene Significance (GS) was quantified by the absolute value of the association between the gene expression and sample trait. In every module, measurement of module membership (MM) was defined as the correlation of the ME and gene expression profile. Modules with high significance (p-value < 0.05) and relationships (correlation >0.6 or <−0.6) were defined as key modules of AAA and used for hub gene selection.

2.4. Functional Enrichment Analysis of the Key Modules

To understand the biological activities of genes in key modules, we conducted Gene Ontology (GO) function enrichment analysis and Kyoto Encyclopedia of Genes and Genomes (KEGG) pathway analysis with the clusterProfiler R package (version 3.10) [34]. Adjusted p-value < 0.05 was considered a statistically significant difference in enrichment analysis, and the top 10 of each analysis were extracted for visualization.

2.5. Identification of Hub Genes in the Key Modules

Hub genes are those that have a high degree of intramodular connectivity. In this study, hub genes were defined as the top 10% of genes from key modules with the highest connectivity. We uploaded them into the search tool for the retrieval of the interacting genes (STRING) website (accessed on 1 May 2020 from www.string-db.org) for protein–protein interaction analysis, choosing the confidence >0.4 [35]. Cytoscape software (San Diego, CA, USA) was used for network visualization and hub gene selection [36]. The top 10 hub genes in each module were selected with the maximal clique centrality (MCC) method using cytoHubba plugin software in Cytoscape (San Diego, CA, USA) [37].

2.6. Hub Genes Validation and Key Genes Selection

The validation of hub genes was performed by comparing the normalized gene expression value between control and AAA groups. The validated datasets GSE12591, GSE7084, GSE47472, and GSE57691 were downloaded from the GEO database, and data were preprocessed as mentioned before. In the GSE12591 mouse dataset, the gene expression of the selected hub genes in AAA and controls were compared, and genes with $p < 0.05$ were confirmed as the key genes. In the GSE7084, GSE47472, and GSE57691 human datasets, genes were extracted as described for dataset GSE12591. Genes with $p < 0.05$ were confirmed as the key genes. Common genes in both the mouse dataset and human datasets were defined as the final key genes.

2.7. Predication of Drug–Gene Interaction

The Drug–Gene Interaction Database (DGIdb) (accessed on 8 June 2020 from http://www.dgidb.org/) is an online database of drug–gene interaction data aggregated from various sources, including several drug databases (DrugBank, PharmGKB, ChEMBL), clinical trial databases, and literature from PubMed [38]. The selected key genes that were considered the potential pharmaceutical targets for AAA treatment were imported into DGIdb to explore existing drugs or small organic compounds. Results were displayed using the R packages ggplot2 (version 3.2.1) [39] and ggalluvial (version 0.11.1) [40].

2.8. Statistical Analysis

To define the statistical significance of differences between the two groups, we performed analysis using a non-parametric test or t-test based on data distribution characteristics. All analyses were conducted with R software (version 3.5.5). p-value < 0.05 was assigned statistical significance.

3. Results

3.1. Construction of Weighted Gene Co-Expression Network

After cleaning the data in the explore dataset GSE17901 by WGCNA, 5408 genes from 17 samples were analyzed for co-expression network construction. A scale-free network was constructed with a soft-threshold at nine, and a correlation coefficient threshold set at 0.85 (Figure 2A), and 15 related co-expression modules were obtained (Figure 2B).

Four main clusters were observed. The turquoise module (1394 genes) was the biggest cluster, followed by the blue module (897 genes), brown module (793 genes), and yellow module (586 genes). All the ungrouped genes (199 genes) were included in the grey module.

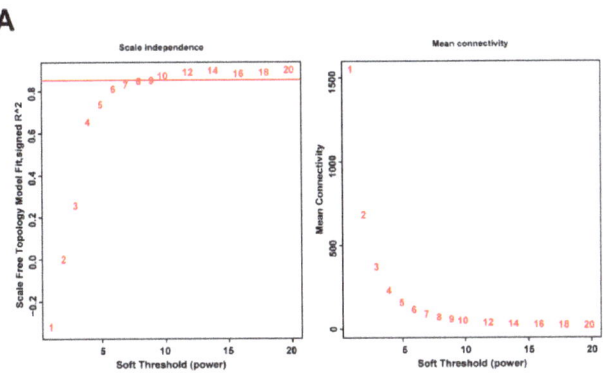

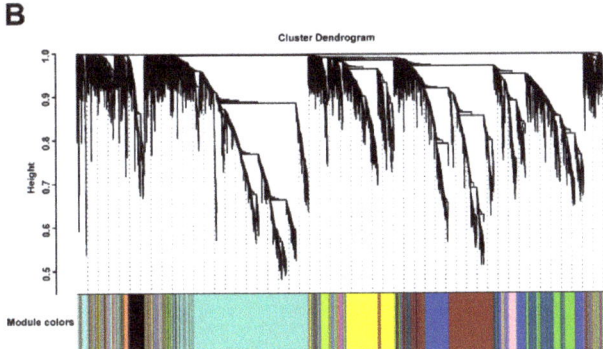

Figure 2. Construction of gene co-expression network by WGCNA. (**A**) Determination of soft-thresholding power for scale-free network construction. Here, we set the coefficient threshold at 0.85, and the soft-threshold was 9; (**B**) cluster analysis of the dendrogram and identification of co-expressed modules. In this study, we got 15 related co-expression modules.

3.2. Construction of Module-Trait Relationships and Detection of Key Modules

The related sample traits (time—day 7, day 14, day 28; dissection of abdominal aorta) were obtained from the sample information in the GSE17901 dataset (Figure S1A). The relationships between these traits and each module were defined by the correlation between ME and sample traits (Figure 3, Figure S1B). These results indicated that three modules (blue, green, and brown) were strongly related to the time trait, representing the progression of AAA (Figure 3, Figure S2A–C). Blue and green modules also significantly correlated with the dissection sample trait (Figure 3, Figure S2D–E). Thus, the blue (897 genes), green (436 genes), and brown (793 genes) modules were defined as the key modules that were highly correlated with AAA.

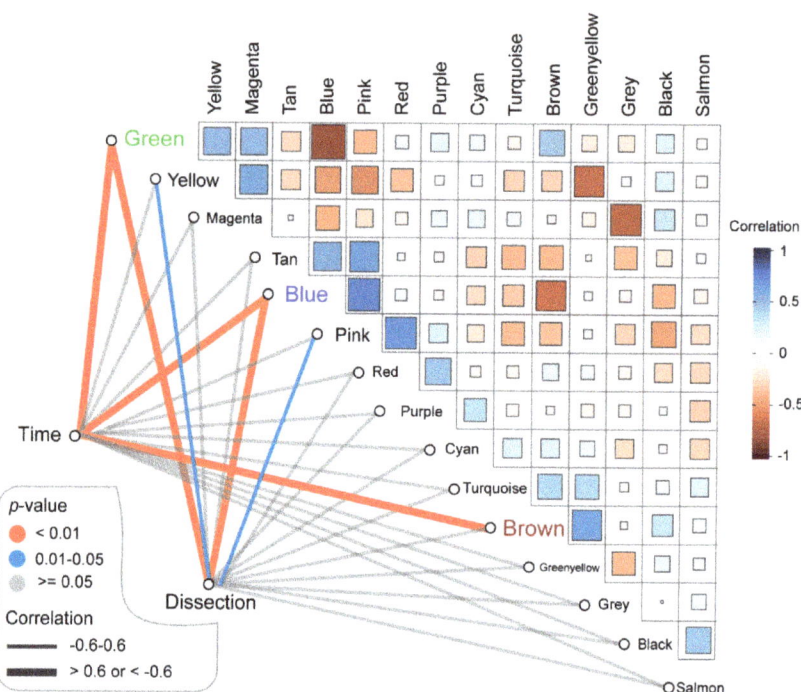

Figure 3. Identification of the key modules associated with AAA progression. Green, blue and brown modules were highly correlated (correlation > 0.6 or −0.6 and *p*-value < 0.01) to the time of sample collecting which stands for AAA progression. Besides, green and blue modules were also related to the dissection happening in the AAA sample (correlation > 0.6 or −0.6 and *p*-value < 0.01). AAA: abdominal aortic aneurysm.

3.3. Functional Enrichment Analysis of Genes in the Module

To investigate the biological functions of key modules related to sample traits, we conducted GO and KEGG enrichment analysis for genes in every key module. The GO analysis showed that genes in the blue modules were mainly involved in the organelle fission, regulation of mitotic cell cycle, and nuclear division related to cell development or differentiation (Figure 4A). The green module was involved in GTPase activity (Figure 4B), and the brown module was clustered in cellular metabolic processes, especially cofactor metabolism, purine-containing compound metabolism, and purine nucleotide metabolism (Figure 4C). The results of the KEGG analysis revealed that the blue module was enriched in fluid shear stress and atherosclerosis pathway, highly related to the progression of AAA (Figure 5A). Genes in the green module were enriched in the regulation of lipolysis in the adipocyte pathway and the pancreatic secretion pathway (Figure 5B). The brown module was enriched in the citrate cycle (TCA cycle) pathway (Figure 5C).

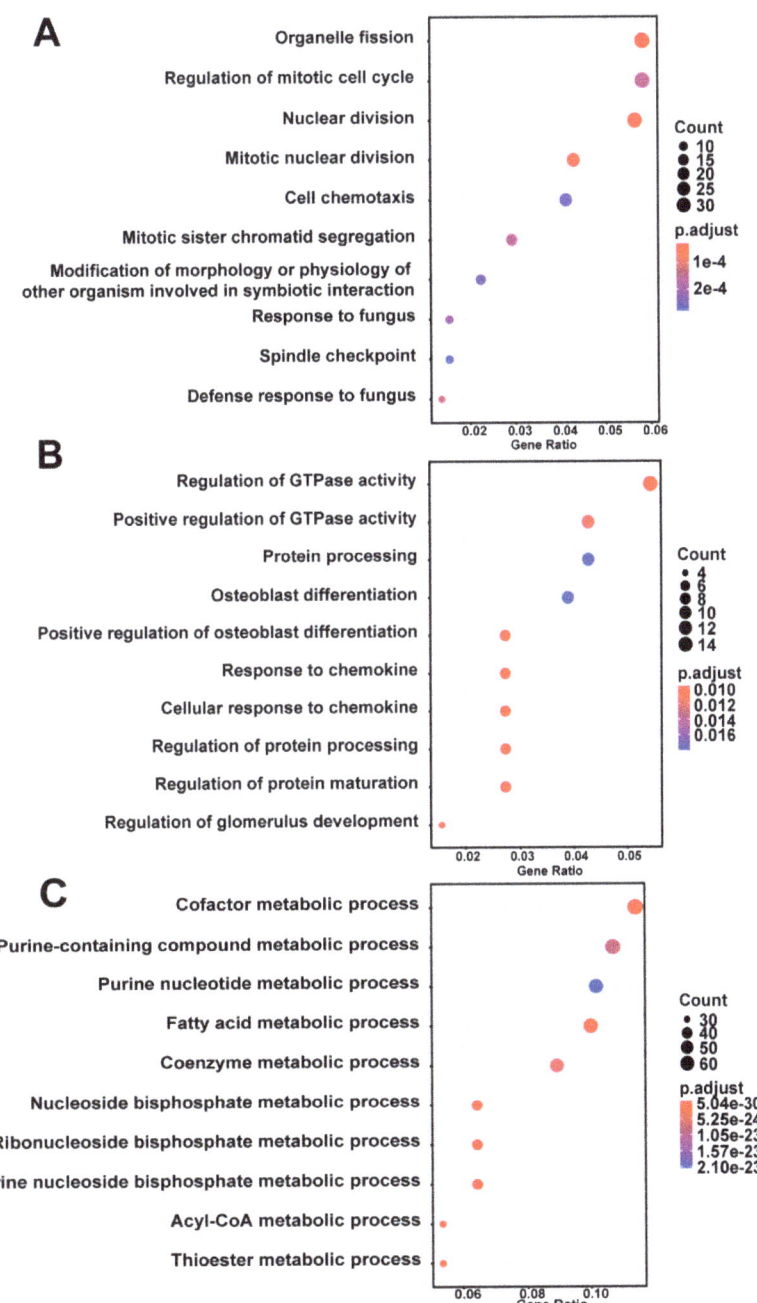

Figure 4. Gene ontology enrichment analysis of key modules of AAA progression. (**A**) blue module; (**B**) green module; (**C**) brown module. Count—the number of genes in the given GO term. Gene ration—the percentage of total genes in the given GO term.

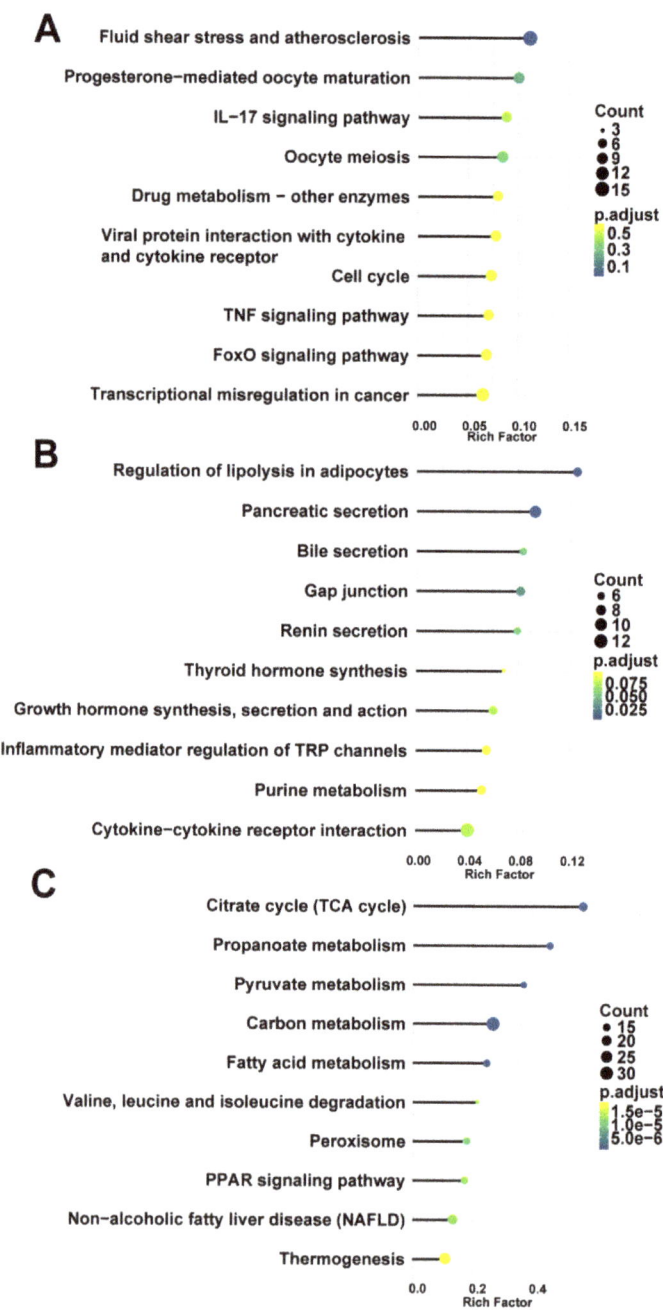

Figure 5. KEGG pathway enrichment analysis of key modules. (**A**) blue module; (**B**) green module; (**C**) brown module. Count—the number of genes in the given KEGG pathway. Rich factor—the ratio of the number of genes annotated in a pathway to the number of all genes annotated in this pathway.

3.4. Identification of Hub Genes in the Key Modules

To explore the hub genes that regulate AAA development, we imported the top 10% of genes with the highest connectivity into the String online database for protein–protein interaction detection, and networks were formed in Cytoscape (San Diego, CA, USA) (the PPI networks were stored in the NDEx: accessed on 11 December 2020 from https://bit.ly/37XZZWh; https://bit.ly/3a7Q2sc; https://bit.ly/38fyckz). With the cytoHubba plugin using the MCC method, the top 10 hub genes were identified in the key modules, namely, in the blue module (Ccr5, Fpr2, Ccr2, Fpr1, P2ry12, Hcar1, Ppbp, Aif1, Sirpb1b, Clec4n), green module (Gnai1, Adcy5, Adcy3, Rnase2a, Cxcl13, Clca1, Ear10, Ear1, Npr1, Ccl11), and brown module (Lpl, Dgat2, Fasn, Acacb, Lpin1, Acsl1, Mogat1, Lep, Ucp3, Pdk4) (Table 2).

Table 2. Top 10 ranked genes in key modules with the MCC method in cytoHubba.

Catalog	Key Modules		
	Blue	Green	Brown
Top 10 Gene	Ccr5	Gnai1	Lpl
	Fpr2	Adcy5	Dgat2
	Ccr2	Adcy3	Fasn
	Fpr1	Rnase2a	Acacb
	P2ry12	Cxcl13	Lpin1
	Hcar1	Clca1	Acsl1
	Ppbp	Ear10	Mogat1
	Aif1	Ear1	Lep
	Sirpb1b	Npr1	Ucp3
	Clec4n	Ccl11	Pdk4

3.5. Hub Genes Validation and Key Genes Selection

To further validate and evaluate the hub genes identified through the above analysis, the mouse dataset GSE12591 was checked using the same mouse angiotensin II-induced AAA model as GSE17901. In the blue module, Ccr5 and P2ry12 were significantly upregulated in the AAA group (Figure 6A), and Hcar1 was significantly down-regulated in the AAA group (Figure 6A). In the green module, Adcy5 and Adcy3 were the two significantly expressed genes (Figure 6B). All significantly expressed genes (Dgat2, Fasn, Acacb, Lpin1, Acsl1, Mogat1, Ucp3, Pdk4) in the brown module were down-regulated in the AAA group (Figure 6C). In the human AAA datasets GSE7084, GSE47472, and GSE57691, all of the significantly expressed genes were identified by comparing organ donors and AAA patients (Table 3). Considering the individual differences within each sample, genes expressed significantly in every human dataset were defined as human key genes. Finally, CCR5, ADCY5, ADCY3, ACACB, LPIN1, ACSL1, and UCP3 were the common genes that showed up both in the mouse AAA dataset and human AAA datasets and these were selected as the key genes in AAA progression.

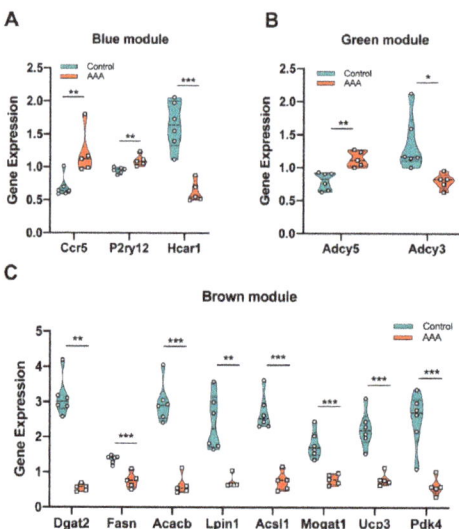

Figure 6. Validation of gene expression from hub genes in mouse dataset GSE12591. (**A**) Ccr5, P2ry12 and Hcar1 were differentially expressed in the blue module; (**B**) Adcy5 and Adcy3 were differentially expressed in the green module; (**C**) Dgat2, Fasn, Acacb, Lpin1, Acsl1, Mogat1, Ucp3 and Pdk4 were differentially expressed in the brown module. *: $p < 0.05$, **: $p < 0.01$, ***: $p < 0.001$ (Wilcoxon rank-sum test).

Table 3. Significantly expressed hub genes in human AAA datasets.

Datasets	Key Modules		
	Blue	Green	Brown
GSE7084	CCR5, CCR2, FPR2, FPR1, AIF1	GNAI1, RNASE2, NPR1	NA
GSE47472	CCR2, FPR2, PPBP	GNAI1, RNASE2, CLCA1, LYVE1	LPIN1, UCP3
GSE57691	CCR2, FPR2, PPBP, CLEC6A, SIRPB1	ADCY5, ADCY3, CXCL13, CLCA1, CCL11	ACACB, LPIN1, ACSL1, LEP
Human	CCR5, CCR2, FPR2, PPBP, AIF1, CLEC6A, SIRPB1, FPR1	GNAI1, RNASE2, NPR1, CLCA1, LYVE1, ADCY5, ADCY3, CXCL13, CCL11	ACACB, LPIN1, ACSL1, LEP, UCP3

3.6. Predication of Drug-Gene Interaction

The seven key genes CCR5, ADCY5, ADCY3, ACACB, LPIN1, ACSL1, and UCP3 were used as the potential druggable targets for AAA treatment. The drug–gene interaction results from the DGIdb database revealed 35 potential target drugs/compounds for AAA treatment. Of these, 23 drugs targeted CCR5, among which maraviroc had the highest score of prediction; seven drugs targeted ACACB, two drugs each targeted ACSL1 and ADCY5, and one drug targeted LPIN1 (Figure 7, Table S1). No potential drugs could be identified for ADCY3 and UCP3

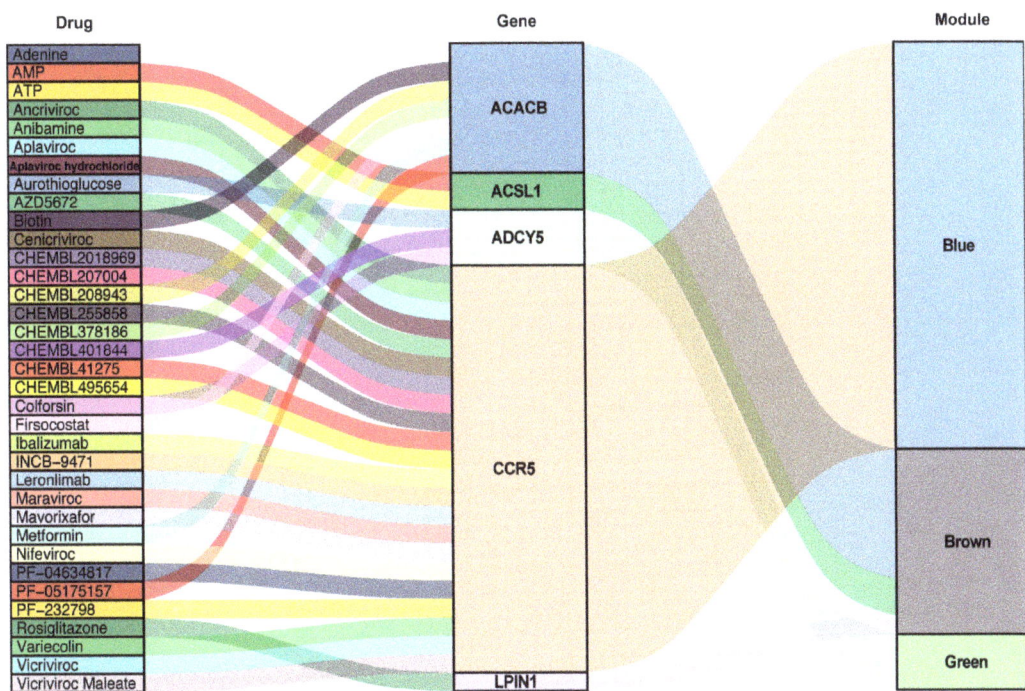

Figure 7. Drug–gene interaction prediction of key genes. Five key genes—ACACB, ACSL1, ADCY5, CCR5 and LPIN1 were targeted in the DGIdb database. A total of 35 potential target drugs/compounds were predicted from the database. AMP: Adenosine monophosphate; ATP: Adenosine triphosphate.

4. Discussion

In the present study, we used WGCNA analysis to identify the key genes involved in AAA progression and the drugs that target these genes, which could be potentially effective for the repression of AAA growth. WGCNA was performed on the available mouse dataset (GSE17901), where AAA samples were obtained at day 7, day 14, and day 28 from ApoE$^{-/-}$ mice treated by angiotensin II or saline. We identified three modules (blue, green, and brown) as key modules that correlated closely with AAA growth. In these three modules, we further identified hub genes using Cytoscape software (San Diego, CA, USA) and validated the model in mouse and human datasets. Seven genes—CCR5, ADCY5, ADCY3, ACACB, LPIN1, ACSL1, and UCP3 were identified as the key genes in AAA progression. Finally, using the DGIdb database, we identified 35 drugs as potential candidates/compounds that could target the key genes and yield beneficial effects in treating AAA.

WGCNA is a systematic biological method that describes the gene co-expression pattern between different samples. It identifies gene sets with highly coordinated variations. The candidate biomarkers or targets of the disease are based on the connectivity between gene modules and sample traits. Compared to the traditional differential gene expression analyses, which focus solely on genes characterizing the difference between groups, WGCNA groups co-expressed genes in an unbiased manner into modules that can be connected to sample traits.

Among the 15 co-expression modules obtained by WGCNA, the blue, green, and brown modules were mostly related to the AAA progression. The enrichment analysis of these key modules' biological functions and pathways revealed that genes in the blue module were mainly enriched in the cellular process, particularly the regulation of the mitotic cell cycle. This has also been reported in several studies. For instance, Butt et al. performed peripheral blood transcriptome profiling of individuals with AAA and healthy donors. They described that significantly expressed genes were enriched in this GO term [41]. Another study showed that the mitotic cell cycle was also significantly associated with dilated aortic perivascular adipose tissue [16]. The most enriched pathway of the blue module in KEGG was fluid shear stress and atherosclerosis. Several studies have shown the association of atherosclerosis disease with AAA [1,42]. Shear stress induced by abnormal blood flow was also previously reported to contribute to the growth or rupture of AAA [43,44]. The GO analysis of the green module showed that the biological process of GTPase activity was involved in AAA development. Dysregulation of GTPase activity would influence normal functions of endothelial cells and vascular smooth cells, including re-endothelialization, cell migration, and proliferation [45,46]. KEGG pathway enrichment of genes in the green module demonstrated that the regulation of lipolysis in the adipocyte pathway is also engaged in AAA growth. Adventitia of the aorta which contains the mass of adipocytes is a new direction of AAA research. One recent study revealed the key regulatory factors in perivascular adipose tissue of AAA [19]. Another study further proved that the increase in AAA diameter was correlated with lipid-related processes in the adventitia [18]. Results from functional enrichment analysis of the brown module indicated that some metabolic processes or pathways are also involved in AAA progression. In our study, cofactor metabolism was the most enriched process. This is in agreement with previously published studies that have shown that cofactors like cobalamin (vitamin B12) and glutathione could slow down the progression of AAA to some extent [47,48]. These findings confirm the involvement of the mitotic cell cycle, GTPase activity, and metabolic process in the pathogenesis of AAA.

The hub genes in the present study were selected by a combined analysis of gene intramodular connectivity and protein–protein interaction in the STRING database and Cytoscape software (San Diego, CA, USA). These selected hub genes were further confirmed in mouse and human datasets with gene differential expression analysis. Seven key genes were eventually identified—CCR5 from the blue module, ADCY5 and ADCY3 from the green module, ACACB, LPIN1, ACSL1, and UCP3 from the brown module. The vital role of CCR5, C-C motif chemokine receptor 5, in HIV-1 infection has been accepted since the discovery of this receptor [49]. It is expressed in many immune cells, including macrophages, T cells, and natural killer cells. CCR5 and its ligands regulate the inflammatory response by affecting the biological activities of the above-mentioned immune cells [50]. The results from GSE12591 identifying Ccr5 as a differential gene upregulated in the mouse aortas with aneurysms [25]. CCR5 signaling in the macrophage pathway was enriched by functional analyses of differential genes in GSE7084 [24]. Furthermore, patients with AAA frequently have CCR5 Delta 32 deletion mutations and are vulnerable to rupture of aneurysms [51]. Thus, CCR5 may be a potential biomarker for AAA progression and an indication of rupture. The hub gene ADCY5 (mouse—Adcy5) in the green module was related to mouse AAA progression and dissection. This was consistent with the findings by Phillips et al. which showed Adcy5 was one of the differentially expressed genes in the murine dissecting AAA [52]. ADCY3 is an enzyme that regulates the cyclic adenosine monophosphate (cAMP). Besides its role in AAA progression, loss of ADCY3 increases the risk of obesity and type 2 diabetes [53], and the single nucleotide polymorphisms of this gene are related to hypertension [54], which are the risk factors leading to the initiation of AAA [55]. LPIN1, ACSL1, and UCP3 were related to adipocyte differentiation and muscle growth [56–60], so dysregulation of these three genes may lead to AAA initiation, growth or rupture, as adipocytes residing in the perivascular tissue, and vascular smooth muscle cells play an important role in the development of AAA [19,60]. According to the reviewed literature, the remaining key gene ACACB had no apparent connection with AAA. This, however, requires further investigation to clarify its function in AAA progression.

So far, there is no effective drug therapy for the prevention of AAA progression or rupture. In this study, seven key genes were identified and used for predicting drug-gene interactions. A total of potential 35 drugs or compounds were presented in the DGIdb database. Most of these targeted the CCR5 gene. We checked these 35 candidates from the literature and ClinicalTrials.gov (accessed on 18 July 2020 from https://clinicaltrials.gov/), the largest clinical trials database containing over 329,000 trials worldwide. Five targetable drugs (PF-05175157, firsocostat, and metformin targeting ACACB; maraviroc targeting CCR5; rosiglitazone targeting LPIN1) were found to be used for AAA treatment. PF-05175157 and firsocostat are two novel acetyl-CoA carboxylase (ACC) inhibitors for lipid disorders [61,62], which could potentially rebalance dysregulated lipid metabolism in AAA to limit the development of the disease. Metformin is the first-line oral antidiabetic drug [63]. It also has proven effects on cardiovascular diseases through the reduction of inflammation and oxidative stress [64–66]. Several epidemiological studies have indicated that the use of metformin use could decrease yearly AAA growth [67,68]. Though maraviroc is a CCR5 antagonist prescribed for HIV-1 treatment, it could also be applied for AAA treatment since it was reported that maraviroc could reduce cardiovascular risk by modulation of atherosclerotic progression in vivo and in vitro [69,70]. Rosiglitazone (RGZ) is a potent peroxisome proliferator-activated receptor-γ (PPAR-γ) agonist that can protect against ischemia/reperfusion injury due to its anti-inflammatory effects [71]. It has been reported that RGZ reduces stent-induced neointimal formation by decreasing the inflammatory responses and vascular smooth muscle hyperplasia [72]. Through the same anti-inflammatory effect, RGZ could also inhibit the growth and rupture of mouse aortic aneurysms induced by angiotensin II and high cholesterol [73]. No drugs could be predicted for the ADCY3 and UCP3 genes. These two gene candidates will have to be evaluated as potential targets in AAA treatment in further studies.

Though our study is the first that performed WGCNA analysis with samples collected at different points of time in AAA growth, this study still has some limitations. Firstly, upon screening of the public database mouse dataset, GSE17901 was the only dataset available that allowed us to follow gene function over time and was used as an exploration dataset for WGCNA analysis. As a result, the sample size used for WGCNA analysis ($n = 17$) just passed the minimum official criteria ($n = 15$), therefore there may be noise for the biological network construction. The angiotensin II-induced AAA in mice may share similar features with human AAA, but the inherent pathology is different and thus, our results should be interpreted with caution. This study has indeed predicted interesting key genes involved in the progression of AAA and potentially useful drugs, however these findings should be validated further with in vitro and in vivo models of AAA.

In summary, this study identified key co-expression modules, key genes, and several critical biological processes related to AAA progression. With drug–gene interaction prediction, target drugs or compounds may provide the possibility of developing a medical treatment for AAA.

5. Conclusions

Our study using WGCNA analyses revealed seven key genes (CCR5, ADCY5, ADCY3, ACACB, LPIN1, ACSL1, UCP3) in three modules correlated to AAA progression. Mitotic cell cycle, GTPase activity, and metabolic process were involved in the pathogenesis of AAA. The therapeutic potential of several predicted drugs for the treatment of AAA could be further explored.

Supplementary Materials: The following are available online at https://www.mdpi.com/article/10.3390/biomedicines9050546/s1, Figure S1: Sample clustering and module relations to sample traits. (A) Sample dendrogram and trait heatmap. The color intensity of time was proportional to the day of the sample collected. The red color in dissected represents the occurrence of dissection in the sample; (B) Module trait relationships. Each row corresponds to a module eigengene (ME) and each column to a sample trait, Figure S2: Correlation of the module membership and the gene significance. (A–C) The relationship between gene significance of time and module membership; (D–E) The relationship between gene significance of dissection and module membership. The color indicates the module, and the dot indicates the gene within the module., Table S1: Potential target agents identified based on drug-gene interaction in DGIdb database.

Author Contributions: Conceptualization, K.-J.K. and F.G.; methodology, K.-J.K. and F.G.; validation, K.-J.K. and F.G. and L.Z.; formal analysis, K.-J.K., F.G., P.P.; investigation, K.-J.K. and F.G. and L.Z.; data curation, K.-J.K. and F.G.; writing—original draft preparation, K.-J.K. and F.G.; writing—review and editing, P.P., M.S., M.K.; visualization, K.-J.K. and F.G.; supervision, M.S., M.K. All authors have read and agreed to the published version of the manuscript.

Funding: K.J.K., F.G. and L.Z. were supported by the China Scholarship Council (CSC), No. 201706230257, No. 201808080101 and No. 201908080072.

Institutional Review Board Statement: Not applicable.

Informed Consent Statement: Not applicable.

Data Availability Statement: All datasets of this study are available in the GEO database (https://www.ncbi.nlm.nih.gov/geo/, accessed on 13 May 2021).

Acknowledgments: We thank "Guotosky", "Shengxinxingqiu", and "Biotrainee" for sharing the knowledge of bioinformatics analysis.

Conflicts of Interest: The authors declare no conflict of interest.

References

1. Golledge, J.; Muller, J.; Daugherty, A.; Norman, P. Abdominal Aortic Aneurysm: Pathogenesis and Implications for Management. *Arterioscler. Thromb. Vasc. Biol.* **2006**, *26*, 2605–2613. [CrossRef]
2. Lucas, R.; Banerjee, A.; Barquera, S.; Blyth, F.M.; Cowie, B.C.; Ding, E.L.; Gunnell, D.; Lan, Q.; J, M.J.; Patton, G.C.; et al. Global, regional, and national age–sex specific all-cause and cause-specific mortality for 240 causes of death, 1990–2013: a systematic analysis for the Global Burden of Disease Study 2013. *Lancet* **2015**, *385*, 117–171. [CrossRef]
3. Sampson, U.K.A.; Norman, P.E.; Fowkes, F.G.R.; Aboyans, V.; Song, Y.; Harrell, F.E.; Forouzanfar, M.H.; Naghavi, M.; Denenberg, J.O.; McDermott, M.M.; et al. Global and Regional Burden of Aortic Dissection and Aneurysms: Mortality Trends in 21 World Regions, 1990 to 2010. *Glob. Heart* **2014**, *9*, 171–180.e10. [CrossRef]
4. Toghill, B.J.; Saratzis, A.; Bown, M.J. Abdominal Aortic Aneurysm—an Independent Disease to Atherosclerosis? *Cardiovasc. Pathol.* **2017**, *27*, 71–75. [CrossRef]
5. Chaikof, E.L.; Dalman, R.L.; Eskandari, M.K.; Jackson, B.M.; Lee, W.A.; Mansour, M.A.; Mastracci, T.M.; Mell, M.; Murad, M.H.; Nguyen, L.L.; et al. The Society for Vascular Surgery Practice Guidelines on the Care of Patients with an Abdominal Aortic Aneurysm. *J. Vasc. Surg.* **2018**, *67*, 2–77.e2. [CrossRef] [PubMed]
6. Wanhainen, A.; Verzini, F.; Van Herzeele, I.; Allaire, E.; Bown, M.; Cohnert, T.; Dick, F.; van Herwaarden, J.; Karkos, C.; Koelemay, M.; et al. Editor's Choice - European Society for Vascular Surgery (ESVS) 2019 Clinical Practice Guidelines on the Management of Abdominal Aorto-Iliac Artery Aneurysms. *Eur. J. Vasc. Endovasc. Surg.* **2019**, *57*, 8–93. [CrossRef]
7. Kokje, V.B.C.; Hamming, J.F.; Lindeman, J.H.N. Pharmaceutical Management of Small Abdominal Aortic Aneurysms: A Systematic Review of the Clinical Evidence. *J. Vasc. Surg.* **2015**, *62*, 1680. [CrossRef]
8. Rughani, G.; Robertson, L.; Clarke, M. Medical Treatment for Small Abdominal Aortic Aneurysms. *Cochrane Datab. Syst. Rev.* **2012**, CD009536. [CrossRef]
9. Daugherty, A.; Cassis, L.A. Mouse Models of Abdominal Aortic Aneurysms. *Arterioscler. Thromb. Vasc. Biol.* **2004**, *24*, 429–434. [CrossRef] [PubMed]
10. Golledge, J. Abdominal aortic aneurysm: update on pathogenesis and medical treatments. *Nat. Rev. Cardiol.* **2019**, *16*, 225–242. [CrossRef]
11. Moran, C.S.; Biros, E.; Krishna, S.M.; Wang, Y.; Tikellis, C.; Morton, S.K.; Moxon, J.V.; Cooper, M.E.; Norman, P.E.; Burrell, L.M.; et al. Resveratrol Inhibits Growth of Experimental Abdominal Aortic Aneurysm Associated With Upregulation of Angiotensin-Converting Enzyme 2. *Arterioscler. Thromb. Vasc. Biol.* **2017**, *37*, 2195–2203. [CrossRef] [PubMed]
12. Trachet, B.; Piersigilli, A.; Fraga-Silva, R.A.; Aslanidou, L.; Sordet-Dessimoz, J.; Astolfo, A.; Stampanoni, M.F.M.; Segers, P.; Stergiopulos, N. Ascending Aortic Aneurysm in Angiotensin II-Infused Mice: Formation, Progression, and the Role of Focal Dissections. *Arterioscler. Thromb. Vasc. Biol.* **2016**, *36*, 673–681. [CrossRef]
13. Rateri, D.L.; Howatt, D.A.; Moorleghen, J.J.; Charnigo, R.; Cassis, L.A.; Daugherty, A. Prolonged Infusion of Angiotensin II in apoE−/− Mice Promotes Macrophage Recruitment with Continued Expansion of Abdominal Aortic Aneurysm. *Am. J. Pathol.* **2011**, *179*, 1542–1548. [CrossRef] [PubMed]
14. Wang, S.; Zhang, C.; Zhang, M.; Liang, B.; Zhu, H.; Lee, J.; Viollet, B.; Xia, L.; Zhang, Y.; Zou, M.-H. Activation of AMP-Activated Protein Kinase A2 by Nicotine Instigates Formation of Abdominal Aortic Aneurysms in Mice in Vivo. *Nat. Med.* **2012**, *18*, 902–910. [CrossRef] [PubMed]

15. Daugherty, A.; Manning, M.W.; Cassis, L.A. Angiotensin II promotes atherosclerotic lesions and aneurysms in apolipoprotein E–deficient mice. *J. Clin. Investig.* **2000**, *105*, 1605–1612. [CrossRef]
16. Piacentini, L.; Chiesa, M.; Colombo, G.I. Gene Regulatory Network Analysis of Perivascular Adipose Tissue of Abdominal Aortic Aneurysm Identifies Master Regulators of Key Pathogenetic Pathways. *Biomedicines* **2020**, *8*, 288. [CrossRef]
17. Coscas, R.; Dupont, S.; Mussot, S.; Louedec, L.; Etienne, H.; Morvan, M.; Chiocchia, G.; Massy, Z.; Jacob, M.-P.; Michel, J.-B. Exploring antibody-dependent adaptive immunity against aortic extracellular matrix components in experimental aortic aneurysms. *J. Vasc. Surg.* **2018**, *68*, 60S–71S.e3. [CrossRef]
18. Liljeqvist, M.L.; Hultgren, R.; Bergman, O.; Villard, C.; Kronqvist, M.; Eriksson, P.; Roy, J. Tunica-Specific Transcriptome of Abdominal Aortic Aneurysm and the Effect of Intraluminal Thrombus, Smoking, and Diameter Growth Rate. *Arter. Thromb. Vasc. Biol.* **2020**, *40*, 2700–2713. [CrossRef]
19. Piacentini, L.; Werba, J.P.; Bono, E.; Saccu, C.; Tremoli, E.; Spirito, R.; Colombo, G.I. Genome-Wide Expression Profiling Unveils Autoimmune Response Signatures in the Perivascular Adipose Tissue of Abdominal Aortic Aneurysm. *Arterioscler. Thromb. Vasc. Biol.* **2019**, *39*, 237–249. [CrossRef]
20. Dale, M.A.; Ruhlman, M.K.; Baxter, B.T. Inflammatory Cell Phenotypes in AAAs. *Arter. Thromb. Vasc. Biol.* **2015**, *35*, 1746–1755. [CrossRef]
21. Kuivaniemi, H.; Ryer, E.J.; Elmore, J.R.; Tromp, G. Understanding the pathogenesis of abdominal aortic aneurysms. *Expert Rev. Cardiovasc. Ther.* **2015**, *13*, 975–987. [CrossRef]
22. Raffort, J.; Lareyre, F.; Clément, M.; Hassen-Khodja, F.L.R.; Chinetti, J.R.F.L.R.H.-K.G.; Mallat, J.R.F.L.M.C.Z. Monocytes and macrophages in abdominal aortic aneurysm. *Nat. Rev. Cardiol.* **2017**, *14*, 457–471. [CrossRef] [PubMed]
23. Weintraub, N.L. Understanding Abdominal Aortic Aneurysm. *N. Engl. J. Med.* **2009**, *361*, 1114–1116. [CrossRef]
24. Pahl, M.C.; Erdman, R.; Kuivaniemi, H.; Lillvis, J.H.; Elmore, J.R.; Tromp, G. Transcriptional (ChIP-Chip) Analysis of ELF1, ETS2, RUNX1 and STAT5 in Human Abdominal Aortic Aneurysm. *Int. J. Mol. Sci.* **2015**, *16*, 11229–11258. [CrossRef]
25. Rush, C.; Nyara, M.; Moxon, J.V.; Trollope, A.; Cullen, B.; Golledge, J. Whole genome expression analysis within the angiotensin II-apolipoprotein E deficient mouse model of abdominal aortic aneurysm. *BMC Genom.* **2009**, *10*, 298. [CrossRef]
26. Spin, J.M.; Hsu, M.; Azuma, J.; Tedesco, M.M.; Deng, A.; Dyer, J.S.; Maegdefessel, L.; Dalman, R.L.; Tsao, P.S. Transcriptional profiling and network analysis of the murine angiotensin II-induced abdominal aortic aneurysm. *Physiol. Genom.* **2011**, *43*, 993–1003. [CrossRef]
27. Zhang, B.; Horvath, S. A General Framework for Weighted Gene Co-Expression Network Analysis. *Stat. Appl. Genet. Mol. Biol.* **2005**, *4*, 17. [CrossRef] [PubMed]
28. Guo, N.; Zhang, N.; Yan, L.; Lian, Z.; Wang, J.; Lv, F.; Wang, Y.; Cao, X. Weighted gene co-expression network analysis in identification of key genes and networks for ischemic-reperfusion remodeling myocardium. *Mol. Med. Rep.* **2018**, *18*, 1955–1962. [CrossRef] [PubMed]
29. Nagenborg, J.; Jin, H.; Brennan, E.; Goossens, P.; Donners, M.; Biessen, E. Re-Programming Atherosclerotic Plaque Macrophages Towards An Anti-Atherogenic Phenotype. *Atheroscler.* **2019**, *287*, e79. [CrossRef]
30. Wang, C.-H.; Shi, H.-H.; Chen, L.-H.; Li, X.-L.; Cao, G.-L.; Hu, X.-F. Identification of Key lncRNAs Associated With Atherosclerosis Progression Based on Public Datasets. *Front. Genet.* **2019**, *10*, 123. [CrossRef]
31. Biros, E.; Gäbel, G.; Moran, C.S.; Schreurs, C.; Lindeman, J.H.N.; Walker, P.J.; Nataatmadja, M.; West, M.; Holdt, L.M.; Hinterseher, I.; et al. Differential gene expression in human abdominal aortic aneurysm and aortic occlusive disease. *Oncotarget* **2015**, *6*, 12984–12996. [CrossRef] [PubMed]
32. Ritchie, M.E.; Phipson, B.; Wu, D.; Hu, Y.; Law, C.W.; Shi, W.; Smyth, G.K. limma powers differential expression analyses for RNA-sequencing and microarray studies. *Nucl. Acids Res.* **2015**, *43*, e47. [CrossRef] [PubMed]
33. Kassambara, A. Ggcorrplot: Visualization of a Correlation Matrix Using "Ggplot2". 2019. Available online: https://github.com/kassambara/ggcorrplot (accessed on 13 September 2020).
34. Yu, G.; Wang, L.-G.; Han, Y.; He, Q.-Y. clusterProfiler: An R Package for Comparing Biological Themes Among Gene Clusters. *OMICS: A J. Integr. Biol.* **2012**, *16*, 284–287. [CrossRef] [PubMed]
35. Szklarczyk, D.; Morris, J.H.; Cook, H.; Kuhn, M.; Wyder, S.; Simonovic, M.; Santos, A.; Doncheva, N.T.; Roth, A.; Bork, P.; et al. The STRING database in 2017: quality-controlled protein–protein association networks, made broadly accessible. *Nucl. Acids Res.* **2017**, *45*, D362–D368. [CrossRef] [PubMed]
36. Shannon, P.; Markiel, A.; Ozier, O.; Baliga, N.S.; Wang, J.T.; Ramage, D.; Amin, N.; Schwikowski, B.; Ideker, T. Cytoscape: A Software Environment for Integrated Models of Biomolecular Interaction Networks. *Genome Res.* **2003**, *13*, 2498–2504. [CrossRef]
37. Chin, C.-H.; Chen, S.-H.; Wu, H.-H.; Ho, C.-W.; Ko, M.-T.; Lin, C.-Y. cytoHubba: identifying hub objects and sub-networks from complex interactome. *BMC Syst. Biol.* **2014**, *8*, S11. [CrossRef]
38. Cotto, K.C.; Wagner, A.H.; Feng, Y.-Y.; Kiwala, S.; Coffman, A.C.; Spies, G.; Wollam, A.; Spies, N.C.; Griffith, O.L.; Griffith, M. DGIdb 3.0: a redesign and expansion of the drug–gene interaction database. *Nucl. Acids Res.* **2018**, *46*, D1068–D1073. [CrossRef] [PubMed]
39. Wickham, H.; Chang, W.; Henry, L.; Pedersen, T.L.; Takahashi, K.; Wilke, C.; Woo, K.; Yutani, H.; Dunnington, D. RStudio Ggplot2: Create Elegant Data Visualisations Using the Grammar of Graphics. 2020. Available online: https://ggplot2.tidyverse.org/ (accessed on 10 September 2020).

40. Brunson, J.C. Ggalluvial: Alluvial Plots in "Ggplot2". 2019. Available online: https://cran.r-project.org/web/packages/ggalluvial/index.html (accessed on 16 September 2020).
41. Butt, H.; Sylvius, N.; Salem, M.; Wild, J.; Dattani, N.; Sayers, R.; Bown, M. Microarray-based Gene Expression Profiling of Abdominal Aortic Aneurysm. *Eur. J. Vasc. Endovasc. Surg.* **2016**, *52*, 47–55. [CrossRef]
42. Cornuz, J.; Pinto, C.S.; Tevaearai, H.; Egger, M. Risk factors for asymptomatic abdominal aortic aneurysm: systematic review and meta-analysis of population-based screening studies. *Eur. J. Public Heal.* **2004**, *14*, 343–349. [CrossRef]
43. Lin, S.; Han, X.; Bi, Y.; Ju, S.; Gu, L. Fluid-Structure Interaction in Abdominal Aortic Aneurysm: Effect of Modeling Techniques. *BioMed Res. Int.* **2017**, *2017*, 1–10. [CrossRef]
44. Sheidaei, A.; Hunley, S.; Zeinali-Davarani, S.; Raguin, L.; Baek, S. Simulation of abdominal aortic aneurysm growth with updating hemodynamic loads using a realistic geometry. *Med Eng. Phys.* **2011**, *33*, 80–88. [CrossRef] [PubMed]
45. Tanaka, S.-I.; Fukumoto, Y.; Nochioka, K.; Minami, T.; Kudo, S.; Shiba, N.; Takai, Y.; Williams, C.L.; Liao, J.K.; Shimokawa, H. Statins Exert the Pleiotropic Effects Through Small GTP-Binding Protein Dissociation Stimulator Upregulation With a Resultant Rac1 Degradation. *Arter. Thromb. Vasc. Biol.* **2013**, *33*, 1591–1600. [CrossRef]
46. Yu, D.; Makkar, G.; Strickland, D.K.; Blanpied, T.A.; Stumpo, D.J.; Blackshear, P.J.; Sarkar, R.; Monahan, T.S. Myristoylated Alanine-Rich Protein Kinase Substrate (MARCKS) Regulates Small GTPase Rac1 and Cdc42 Activity and Is a Critical Mediator of Vascular Smooth Muscle Cell Migration in Intimal Hyperplasia Formation. *J. Am. Heart Assoc.* **2015**, *4*, e002255. [CrossRef] [PubMed]
47. Lindqvist, M.; Hellström, A.; Henriksson, A.E. Abdominal Aortic Aneurysm and the Association with Serum Levels of Homocysteine, Vitamins B6, B12 and Folate. *Am. J. Cardiovasc. Dis.* **2012**, *2*, 318–322.
48. Wiernicki, I.; Parafiniuk, M.; Kolasa-Wołosiuk, A.; Gutowska, I.; Kazimierczak, A.; Clark, J.; Baranowska-Bosiacka, I.; Szumilowicz, P.; Gutowski, P. Relationship between aortic wall oxidative stress/proteolytic enzyme expression and intraluminal thrombus thickness indicates a novel pathomechanism in the progression of human abdominal aortic aneurysm. *FASEB J.* **2018**, *33*, 885–895. [CrossRef]
49. Berger, E.A.; Murphy, P.M.; Farber, J.M. CHEMOKINE RECEPTORS AS HIV-1 CORECEPTORS: Roles in Viral Entry, Tropism, and Disease. *Annu. Rev. Immunol.* **1999**, *17*, 657–700. [CrossRef]
50. Kohlmeier, J.E.; Reiley, W.W.; Perona-Wright, G.; Freeman, M.L.; Yager, E.J.; Connor, L.M.; Brincks, E.L.; Cookenham, T.; Roberts, A.D.; Burkum, C.E.; et al. Inflammatory chemokine receptors regulate CD8+ T cell contraction and memory generation following infection. *J. Exp. Med.* **2011**, *208*, 1621–1634. [CrossRef]
51. Ghilardi, G.; Biondi, M.L.; Battagliolí, L.; Zambon, A.; Guagnellini, E.; Scorza, R. Genetic risk factor characterizes abdominal aortic aneurysm from arterial occlusive disease in human beings: CCR5 Δ32 deletion. *J. Vasc. Surg.* **2004**, *40*, 995–1000. [CrossRef]
52. Phillips, E.H.; Lorch, A.H.; Durkes, A.C.; Goergen, C.J. Early pathological characterization of murine dissecting abdominal aortic aneurysms. *APL Bioeng.* **2018**, *2*, 046106. [CrossRef]
53. Grarup, N.; Moltke, I.; Andersen, M.K.; Dalby, M.; Vitting-Seerup, K.; Kern, T.; Mahendran, Y.; Jørsboe, E.; Larsen, C.V.L.; Dahl-Petersen, I.K.; et al. Loss-of-function variants in ADCY3 increase risk of obesity and type 2 diabetes. *Nat. Genet.* **2018**, *50*, 172–174. [CrossRef] [PubMed]
54. Chen, Y.; Gong, Y.W.; Zhou, X.Q.; Xu, H.X.; Yang, L.; Wu, Y.Y. [Association between single nucleotide polymorphism of adenylyl cyclase 3 and essential hypertension]. *Zhonghua Xin Xue Guan Bing Za Zhi* **2016**, *44*, 594–599.
55. Thompson, A.; Drenos, F.; Hafez, H.M.; E Humphries, S. Candidate Gene Association Studies in Abdominal Aortic Aneurysm Disease: A Review and Meta-Analysis. *Eur. J. Vasc. Endovasc. Surg.* **2008**, *35*, 19–30. [CrossRef]
56. Reue, K.; Xu, P.; Wang, X.-P.; Slavin, B.G. Adipose tissue deficiency, glucose intolerance, and increased atherosclerosis result from mutation in the mouse fatty liver dystrophy (fld) gene. *J. Lipid Res.* **2000**, *41*, 1067–1076. [CrossRef]
57. Jama, A.; Huang, D.; A Alshudukhi, A.A.; Chrast, R.; Ren, H. Lipin1 is required for skeletal muscle development by regulating MEF2c and MyoD expression. *J. Physiol.* **2019**, *597*, 889–901. [CrossRef]
58. Koh, J.-H.; Kim, K.-H.; Park, S.-Y.; Kim, Y.-W.; Kim, J.-Y. PPARδ Attenuates Alcohol-Mediated Insulin Resistance by Enhancing Fatty Acid-Induced Mitochondrial Uncoupling and Antioxidant Defense in Skeletal Muscle. *Front. Physiol.* **2020**, *11*, 749. [CrossRef]
59. Silvestri, E.; Senese, R.; De Matteis, R.; Cioffi, F.; Moreno, M.; Lanni, A.; Gentile, A.; Busiello, R.A.; Salzano, A.M.; Scaloni, A.; et al. Absence of uncoupling protein 3 at thermoneutrality influences brown adipose tissue mitochondrial functionality in mice. *FASEB J.* **2020**, *34*, 15146–15163. [CrossRef]
60. Stierwalt, H.D.; Ehrlicher, S.E.; Robinson, M.M.; Newsom, S.A. Skeletal Muscle ACSL Isoforms Relate to Measures of Fat Metabolism in Humans. *Med. Sci. Sports Exerc.* **2020**. [CrossRef]
61. Alkhouri, N.; Lawitz, E.; Noureddin, M.; DeFronzo, R.; Shulman, G.I. GS-0976 (Firsocostat): an investigational liver-directed acetyl-CoA carboxylase (ACC) inhibitor for the treatment of non-alcoholic steatohepatitis (NASH). *Expert Opin. Investig. Drugs* **2020**, *29*, 135–141. [CrossRef]
62. Huard, K.; Smith, A.C.; Cappon, G.D.; Dow, R.L.; Edmonds, D.J.; El-Kattan, A.; Esler, W.P.; Fernando, D.P.; Griffith, D.A.; Kalgutkar, A.S.; et al. Optimizing the Benefit/Risk of Acetyl-CoA Carboxylase Inhibitors through Liver Targeting. *J. Med. Chem.* **2020**, *63*, 10879–10896. [CrossRef]

63. Chaudhury, A.; Duvoor, C.; Dendi, V.S.R.; Kraleti, S.; Chada, A.; Ravilla, R.; Marco, A.; Shekhawat, N.S.; Montales, M.T.; Kuriakose, K.; et al. Clinical Review of Antidiabetic Drugs: Implications for Type 2 Diabetes Mellitus Management. *Front. Endocrinol.* **2017**, *8*, 6. [CrossRef]
64. Isoda, K.; Young, J.L.; Zirlik, A.; Macfarlane, L.A.; Tsuboi, N.; Gerdes, N.; Schoönbeck, U.; Libby, P. Metformin Inhibits Proinflammatory Responses and Nuclear Factor-κB in Human Vascular Wall Cells. *Arter. Thromb. Vasc. Biol.* **2006**, *26*, 611–617. [CrossRef]
65. Esfahanian, N.; Shakiba, Y.; Nikbin, B.; Soraya, H.; Maleki-Dizaji, N.; Ghazi-Khansari, M.; Garjani, A. Effect of metformin on the proliferation, migration, and MMP-2 and -9 expression of human umbilical vein endothelial cells. *Mol. Med. Rep.* **2012**, *5*, 1068–1074. [CrossRef] [PubMed]
66. Kim, S.A.; Choi, H.C. Metformin inhibits inflammatory response via AMPK–PTEN pathway in vascular smooth muscle cells. *Biochem. Biophys. Res. Commun.* **2012**, *425*, 866–872. [CrossRef]
67. Fujimura, N.; Xiong, J.; Kettler, E.B.; Xuan, H.; Glover, K.J.; Mell, M.W.; Xu, B.; Dalman, R.L. Metformin treatment status and abdominal aortic aneurysm disease progression. *J. Vasc. Surg.* **2016**, *64*, 46–54.e8. [CrossRef]
68. Itoga, N.K.; Rothenberg, K.A.; Suarez, P.; Ho, T.-V.; Mell, M.W.; Xu, B.; Curtin, C.M.; Dalman, R.L. Metformin prescription status and abdominal aortic aneurysm disease progression in the U.S. veteran population. *J. Vasc. Surg.* **2019**, *69*, 710–716.e3. [CrossRef] [PubMed]
69. Afonso, P.; Auclair, M.; Caron-Debarle, M.; Capeau, J. Impact of CCR5, integrase and protease inhibitors on human endothelial cell function, stress, inflammation and senescence. *Antivir. Ther.* **2017**, *22*, 645–657. [CrossRef] [PubMed]
70. Francisci, D.; Pirro, M.; Schiaroli, E.; Mannarino, M.R.; Cipriani, S.; Bianconi, V.; Alunno, A.; Bagaglia, F.; Bistoni, O.; Falcinelli, E.; et al. Maraviroc Intensification Modulates Atherosclerotic Progression in HIV-Suppressed Patients at High Cardiovascular Risk. A Randomized, Crossover Pilot Study. *Open Forum Infect. Dis.* **2019**, *6*, ofz112. [CrossRef]
71. Yue, T.-L.; Chen, J.; Bao, W.; Narayanan, P.K.; Bril, A.; Jiang, W.; Lysko, P.G.; Gu, J.-L.; Boyce, R.; Zimmerman, D.M.; et al. In Vivo Myocardial Protection From Ischemia/Reperfusion Injury by the Peroxisome Proliferator–Activated Receptor-γ Agonist Rosiglitazone. *Circulation* **2001**, *104*, 2588–2594. [CrossRef]
72. Wu, H.; Yang, Y.; Zheng, B.; Chen, K. Decreased PPAR-γ expression after internal carotid artery stenting is associated with vascular lesions induced by smooth muscle cell proliferation and systemic inflammation in a minipig model. *Int. J. Clin. Exp. Pathol.* **2017**, *10*, 7375–7383.
73. Jones, A.; Deb, R.; Torsney, E.; Howe, F.; Dunkley, M.; Gnaneswaran, Y.; Gaze, D.; Nasr, H.; Loftus, I.M.; Thompson, M.M.; et al. Rosiglitazone Reduces the Development and Rupture of Experimental Aortic Aneurysms. *Circulation* **2009**, *119*, 3125–3132. [CrossRef]

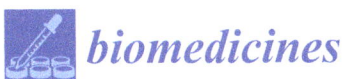

Article

Gene Regulatory Network Analysis of Perivascular Adipose Tissue of Abdominal Aortic Aneurysm Identifies Master Regulators of Key Pathogenetic Pathways

Luca Piacentini *, Mattia Chiesa and Gualtiero Ivanoe Colombo

Immunology and Functional Genomics Unit, Centro Cardiologico Monzino, IRCCS, 20138 Milan, Italy; mattia.chiesa@cardiologicomonzino.it (M.C.); gualtiero.colombo@cardiologicomonzino.it (G.I.C.)
* Correspondence: luca.piacentini@cardiologicomonzino.it

Received: 1 July 2020; Accepted: 12 August 2020; Published: 14 August 2020

Abstract: The lack of medical therapy to treat abdominal aortic aneurysm (AAA) stems from our inadequate understanding of the mechanisms underlying AAA pathogenesis. To date, the only available treatment option relies on surgical intervention, which aims to prevent AAA rupture. Identifying specific regulators of pivotal pathogenetic mechanisms would allow the development of novel treatments. With this work, we sought to identify regulatory factors associated with co-expressed genes characterizing the diseased perivascular adipose tissue (PVAT) of AAA patients, which is crucially involved in AAA pathogenesis. We applied a reverse engineering approach to identify cis-regulatory elements of diseased PVAT genes, the associated transcription factors, and upstream regulators. Finally, by analyzing the topological properties of the reconstructed regulatory disease network, we prioritized putative targets for AAA interference treatment options. Overall, we identified NFKB1, SPIB, and TBP as the most relevant transcription factors, as well as MAPK1 and GSKB3 protein kinases and RXRA nuclear receptor as key upstream regulators. We showed that these factors could regulate different co-expressed gene subsets in AAA PVAT, specifically associated with both innate and antigen-driven immune response pathways. Inhibition of these factors may represent a novel option for the development of efficient immunomodulatory strategies to treat AAA.

Keywords: gene regulatory network; transcription factors; perivascular adipose tissue; immune response; inflammation; abdominal aortic aneurysm; vascular diseases

1. Introduction

Despite intensive efforts over the last decades, abdominal aortic aneurysm (AAA) remains an elusive disease for which no effective treatment aiming to hinder or reduce its growth is yet available [1,2]. This reflects our incomplete understanding of the etiology and pathogenetic mechanisms leading to the development and evolution of AAA. Mechanistic studies mainly rely on animal models, which despite the large number of different methods available to induce an "acute" form of AAA, have not been individually able to thoroughly elucidate the pathogenesis of the disease, which instead presents a natural history characterized by a multifactorial, slow, and chronic process [3]. Thus, integration of in vivo models with knowledge from preclinical research on human patients is needed for a greater understanding of the processes underlying AAA [2].

A successful approach to dissecting complex phenotypes is molecular profiling, which allows a large-scale exploration of pathological processes in diseased tissues without the need for an a priori selection of the factors to be tested; therefore, it is potentially capable of uncovering new and unrecognized causes of disease onset or progression [4,5]. We have recently used this approach to explore the transcriptome of the perivascular adipose tissue (PVAT) in patients with abdominal aortic diseases [6,7]. PVAT has received growing interest in the study of large artery diseases, either because it has a fundamental role in the regulation of vascular physiology [8–10] or because its dysfunction is recognized to affect the development of both dilated and atherosclerotic aortic diseases [11]. Indeed, by comparing the adipose layer of a dilated abdominal aorta with that of a non-dilated aortic neck in each patient, we revealed locally restricted gene expression patterns characterizing the dilated PVAT of AAA. Overall, these genes were functionally associated with inflammatory and innate or adaptive immune responses, which along with other relevant pathways, including cell-death and extracellular matrix degradation, led us to hypothesize that AAA is an immunological disease with a possible underlying autoimmune component [6]. However, the regulatory elements underlying the pivotal pathogenetic processes associated with PVAT in AAA patients remained to be defined.

Reverse engineering from RNA expression data is a valuable and grounded approach that allows reconstruction of gene regulatory networks by identifying cis-regulatory elements, which are the targets of sequence-specific transcription factors (TFs) [12,13]. TFs are often defined as the master regulators of cellular processes because they can control the simultaneous expression of many genes at once [14]. TFs regulate the transcription of their target genes by interacting with other TFs and co-factors to constitute transcriptional complexes, but can also be directly targeted by other regulators acting upstream of the TFs, e.g., protein kinases. Identifying cis-regulatory elements and their respective TFs from co-expressed genes can, thus, provide important insights into the regulatory mechanism affecting a specific biological process.

In the present work, we aimed to identify the regulators that may control the most prominent pathogenetic processes we found associated with PVAT in AAA patients. For this purpose, we first applied a reverse engineering approach on co-expressed genes, distinguishing the dilated PVAT (diseased) from the non-dilated (healthy) aortic neck to find cis-regulatory elements and associated TFs. Then, we sought upstream regulators that could directly affect (e.g., activate) the TFs identified above or help form transcriptional complexes. Finally, exploring the topological properties of the resulting regulatory network, we outlined the most likely putative targets for AAA interference treatment options.

2. Materials and Methods

2.1. Study Population and Gene Expression Data

This study relies on the cohort of 30 AAA patients characterized in the previous study by Piacentini et al. [6]. Patient features, including demographic data, risk factors, medications, and exclusion criteria, have been extensively described in the aforementioned work. AAA patients enrolled in the study underwent elective surgery at the Centro Cardiologico Monzino IRCCS, Milan, Italy, between 2010 and 2014. Elective repair of AAA was done in compliance with the international and national guidelines for the care and treatment of AAA [15,16]. From each patient, adipose tissue specimens were collected at the time of surgery, which included the periaortic adipose tissue obtained from the aortic neck proximal to the aneurismal sac (non-dilated PVAT) and periaortic adipose tissue surrounding the aneurysmal sac (dilated PVAT).

The expression data produced in the study have been made publicly available at the NCBI's GEO repository and can be accessed at https://www.ncbi.nlm.nih.gov/geo/query/acc.cgi?acc=GSE119717.

2.2. Selection of Differentially Expressed (DE) Genes in Dilated PVAT of AAA

Based on our previous results, we selected 172 unique genes positively associated with dilated AAA, corresponding to the most significant set of DE probes (transcripts), which distinguished dilated (diseased) from non-dilated (healthy) PVAT. Supplementary Data 1a shows the annotation of these 172

DE genes. We used these DE genes as the seed gene list for the identification of cis-regulatory elements and candidate TFs.

2.3. Identification of Cis-Regulatory Elements and TFs

To identify regulatory elements, we relied on a reverse engineering approach to infer transcriptional regulatory network underlying the 172 DE genes by cis-regulatory sequence analysis. This analysis was performed in the Cytoscape environment v3.7.1 [17] through the iRegulon software v1.3 [18]. Briefly, iRegulon performs a "rank-and-recovery" procedure. The ranking step allows genes (RefSeq annotation) to be ranked for a library of positional weight matrices (PWMs), which represent matrices of regulatory motifs. Then, for each gene a regulatory search space around the transcription start site (TSS) is scanned for homotypic cis-regulatory modules (CRM) using a hidden Markov model across multiple vertebrate species. A ranked list of genes is generated, with the most likely genomic target of a specific motif at the top of the ranking. In the recovery step, the enrichment of genes from the input gene list (i.e., DE genes) is tested against the gene rankings by calculating the area under the cumulative recovery curve (AUC) in the top of the ranking (3%), which is then normalized into a normalized enrichment score (NES). The method exploits a wide collection of 18 databases of 9713 non-redundant TF motifs and 3 databases of 1120 chromatin immunoprecipitation sequencing (ChIP-seq) signals along the genome (i.e., tracks).

Parameters used for the ranking step were: motive collection: "10K (9713 PWMs)" (i.e., the most extensive motif collections); track collection: "1120 ChIP-seq tracks (ENCODE raw signals)" (i.e., full collection of ChIP-seq data against TFs); putative regulatory region: "20 kb centered around TSS" (i.e., it may return promoter-based and/or distal regulators); motif rankings database: "20 kb centered around TSS (7 species)" (including the mammalian species *Bos taurus*, *Canis familiaris*, *Mus musculus*, *Monodelphis domestica*, *Pan troglodytes*, *Macaca mulatta*, and *Rattus norvegicus*, as well as considering the conservation among them).

Parameters for the recovery step were: enrichment score threshold = "3.0" (raising the post-hoc threshold to 3.5); receiver operating characteristic (ROC) threshold for AUC calculation = "0.03"; rank threshold = "5000"; minimum identity between orthologous genes = "0"; maximum false discovery rate (FDR) on motif similarity = "0.001".

Resulting motifs and tracks were ranked according to NES and labeled with the motif or track identifier (ID) of their original database. Motifs that shared a higher level of similarity were grouped into clusters using the default method (see [19]). The motif-to-TF association procedure for the algorithm, based on motif similarity and orthology, returns the TFs that more likely bind to the enriched motif. The TFs with the highest levels of confidence (i.e., TFs recorded as having a direct annotation, meaning that the PWM was determined for a certain TF in that species) were selected as the most reliable candidate TFs for each cluster of motifs or tracks.

2.4. Inferring the TFs' Upstream Regulatory Factors

To infer regulatory modules upstream of the "hub" candidate TFs, additional proteins that directly connect to TFs were firstly identified (i) by using experimentally reported protein–protein interactions (PPI) or protein complexes; and then (ii) by identifying protein kinases regulating the above extended transcriptional complexes. The Expression2kinase (X2K) software v1.6.1207 [20] was used with default parameters for both protein network expansion and kinase retrieval, except for the "allow a maximum of 10,000 node links from a node", "allow a maximum of 100,000 interactions from an article", and "allow a minimum of 1 article reporting a specific interaction" options, which were enabled to ensure a higher quality of interactions in outputted additional proteins. The method for drawing PPI exploits experimentally validated mammalian interactions from 18 databases containing more than 24,000 proteins and almost 390,000 interactions. The kinase–substrate interactions are instead from other sources for a consolidated dataset of 14,374 interactions from more than 3400 publications on 436 kinases (see [20] for details).

2.5. Topological Analysis

Topological analysis was performed on two different networks through Network Analyzer v3.3.2 [21] and CentiScape 2.2 software [22] into the Cytoscape environment v3.7.1. The first analyzed network was the whole regulatory network (cf. Figure 2) drawn to connect candidate TFs (regulators; source nodes) with their target DE genes (regulated; target nodes). This facilitated visual inspection of clusters of shared and unique target regulated genes and their relationships. To disentangle the complexity of the network and to find the most relevant "hub" TFs, three centrality measures, i.e., connectivity degree (aka degree), betweenness, and radiality, were evaluated. The higher the values of these topological indexes among nodes, the higher the relevance of a specific node in the network in relation to the others [23]. TFs ranked in the upper tertile for the three centrality measures were selected as the "hub" master regulators.

The second topological analysis was performed on the regulatory transcriptional complex network made of "hub" TFs, additional or intermediate proteins, and upstream kinases (cf. Figure 3). The network was treated as a directed network because the regulator–regulated target relationships were highlighted by directed edges. Measures of in-going and out-going direct connections (edges) of a node were defined as the in-degree and out-degree, respectively. Additionally, radiality, stress, betweenness, bridging, centroid, closeness, eccentricity, eigenvector centralities were also assessed. The relevance of the topological index for each node was weighted through the z-score calculation, which assesses how a specific observation (node) moves away from the mean of the total observations, measured in terms of standard deviations from the mean. A node with a z-score ≥2 was deemed as very relevant for that topological index.

For an easier interpretation of topological indexes [22,23], it should be considered that nodes with a large degree of connectivity are defined as "hubs", since they are likely crucial factors that might play key (e.g., causative) roles in the biological context (e.g., disease) of interest [24,25]. Nodes with high betweenness (and with similar but not equal stress, bridging, closeness, and eigenvector values) are defined as "bottlenecks", which are likely important factors that can hold together communicating proteins or genes and which might be relevant as organizing (or very central) regulatory molecules [26]. Nodes with high eccentricity show how easily a protein or gene can be functionally influenced by all other proteins or genes in the network. High centroid values instead show those nodes that are functionally able to organize subclusters of proteins or genes, thus possibly coordinating the activity of nodes with high connectivity. A node with high radiality, high eccentricity, and high closeness provides a consistent indication that it plays a central position in the network.

2.6. Linking Transcriptional Complex Clusters with AAA Pathogenetic Biological Functions

Functional association of transcriptional complex clusters (each including a subset of the seed list of DE genes and additional or intermediate proteins and kinases) with AAA pathogenetic biological processes or pathways was performed by measuring the overlap of the transcriptional complex cluster gene sets with the results of the original gene set enrichment analysis (GSEA; see Supplementary Materials of [6]). The collection of transcriptional complex cluster gene sets was generated in the Gene Matrix Transposed file format (*.gmt) and imported into the Enrichment Map software v3.2.1 [27] to visualize and measure the overlap of these gene sets with the enrichment network drawn from GSEA, which displayed all of the significant Gene Ontology–biological process (GO-BP) orpathway gene sets that were suggested to be pathogenically associated with dilated PVAT in AAA. The consistency of the overlap was tested through a hypergeometric test. Associations were deemed to be significant for adjusted p-values < 0.01 (Benjamini–Hochberg method for multiple testing correction) and with a gene set overlap corresponding to ≥5% of the genes for each specific transcriptional complex cluster. To facilitate visualization of the most significant relationships of each transcriptional complex cluster with their associated GO-BP or pathways, an enrichment subnetwork was subsequently generated.

3. Results

For this work, we selected the 172 unique genes we found overexpressed in dilated PVAT compared with non-dilated PVAT in AAA patients (see Supplementary Materials of [6]). Gene annotation is reported in Data Supplement 1a. These genes were positively associated with the layer of adipose tissue surrounding the dilated (diseased) abdominal aorta and included several factors of the inflammatory and immune responses, which were claimed as being the most relevant for the pathogenesis of AAA [28,29]. We, thus, sought the regulatory sequence motifs (i.e., target gene nucleotide sequences used to control its expression) and tracks (i.e., ChIP-seq signals along the genome) for these 172 genes and reconstructed a gene regulatory network.

3.1. Identification of Motifs and Tracks of Genes Over-Expressed in Dilated PVAT of AAA Patients

By cis-regulatory sequence analysis, which leverages the use of combined multiple collections of motifs and tracks, we identified 30 motifs and 1 track with NES values >3.5 and AUC values >0.06. The selected NES and AUC thresholds were chosen to reduce the probability of recovering false-positive associations, which would, therefore, ensure more robust and accurate results [18]. Exploring the motif enrichment results, we observed that subgroups of the 30 motifs showed a high sequence overlap, which were, thus, grouped into 8 different clusters based on similarity (M1 to 8; Data Supplement 1b). Notably, each cluster included one TF with a direct annotation, which represents the highest level of confidence for a motif-to-TF association. Thus, we ranked the TF with the direct annotation as the most reliable candidate TF for each related motif or track cluster (Table 1, Figure 1, and Data Supplement 1b).

Table 1. Summary of enriched motifs and tracks aggregated in clusters.

Cluster	TF	NES	AUC	# Targets	# Motifs/Tracks
M1	TBP	6.20	0.098	74	5
M2	NFKB1	5.91	0.095	91	7
T1	CHD1	5.23	0.130	29	1
M3	SPIB	5.12	0.085	104	4
M4	SRF	4.66	0.080	53	6
M5	BCL6	4.14	0.074	55	3
M6	PAX3	4.07	0.073	48	2
M7	ATF2	3.58	0.068	46	1
M8	CEBPE	3.53	0.067	50	2

Transcription factors (TFs) with direct annotation, normalized enrichment score (NES), and area under the cumulative recovery curve (AUC) values refer to the highest enriched motif or track of each cluster. Motif (M) and track (T) clusters are ordered by NES. #, number of.

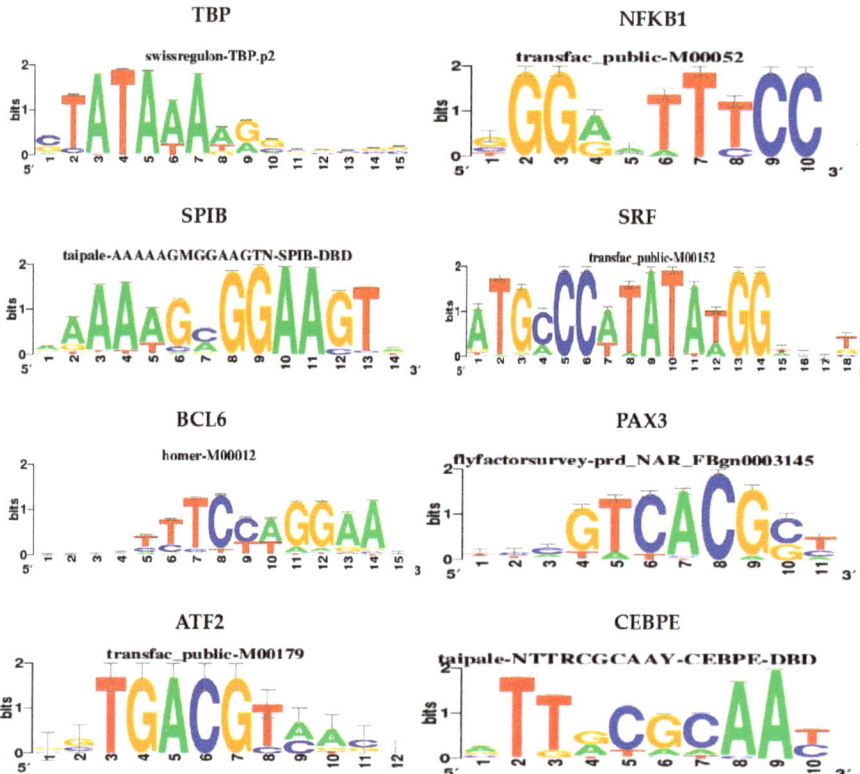

Figure 1. Target nucleotide sequences. Logos of cis-regulatory elements corresponding to the highest enriched motif of each cluster are shown. Motif IDs are reported on top of each sequence. The logo for tracks, i.e., CHD1, is not available.

3.1.1. Regulatory Network of TFs and Over-Expressed Genes in Dilated PVAT

To visually explore the relationships between candidate TFs and their relative target genes, we drew a gene regulatory network consisting of TFs as source nodes, presenting direct evidence for significant motifs with the highest NES values, as well as the DE genes as target nodes (Figure 2). The network shows the complex relationships between TFs and their targets, with TFs displaying both shared and unique target genes.

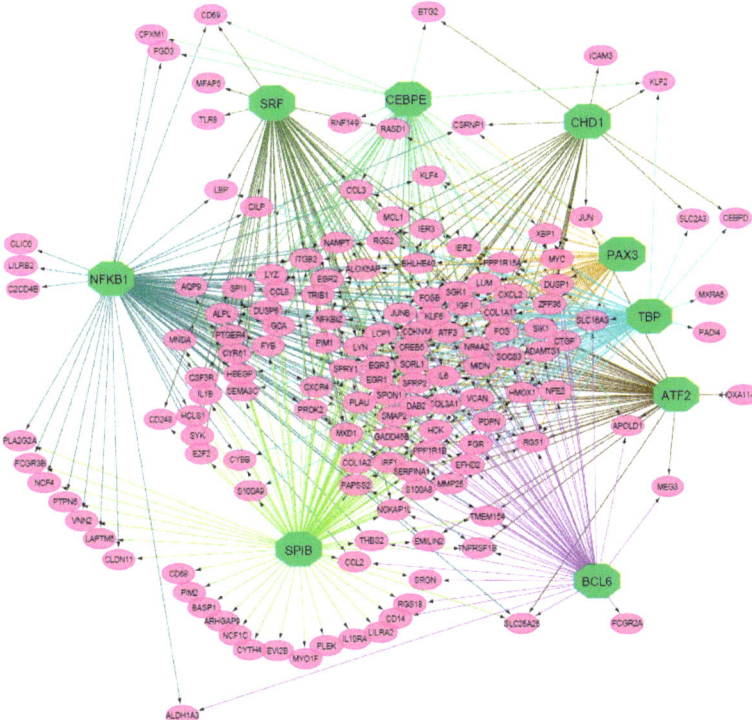

Figure 2. Gene regulatory network. The network shows the connectivity between candidate transcription factors (source nodes; green hexagons) and differentially expressed (DE) genes (target nodes; pink ovals). Edge color refers to clusters of DE genes based on the connections to a specific TF.

3.1.2. Selection of "hub" TFs through Topological Analysis

Although all of the identified TFs presented a significant association with DE genes, we tried to figure out the regulatory elements that more likely associate with the most relevant pathogenetic processes in dilated PVAT of AAA. For this purpose, we applied a network topology analysis to identify TFs representing the most relevant "hub" in the whole regulatory network. With this approach, we found that three TFs, i.e., TBP, NFKB1, and SPIB, displayed the highest values for all the assessed topological centrality measures (Table 2). The advantage of this approach is that we could extract key TFs by taking into account both the statistics of motif and track identification and TF "centrality" ranking in a complex gene regulatory network. In particular, the degree index indicates the relevance that SPIB, NFKB1, and TBP have within the network—they displayed the highest connectivity by interacting with large numbers of the 172 DE genes (104, 91, and 74, respectively), suggesting a central regulatory role.

Table 2. Summary of topological indexes used to evaluate the centrality of each candidate TF in the reconstructed gene regulatory network.

TF (Cluster)	Degree	Betweenness Centrality	Radiality
SPIB (M3)	104	0.36	3.41
NFKB1 (M2)	91	0.22	3.24
TBP (M1)	74	0.14	3.02
BCL6 (M5)	55	0.08	2.77
SRF (M4)	53	0.08	2.75
CEBPE (M8)	50	0.08	2.71
PAX3 (M6)	48	0.05	2.68
ATF2 (M7)	46	0.06	2.65
CHD1 (T1)	29	0.04	2.43

Candidate transcription factors (TFs) of each cluster are ranked by degree. The selected "hub" TFs are highlighted with bold characters.

3.2. Identification of Transcriptional Complexes and Upstream Regulators

We refined our search for regulatory molecules by including those that physically connect to and act on the identified "hub" TFs. To this end, we first extended the regulatory network by retrieving intermediate direct interactors of SPIB, NFKB1, and TBP, and by drawing putative transcriptional complexes. Then, we inferred upstream protein kinases that could regulate those transcriptional complexes.

3.2.1. Connecting Additional Proteins to TFs through Protein–Protein Interactions (PPI)

By leveraging experimentally validated PPI, we identified 28 intermediate proteins (annotated in Data Supplement 1d) directly linked to SPIB, NFKB1, and TBP. Then, we drew a directional network to show the relationships (i.e., from regulator-to-regulated target) among the "hub" TFs and all the retrieved intermediate proteins (Figure 3). NKFB1 and TBP displayed the highest direct connections, with 8 out-degree (outcoming connections) and 19 in-degree (incoming connections) and with 12 out-degree and 15 in-degree connections, respectively. SPIB presented 4 out- and 3 in-degree connections but displayed a direct edge towards TBP, suggesting that their possible interaction constitutes a transcriptional complex together with other proteins. Notably, we found 18 other TFs among the additional proteins (i.e., AR, BCL3, CEBPB, CREBBP, E2F1, ELF3, ESR1, FOS, JUN, KLF5, NCOA1, NCOA6, NR3C1, REL, RELA, RXRA, SP1, and SPI1), which may participate in forming such transcriptional complexes (Figure 3; green ovals). Consistently, some of them were also predicted to associate with motif clusters M2 (i.e., BCL3, E2F1, REL, RELA), M3 (i.e., SPI1), and M8 (i.e., CEBPB; cf. Data Supplement 1b), strengthening the idea that these TFs may cooperate with "hub" TFs to target common sequence motifs and coordinate transcription of DE genes. Furthermore, relying on the Transcription co-Factor DataBase (TcoF-DB) [30], we could annotate 7 proteins that act as transcriptional co-factors (i.e., that may regulate transcription by interacting with TFs), but in contrast to TFs these do not bind directly to regulatory DNA regions (Figure 3; orange ovals). Six of them (i.e., CTNNB1, HDAC1, HMGB1, RUVBL2, SIN3A, and TRIP4) have experimental evidence for both involvement in transcriptional regulation and for presence in the cell nucleus (classified as class high-confidence); RUVBL1 has evidence: inferred from electronic annotation" (classified as class 2) for involvement in transcriptional regulation.

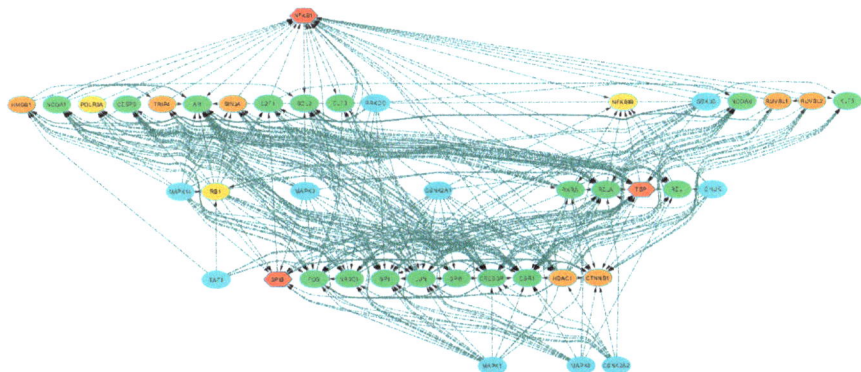

Figure 3. Extended regulatory network. The network shows the relationships (directed dashed edges) among the hub transcriptional factors, the additional proteins inferred by protein–protein interactions, and the most significant kinases identified by kinase enrichment analysis. Node shapes distinguish hub TFs (hexagon) from all the other inferred proteins (ovals). Node colors reflect node types or functions: hub TFs = red; inferred TFs = green; kinases = light blue; TcoFs = orange; inferred molecules with other functions = light orange. Also see Data Supplement 1d for detailed annotation.

3.2.2. Identification of Protein Kinases Upstream Transcriptional Complexes.

The expansion of the network to protein–TF interactions allowed an increase of the number of possible regulatory molecules that can influence specific functions in the dilated PVAT of AAA. The search for further kinase–substrate interactions can add an upstream level of control of gene expression and helps to identify key target regulators. Indeed, by kinase enrichment analysis, we found 42 associations with protein kinases (nominal p-values < 0.01), of which 28 stood correction for multiple testing (adjusted p-values < 0.01; Data Supplement 1c). To focus on the most significant kinases, we selected those that were ranked in the upper tertile of the distribution according to the "combined score", i.e., CHUK, CSNK2A1, CSNK2A2, GSK3B, MAPK1, MAPK14, MAPK3, MAPK8, PRKDC, and TAF1 (Figure 3, light blue ovals; annotation in Data Supplement 1d).

Network analysis showed that CHUK, CSNK2A1, GSK3B, and PRKDC were directly associated with NFKB1; TAF1 targeted TBP; and CSNK2A1, CSNK2A2, GSK3B, MAPK3, MAPK8, and MAPK14 interacted with SPIB. Specifically, GSK3B, MAPK1, and CSNK2A1 displayed the highest out-degree values (17, 15, and 13, respectively), which suggests that they can be functionally relevant for most of the protein–TF interactions in the regulatory network.

3.2.3. Topological Analysis of Regulatory Transcriptional-Complex

Topological analysis of the regulatory transcriptional complex network (cf. Figure 3), inferred the relative importance that specific proteins and genes may have as regulators in the network (Data Supplement 1e). First, we observed that centrality measures with similar meanings were highly correlated, indicating their consistency (Figure 4). Indeed, out-degree, radiality, and closeness, which indicate the possibility that a node is functionally relevant for several others, showed high positive correlations, with Pearson's coefficient r values ranging from 0.89 to 0.99 (p-values < 0.001). Similarly, betweenness, bridging, and stress indexes, whose values if elevated suggest that a gene or protein likely connects (i.e., holds together) pivotal regulatory molecules, were positively correlated, with r values ranging from 0.65 to 0.97 (p-values < 0.001).

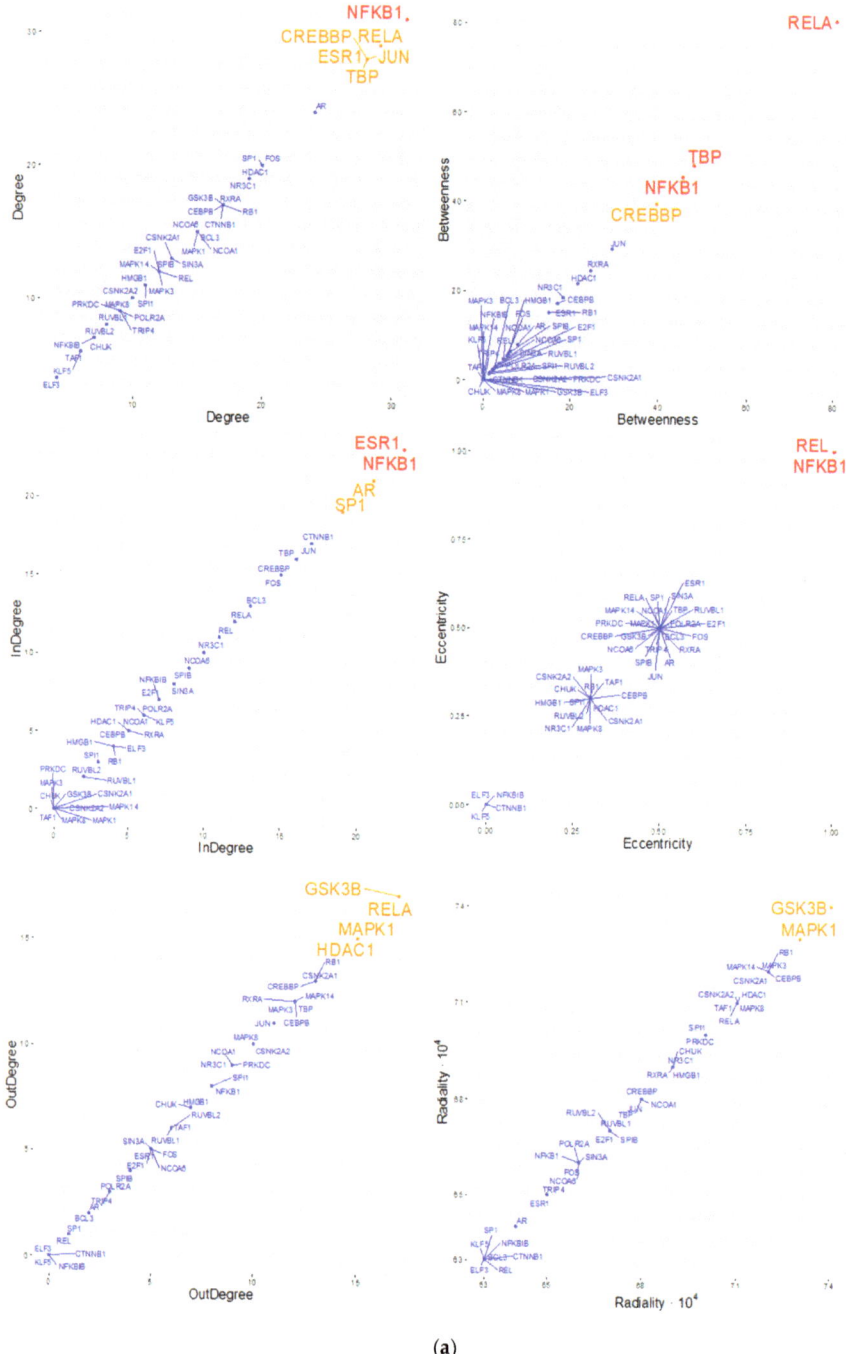

(a)

Figure 4. Cont.

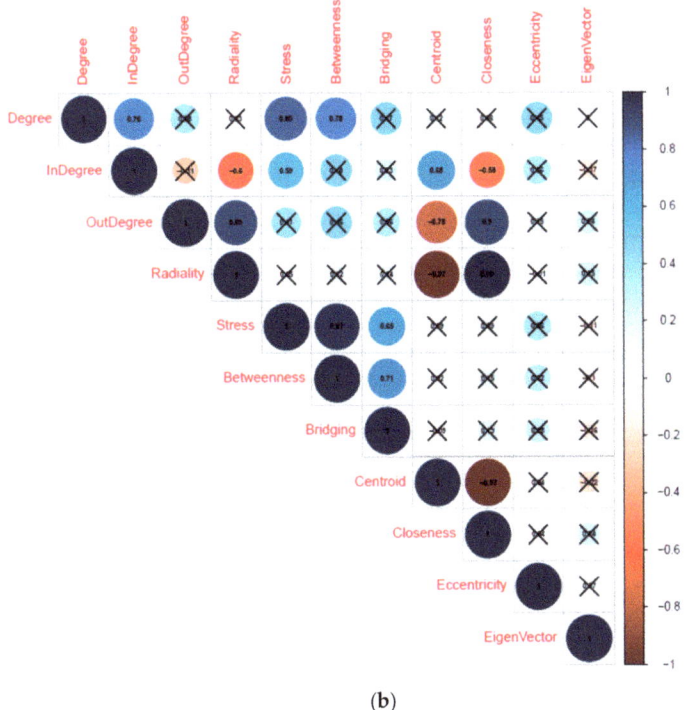

(b)

Figure 4. (a) Topological analysis of the extended regulatory network. Each panel represents the scatterplot of the index-over-index topological measures calculated for the extended regulatory network. To draw the representative scatterplots, only one index was chosen among those that were highly correlated and with very similar meanings. The presence of a non-uniform distribution of nodes, with most nodes having a low index and a few having a high index, identifies those nodes that clearly differ from the average measure of the index throughout the network (red and orange dots or labels). Red, orange, and blue colors, respectively, refer to nodes with z-scores > 2.0, between 1.5 and 2.0, and <1.5. Detailed results are reported in Data Supplement 1e. (b) Correlation plot of the topological indexes. Indexes with similar meanings show a highly significant Pearson's correlation (p-values < 0.001). Numbers and circle sizes (from smaller to bigger) refer to correlation coefficient r values. Positive and negative correlations are displayed by a gradient color from white (low) to blue (high) and from white (low) to red (high), respectively. To simplify visualization, crosses mark non-significant correlations.

Specifically, we showed that NFKB1 showed the highest degree (total connectivity), in-degree, and eccentricity, suggesting that it is likely affected by the activity of many other proteins. Interestingly, REL, which is part of the well-known NK-kB complex together with NFKB1, has high eccentricity as well, although with lower global connectivity. NFKB1 also presents high betweenness and stress, suggesting the capability to hold together communicating proteins and to play a role as an organizing regulatory molecule. Similarly, RELA, which is also a subunit of the NF-kB complex, has the highest betweenness, stress, and bridging centrality values, leading to the hypothesis that it can serve in an organizing module along with NFKB1, "bridging" another possible set of regulatory proteins. For example, RELA targets TBP, which also displays very high betweenness and stress indexes and may serve as a central regulatory protein. Another remarkable finding concerns the role of MAPK1. Indeed, we can postulate that MAPK1 could be functionally essential for several other proteins, as indicated by its eigenvector index, out-degree (n = 15), and high closeness and radiality values compared to the mean of the network, which overall suggests a prominent regulatory role for this kinase in the network. Similarly, GSK3B showed a high out-degree ($n = 17$), radiality, and closeness over the network mean. Together these results provide a consistent suggestion that both MAPK1 and GSK3B kinases might have central regulatory roles in the network. CREBBP, as with NFKB1, RELA, and TBP, showed a high-stress index, indicating that it may be functionally relevant in connecting other regulatory molecules. CREBBP presents a high total degree of connectivity (15 in-degree and 13 out-degree connections), with a direct connection towards NFKB1 and incoming connections from RELA and SPIB. TBP displayed high stress and betweenness, which underlie its important roles as a "hub" TF and an organizing regulatory protein. Finally, RXRA showed the most consistent bridging index together with RELA, indicating its possible role as a connector of other central regulatory proteins. Indeed, RXRA is directly linked to very central proteins, such as the TFs NFKB1, RELA, and TBP, and the kinases MAPK1 and GSK3B. In line with this, we observed that the connection between RELA and RXRA showed the highest "edge-betweenness" value (33; with network mean ± SD = 8 ± 5, over 311 total edges), which indicates that this connection separates highly interconnected subgraph clusters.

3.3. Association of Regulatory Subnetworks with AAA Pathogenetic Pathways

We eventually built the entire regulatory network obtained by reverse engineering, including DE genes, candidate TFs, intermediate protein interactors, and upstream kinase regulators. By selecting the first neighbors of each "hub" TF throughout the network, we generated three "transcriptional clusters" to infer specific functional association with AAA-related pathways. This approach allowed matching each transcriptional cluster with those GO-BP or pathways associated with dysfunctional PVAT that could have a pathogenetic role in the development or progression of AAA (see Supplementary Materials in [6]). The significance of the overlapping genes, which measure the consistency of the association between each transcriptional cluster and specific GO-BP pathways, was estimated through a hypergeometric test. We found 69, 54, and 32 GO-BP pathways with a significant number of genes overlapping those of the transcriptional clusters of NFKB1, SPIB, and TBP, respectively (adjusted I-values < 0.01 and overlap size threshold ≥ 5% for the genes of the transcriptional cluster; Data Supplement 2). Interestingly, the 3 transcriptional clusters presented both shared unique associations with pathogenetic GO-BP pathways. To summarize results and reduce redundancy of the overlapping GO-BP pathways, we drew an enrichment network (Figure 5). We found that the NFKB1 transcriptional cluster was uniquely associated with "regulation of lymphocytes proliferation" (specifically T-cells), "regulation of protein secretion", and "vasculature development". The SPIB transcriptional cluster was univocally associated with "regulation of phagocytosis", "granulocyte or neutrophil chemotaxis", "humoral immune response", and "Fc receptor-mediated signaling". TBP displayed a distinctive association with "regulation of cytokine's biosynthetic process". NFKB1 and TBP transcriptional clusters shared GO-BP pathways involved in TLR signaling (in particular, TRAF6-mediated induction of NFkB and MAP kinases upon endosomal TLR activation) and in the regulation of the JAK/STAT cascade. NFKB1 and SPIB transcriptional clusters shared GO-BP pathways involved in the regulation of lymphocyte activation and differentiation and inflammatory response, as well as in leukocyte cell–cell adhesion. Finally, we found common GO-BP pathways between the three transcriptional clusters, e.g., "response to molecule of bacterial origin", "leukocyte chemotaxis", "regulation of ERK1 and ERK2 cascade", and "IL-4 and IL-13 signaling".

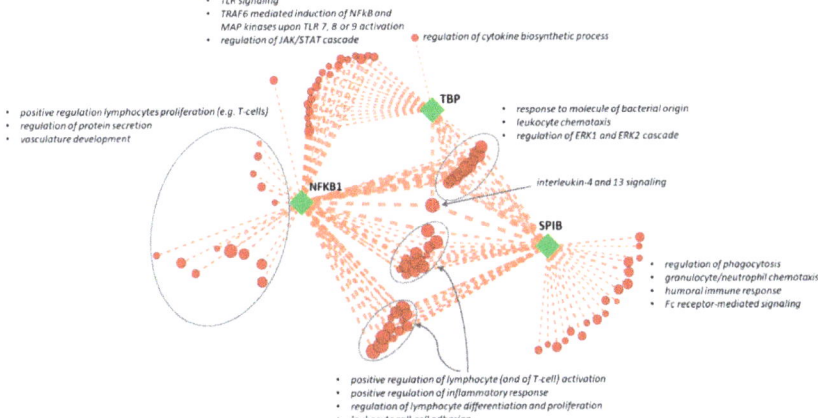

Figure 5. Enrichment network of transcriptional clusters. NFKB1, SPIB, and TBP transcriptional clusters (squared green nodes) and pathogenetic Gene Ontology–biological process (GO-BP) pathways associated with abdominal aortic aneurysm perivascular adipose tissue (red nodes) are connected by dashed orange edges, which indicate significant overlaps between two gene sets. Edge thickness (from thinner to thicker) is proportional to the number of overlapping genes. GO-BP pathway node colors (from lighter to darker) and sizes (from smallest to bigger) are proportional to the original normalized enrichment score calculated by gene set enrichment analysis. Groups of redundant gene sets were manually circled and labeled by relevant overview GO-BP pathways terms.

4. Discussion

The pathogenic mechanisms responsible for AAA formation and expansion are largely unknown. PVAT is a well-known vessel homeostasis regulator that can have a major role in vascular disease pathogenesis [11,31]. Mounting evidence suggests that dysfunctional PVAT may play a role in vascular diseases, including AAA development [32]. To date, large-scale gene expression profiling of AAA has been carried out only on full-thickness aortic walls, excluding the adipose layer of the vessel [33]. Through genome-wide expression studies, we have recently gained insights into the important role that PVAT can play in both atherosclerotic and non-atherosclerotic abdominal aortic diseases in humans [6,7]. In AAA patients, our data suggested that an altered immune response in PVAT, alongside other concurring mechanisms, is a crucial pathogenetic element that leads to the progression of AAA, and ultimately to its rupture, by amplifying inflammation and degenerative mechanisms (e.g., loss of aorta structural integrity) [6].

With this work, we inferred the regulatory molecules that govern the most prominent pathogenetic processes in PVAT of AAA patients. Our study consistently shows that subsets of co-expressed genes characterizing the diseased PVAT in AAA present common cis-regulatory elements, which are the targets of specific TFs.

The reconstruction of regulatory networks proves to be particularly enlightening, as the disease phenotype is only occasionally the result of a single gene or protein effector, but is more commonly the combination of multiple pathobiological effectors acting together in complex relationships [24]. Analyzing molecular networks through their topological properties can help to identify both crucial disease genes (hubs) and potential drug targets [24,34]. However, it is worth noting that pharmacological targets are not necessarily the network "hub nodes", because these are often essential factors with a strong influence on the phenotype of the cell or organism. Hub genes or proteins should be targeted only in particular subsets of cells with a strong and direct pathogenetic role. Otherwise, interference with the activity of essential genes may influence physiological processes that are crucial to the normal functioning of the organism. On the contrary, proteins that act as connectors (or presenting lower degrees of connectivity) have a lower impact on the overall structure of the network, thus resulting in likely safer candidate disease targets [35,36].

We identified SPIB, NFKB1, and TBP (i.e., "hub" TFs) as the master regulators of the resulting gene regulatory network, as they have the largest connectivity with the co-expressed genes associated with diseased PVAT. Therefore, we hypothesized that these TFs could be responsible for regulating the most impactful pathogenetic mechanisms of dysfunctional PVAT in AAA patients. Additionally, we identified additional proteins that can directly interact with the "hub" TFs to form transcriptional complexes, as well as protein kinases that can regulate the state of activation of "hub" TFs and transcriptional complexes.

We showed that the transcriptional clusters of SPIB, NFKB1, and TBP have strong functional associations with mechanisms of the innate and adaptive immune response, which we assumed to be the main drivers of the (auto)immune mechanisms in AAA PVAT. Specifically, we associated the NFKB1 transcriptional cluster with the positive regulation of lymphocyte proliferation, and together with TBP with the expression of genes involved in the innate immune response, i.e., the toll-like receptor (TLR) signaling. This is consistent with the well-known role of NF-kB complex activation in guiding both lymphocyte function, including cell proliferation and differentiation [37], and TLR signaling [38], which ultimately ends in NF-kB-triggered downstream transcription of genes that allow for an effective response to primary stimuli, such as antigens (or self-antigens) and danger- or pathogen-associated molecular patterns [39]. Additionally, NFKB1, REL, and RELA may differently combine to form heterodimers and carry out both unique and overlapping roles in T-cell proliferation during different stages of the cell cycle [40]. The relevance of the NF-kB complex in AAA pathogenesis has already been shown in vivo AAA-induced models. Activation of the NF-kB complex has been proposed as a key factor inducing macrophage infiltration and osteoclastogenic differentiation [41,42] and affecting the inflammatory response in other cell types (e.g., vascular smooth muscle cells and mesenchymal cells) [43,44], ultimately leading to aortic inflammation and vessel wall degeneration. Nonetheless, our data suggest that lymphocyte activation and proliferation mechanisms could be crucial for amplifying the local antigen-driven immune response in the PVAT of AAA patients. Interfering with NK-kB signaling [45] in immune cells may, thus, have a significant impact on the evolution of AAA. Although immune-suppressive treatment should be carefully evaluated [46], selectively inhibiting NF-kB signaling in activated and proliferating lymphocytes in dysfunctional AAA PVAT may be a targeted therapeutic intervention without compromising the healthy effect mediated by NF-kB in other immune cells.

Mechanisms of the innate and adaptive immune response can also be mediated by SPIB and its cognate SPI1, which we found to be directly connected to SPIB in the regulatory network. Both SPIB and SPI1 are required for all of the signaling pathways by which B-lymphocytes sense and respond to local environmental stimuli, including antigens and molecules acting through TLRs [47]. Accordingly, we found that the SPIB transcriptional cluster was associated with response to TLR engagement, humoral immunity, and lymphocyte activation in PVAT of AAA. Interestingly, we also found a significant association with Fcγ receptor signaling, which underlies a localized antigen-specific humoral immune response. This signaling mechanism can be activated by B cells or neutrophils in the presence of immunoglobulin–antigen aggregates [48,49], and has been involved in the pathogenesis of AAA [50]. The downregulation of Fc receptor actions has been proposed as a therapeutic approach for other inflammatory and autoimmune diseases [51]. Targeting Fc receptor signaling regulators by manipulating the SPIB/SPI1 complex could be tested to block or minimize the local self-sustaining chronic inflammation observed in AAA PVAT.

Evaluating topological indexes of the extended regulatory network, we found that the protein kinases MAPK1 and GSK3B and the nuclear receptor RXRA (a type of retinoid X receptor) appear to play key roles in AAA pathogenetic mechanisms, and thus may be intended for interference therapy, as they are "non-hub" connecting proteins that could regulate signaling through the "hub" TFs. Both MAPKs and GSK3s have been recognized as having considerable roles in the immune response. MAPKs are strongly involved in innate immunity, including signaling related to TLRs [52]. Additionally, the

MAPK/ERK pathway is an important modulator of matrix metalloproteinases during AAA formation in in vivo models, and its inhibition could represent a possible therapeutic approach to prevent AAA formation [53]. Consistently, we found that NFKB1, SPIB, and TBP transcriptional clusters were associated with the regulation of ERK1 and ERK2 cascade in the PVAT, reinforcing the concept that specific protein kinases play central roles in the regulation of inflammation and immune response in AAA. A direct role of GSK3s in AAA pathogenesis has not been established, although GSK3s were shown to regulate the production of pro- and anti-inflammatory cytokines and to influence the proliferation, differentiation, and survival of T-cells. GSK3s mainly work through the regulation of critical transcription factors, including NF-kB, the inhibition of which has been proposed for the treatment of several pathological conditions with underlying altered immune responses in animal models [54]. Evidence concerning the roles of retinoid X receptors in AAA is also limited [55]. It has been proposed that RXR activation may have a beneficial role in AAA by inhibiting the angiotensin type 1 receptor in vascular smooth muscle cells, a factor which is known to affect AAA development in angiotensin II–induced AAA models [56]. However, RXRA is also known to be involved in the regulation of innate immunity [57], and thus its inhibition could suppress immune-mediated pathogenetic mechanisms in AAA PVAT.

Since SPIB, TBP, MAPK1, GSK3B, and RXRA have not yet been associated with AAA in humans, they may be considered as newly identified targets for disease treatment.

Other proteins or kinases with less connectivity in the regulatory network may be potential therapeutic targets for AAA [35]. An example is histone deacetylase 1 (HDCA1), which despite its low centrality in our regulatory network, directly interacts with both NFKB1 and TBP, and thus might be considered as a possible target for interference treatments. Consistently, the use of HDACs inhibitors has been demonstrated to be effective in in vivo AAA models and has been proposed for treatment in humans [58]. Notably, HDACs have many TFs as natural substrates, including NF-kB, and are well-known regulators of the T-cell immune response. HDAC inhibition enhances T-regulatory cell survival and immune-modulating functions, and affects the development of T-cell response, including T-cell proliferation in response to antigen stimulation [59].

In summary, innate and adaptive immune responses are characterized by complex crosstalking mechanisms [60] and are both involved in AAA pathogenesis [28]. Additionally, communication between perivascular adipocytes and immune cells may also play a role in these complex relationships. For example, adipocytes secrete soluble factors (e.g., adipokines, chemokine, or pro-inflammatory interleukins), which may trigger signaling pathways in target cells involving the activation of the NF-kB complex, among others. Immune cells, in turn, produce inflammatory molecules and recognize antigens presented by the class I or II human leukocyte antigens (HLAs) expressed on adipocytes [8,61,62].

Innovative strategies for treating AAA may include both immune modulation to stimulate local anti-inflammatory mechanisms and targeting of specific pathogenetic lymphocytes and their interactions with other cells, such as antigen-presenting cells [63–65]. In our previous research, while showing that the activation of several pathways can contribute to the evolution of the disease, we assumed that immune response processes were essential to sustain a chronic inflammatory cycle that characterizes AAA, since they were involved in both the early and later stages of AAA [6]. It is tempting to speculate that interventions on these specific pathogenetic pathways could be therapeutically beneficial, because they could limit the main harmful mechanism that appears to be necessary for all phases of AAA. Notably, an immune phenotyping analysis in human AAA samples recently found that T-lymphocytes are the primary cell leukocyte population in AAA, with the largest concentration in PVAT, and that these PVAT-associated T-lymphocytes correlated with the severity of the disease [66]. Assessing the presence of a locally restricted, antigen-driven clonal expansion in PVAT of AAA could, thus, be the goal of future studies, which will allow for the precise detection of pathogenic lymphocytes for direct interference treatment [45], possibly through the above-suggested disease gene targets.

To our knowledge, this is the first study that describes the regulatory elements that may contribute to controlling the major pathogenetic processes observed in PVAT of AAA patients. Our study takes advantage of a reverse engineering approach that emerged as a valuable tool for elucidating cellular function and dysregulation in pathological contexts, and which promises to increase our ability to identify potential therapeutic targets and disease biomarkers as well [13].

Our work also has limitations. It relies on inferential analysis and suggests putative sensitive AAA target genes, for which formal evidence should still be provided showing that they can be used for effective interference treatments. Furthermore, our work has focused on the potential regulators of the most significant overexpressed genes restricted to the diseased PVAT of our AAA patient cohort, without ruling out the possibility that other regulatory mechanisms may still be important in the development and progression of the disease. Finally, we did not evaluate any possible interactions with genetic variants known to be associated with AAA [67]. However, given their putative relevance in aneurysm diseases, it may be important in future research to explore the existence of specific polymorphisms that could affect gene expression and offer insight into the molecular pathogenesis of AAA.

5. Conclusions

After a long-lasting period of research, our understanding of AAA is still in its "adolescence". Despite a clear knowledge of the pathological hallmarks, the enigmatic "trait" characterizing AAA is still unknown, and is a relentless obstacle to its overall comprehension and the potential for effective care.

The translational gap between preclinical disease models and successful clinical studies prompts the research on AAA to explore and find novel candidates for treatments. Due to its critical role in AAA pathogenesis, PVAT promises to be a reliable target for testing innovative treatment options.

With this work, we identified master regulators of prominent pathogenetic processes associated with PVAT of AAA patients, i.e., altered immune response, including antigen-specific lymphocytes activation or proliferation and TLR signaling. Through the reconstruction of a gene regulatory network and the associated upstream regulators, we also suggested novel possible targets that may be considered for locally restricted interference treatments of AAA.

Supplementary Materials: Supplementary materials can be found at http://www.mdpi.com/2227-9059/8/8/288/s1.

Author Contributions: Conceptualization, L.P.; methodology, L.P., and M.C.; formal analysis, L.P.; writing—original draft preparation, L.P. and G.I.C.; visualization, L.P. and M.C.; supervision, G.I.C.; project administration, L.P. and G.I.C. All authors have read and agreed to the published version of the manuscript.

Funding: This work was supported by the Italian Ministry of Health (Research Projects RC Nos. 2600658, 2627621, and 2631196).

Acknowledgments: We thank Rita Spirito, Claudio Saccu, and José Pablo Werba for providing original specimens.

Conflicts of Interest: The authors declare no conflict of interest.

Abbreviations

AAA	Abdominal aortic aneurysm
AUC	Area under the cumulative recovery curve
ChIP	Chromatin immunoprecipitation
DE	Differentially expressed
GO-BP	Gene Ontology–biological process
GSEA	Gene set enrichment analysis
NES	Normalized enrichment score
PWM	Positional weight matrix
PPI	Protein–protein interaction
PVAT	Perivascular adipose tissue
TcoF	Transcription co-factor
TF	Transcription factor
TLR	Toll-like receptors
TSS	Transcription start site

References

1. Golledge, J. Abdominal aortic aneurysm: Update on pathogenesis and medical treatments. *Nat. Rev. Cardiol.* **2019**, *16*, 225–242. [CrossRef] [PubMed]
2. Lindeman, J.H.; Matsumura, J.S. Pharmacologic Management of Aneurysms. *Circ. Res.* **2019**, *124*, 631–646. [CrossRef] [PubMed]
3. Poulsen, J.L.; Stubbe, J.; Lindholt, J.S. Animal Models Used to Explore Abdominal Aortic Aneurysms: A Systematic Review. *Eur. J. Vasc. Endovasc. Surg.* **2016**, *52*, 487–499. [CrossRef] [PubMed]
4. Tromp, G.; Kuivaniemi, H. Developments in genomics to improve understanding, diagnosis and management of aneurysms and peripheral artery disease. *Eur. J. Vasc. Endovasc. Surg.* **2009**, *38*, 676–682. [CrossRef] [PubMed]
5. Casamassimi, A.; Federico, A.; Rienzo, M.; Esposito, S.; Ciccodicola, A. Transcriptome Profiling in Human Diseases: New Advances and Perspectives. *Int. J. Mol. Sci.* **2017**, *18*, 1652. [CrossRef] [PubMed]
6. Piacentini, L.; Werba, J.P.; Bono, E.; Saccu, C.; Tremoli, E.; Spirito, R.; Colombo, G.I. Genome-Wide Expression Profiling Unveils Autoimmune Response Signatures in the Perivascular Adipose Tissue of Abdominal Aortic Aneurysm. *Arter. Thromb. Vasc. Biol.* **2019**, *39*, 237–249. [CrossRef]
7. Piacentini, L.; Saccu, C.; Bono, E.; Tremoli, E.; Spirito, R.; Colombo, G.I.; Werba, J.P. Gene-expression profiles of abdominal perivascular adipose tissue distinguish aortic occlusive from stenotic atherosclerotic lesions and denote different pathogenetic pathways. *Sci. Rep.* **2020**, *10*, 6245. [CrossRef]
8. Rajsheker, S.; Manka, D.; Blomkalns, A.L.; Chatterjee, T.K.; Stoll, L.L.; Weintraub, N.L. Crosstalk between perivascular adipose tissue and blood vessels. *Curr. Opin. Pharmacol.* **2010**, *10*, 191–196. [CrossRef]
9. Brown, N.K.; Zhou, Z.; Zhang, J.; Zeng, R.; Wu, J.; Eitzman, D.T.; Chen, Y.E.; Chang, L. Perivascular adipose tissue in vascular function and disease: A review of current research and animal models. *Arter. Thromb. Vasc. Biol.* **2014**, *34*, 1621–1630. [CrossRef]
10. Gil-Ortega, M.; Somoza, B.; Huang, Y.; Gollasch, M.; Fernández-Alfonso, M.S. Regional differences in perivascular adipose tissue impacting vascular homeostasis. *Trends Endocrinol. Metab.* **2015**, *26*, 367–375. [CrossRef]
11. Queiroz, M.; Sena, C.M. Perivascular adipose tissue in age-related vascular disease. *Ageing Res. Rev.* **2020**, *59*, 101040. [CrossRef] [PubMed]
12. Emmert-Streib, F.; Dehmer, M.; Haibe-Kains, B. Gene regulatory networks and their applications: Understanding biological and medical problems in terms of networks. *Front. Cell Dev. Biol.* **2014**, *2*, 38. [CrossRef] [PubMed]
13. Lefebvre, C.; Rieckhof, G.; Califano, A. Reverse-engineering human regulatory networks. *Wiley Interdiscip. Rev. Syst. Biol. Med.* **2012**, *4*, 311–325. [CrossRef] [PubMed]
14. Lambert, S.A.; Jolma, A.; Campitelli, L.F.; Das, P.K.; Yin, Y.; Albu, M.; Chen, X.; Taipale, J.; Hughes, T.R.; Weirauch, M.T. The Human Transcription Factors. *Cell* **2018**, *172*, 650–665. [CrossRef] [PubMed]
15. Moll, F.L.; Powell, J.T.; Fraedrich, G.; Verzini, F.; Haulon, S.; Waltham, M.; van Herwaarden, J.A.; Holt, P.J.E.; van Keulen, J.W.; Rantner, B.; et al. Management of abdominal aortic aneurysms clinical practice guidelines of the European society for vascular surgery. *Eur. J. Vasc. Endovasc. Surg.* **2011**, *41*, S1–S58. [CrossRef] [PubMed]
16. Italian Journal of Vascular and Endovascular Surgery 23 March 2016 (1 Suppl 1)—Minerva Medica Journals. Available online: https://www.minervamedica.it/en/journals/vascular-endovascular-surgery/issue.php?cod=R46Y2016S01 (accessed on 30 July 2020).
17. Shannon, P.; Markiel, A.; Ozier, O.; Baliga, N.S.; Wang, J.T.; Ramage, D.; Amin, N.; Schwikowski, B.; Ideker, T. Cytoscape: A Software Environment for Integrated Models of Biomolecular Interaction Networks. *Genome Res.* **2003**, *13*, 2498–2504. [CrossRef] [PubMed]
18. Janky, R.; Verfaillie, A.; Imrichová, H.; Van de Sande, B.V.; Standaert, L.; Christiaens, V.; Hulselmans, G.; Herten, K.; Sanchez, M.N.; Potier, D.; et al. iRegulon: From a Gene List to a Gene Regulatory Network Using Large Motif and Track Collections. *PLoS Comput. Biol.* **2014**, *10*, e1003731. [CrossRef]
19. Verfaillie, A.; Imrichova, H.; Janky, R.; Aerts, S. iRegulon and i-cisTarget: Reconstructing Regulatory Networks Using Motif and Track Enrichment. *Curr. Protoc. Bioinform.* **2015**, *52*, 2.16.1–2.16.39. [CrossRef]
20. Chen, E.Y.; Xu, H.; Gordonov, S.; Lim, M.P.; Perkins, M.H.; Ma'ayan, A. Expression2Kinases: mRNA profiling linked to multiple upstream regulatory layers. *Bioinformatics* **2012**, *28*, 105–111. [CrossRef]

21. Assenov, Y.; Ramírez, F.; Schelhorn, S.-E.; Lengauer, T.; Albrecht, M. Computing topological parameters of biological networks. *Bioinformatics* **2008**, *24*, 282–284. [CrossRef]
22. Scardoni, G.; Petterlini, M.; Laudanna, C. Analyzing biological network parameters with CentiScaPe. *Bioinformatics* **2009**, *25*, 2857–2859. [CrossRef] [PubMed]
23. Doncheva, N.T.; Assenov, Y.; Domingues, F.S.; Albrecht, M. Topological analysis and interactive visualization of biological networks and protein structures. *Nat. Protoc.* **2012**, *7*, 670–685. [CrossRef] [PubMed]
24. Barabási, A.-L.; Gulbahce, N.; Loscalzo, J. Network medicine: A network-based approach to human disease. *Nat. Rev. Genet.* **2011**, *12*, 56–68. [CrossRef] [PubMed]
25. Stelzl, U.; Worm, U.; Lalowski, M.; Haenig, C.; Brembeck, F.H.; Goehler, H.; Stroedicke, M.; Zenkner, M.; Schoenherr, A.; Koeppen, S.; et al. A human protein-protein interaction network: A resource for annotating the proteome. *Cell* **2005**, *122*, 957–968. [CrossRef] [PubMed]
26. Yu, H.; Kim, P.M.; Sprecher, E.; Trifonov, V.; Gerstein, M. The Importance of Bottlenecks in Protein Networks: Correlation with Gene Essentiality and Expression Dynamics. *PLoS Comput. Biol.* **2007**, *3*, e59. [CrossRef] [PubMed]
27. Merico, D.; Isserlin, R.; Stueker, O.; Emili, A.; Bader, G.D. Enrichment map: A network-based method for gene-set enrichment visualization and interpretation. *PLoS ONE* **2010**, *5*, e13984. [CrossRef]
28. Dale, M.A.; Ruhlman, M.K.; Baxter, B.T. Inflammatory cell phenotypes in AAAs: Their role and potential as targets for therapy. *Arter. Thromb. Vasc. Biol.* **2015**, *35*, 1746–1755. [CrossRef]
29. Folkesson, M.; Vorkapic, E.; Gulbins, E.; Japtok, L.; Kleuser, B.; Welander, M.; Länne, T.; Wågsäter, D. Inflammatory cells, ceramides, and expression of proteases in perivascular adipose tissue adjacent to human abdominal aortic aneurysms. *J. Vasc. Surg.* **2017**, *65*, 1171–1179.e1. [CrossRef]
30. Schmeier, S.; Alam, T.; Essack, M.; Bajic, V.B. TcoF-DB v2: Update of the database of human and mouse transcription co-factors and transcription factor interactions. *Nucleic Acids Res.* **2017**, *45*, D145–D150. [CrossRef]
31. Cao, Z.F.H.; Stoffel, E.; Cohen, P. Role of Perivascular Adipose Tissue in Vascular Physiology and Pathology. *Hypertension* **2017**, *69*, 770–777. [CrossRef]
32. Horimatsu, T.; Kim, H.W.; Weintraub, N.L. The Role of Perivascular Adipose Tissue in Non-atherosclerotic Vascular Disease. *Front. Physiol.* **2017**, *8*, 969. [CrossRef] [PubMed]
33. Estrelinha, M.; Hinterseher, I.; Kuivaniemi, H. Gene expression studies in human abdominal aortic aneurysm. *Rev. Vasc. Med.* **2014**, *2*, 77–82. [CrossRef]
34. Hao, T.; Wang, Q.; Zhao, L.; Wu, D.; Wang, E.; Sun, J. Analyzing of Molecular Networks for Human Diseases and Drug Discovery. *Curr. Top. Med. Chem.* **2018**, *18*, 1007–1014. [CrossRef] [PubMed]
35. Safari-Alighiarloo, N.; Taghizadeh, M.; Rezaei-Tavirani, M.; Goliaei, B.; Peyvandi, A.A. Protein-protein interaction networks (PPI) and complex diseases. *Gastroenterol. Hepatol. Bed Bench* **2014**, *7*, 17–31.
36. Rivas, J.D.L.; Prieto, C. Protein Interactions: Mapping Interactome Networks to Support Drug Target Discovery and Selection. In *Bioinformatics and Drug Discovery*; Larson, R.S., Ed.; Methods in Molecular Biology; Humana Press: Totowa, NJ, USA, 2012; pp. 279–296. ISBN 978-1-61779-965-5.
37. Gerondakis, S.; Siebenlist, U. Roles of the NF-κB Pathway in Lymphocyte Development and Function. *Cold Spring Harb. Perspect. Biol.* **2010**, *2*, a000182. [CrossRef]
38. Kawai, T.; Akira, S. Signaling to NF-kappaB by Toll-like receptors. *Trends Mol. Med.* **2007**, *13*, 460–469. [CrossRef]
39. Hayden, M.S.; West, A.P.; Ghosh, S. NF-κB and the immune response. *Oncogene* **2006**, *25*, 6758–6780. [CrossRef]
40. Gerondakis, S.; Grumont, R.; Gugasyan, R.; Wong, L.; Isomura, I.; Wong, H.; Banerjee, A. Unravelling the complexities of the NF-kappaB signalling pathway using mouse knockout and transgenic models. *Oncogene* **2006**, *25*, 6781–6799. [CrossRef]
41. Shiraya, S.; Miwa, K.; Aoki, M.; Miyake, T.; Oishi, M.; Kataoka, K.; Ohgi, S.; Ogihara, T.; Kaneda, Y.; Morishita, R. Hypertension Accelerated Experimental Abdominal Aortic Aneurysm Through Upregulation of Nuclear Factor κB and Ets. *Hypertension* **2006**, *48*, 628–636. [CrossRef]
42. Takei, Y.; Tanaka, T.; Kent, K.C.; Yamanouchi, D. Osteoclastogenic Differentiation of Macrophages in the Development of Abdominal Aortic Aneurysms. *Arterioscler. Thromb. Vasc. Biol.* **2016**, *36*, 1962–1971. [CrossRef]

43. Cui, R.; Tieu, B.; Recinos, A.; Tilton, R.G.; Brasier, A.R. RhoA mediates angiotensin II-induced phospho-Ser536 nuclear factor kappaB/RelA subunit exchange on the interleukin-6 promoter in VSMCs. *Circ. Res.* **2006**, *99*, 723–730. [CrossRef] [PubMed]
44. Ijaz, T.; Sun, H.; Pinchuk, I.V.; Milewicz, D.M.; Tilton, R.G.; Brasier, A.R. Deletion of NF-κB/RelA in Angiotensin II-Sensitive Mesenchymal Cells Blocks Aortic Vascular Inflammation and Abdominal Aortic Aneurysm Formation. *Arter. Thromb. Vasc. Biol.* **2017**, *37*, 1881–1890. [CrossRef] [PubMed]
45. Miyake, T.; Miyake, T.; Kurashiki, T.; Morishita, R. Molecular Pharmacological Approaches for Treating Abdominal Aortic Aneurysm. *Ann. Vasc. Dis.* **2019**, *12*, 137–146. [CrossRef] [PubMed]
46. Lindeman, J.H.N.; Rabelink, T.J.; van Bockel, J.H. Immunosuppression and the abdominal aortic aneurysm: Doctor Jekyll or Mister Hyde? *Circulation* **2011**, *124*, e463–e465. [CrossRef]
47. Willis, S.N.; Tellier, J.; Liao, Y.; Trezise, S.; Light, A.; O'Donnell, K.; Garrett-Sinha, L.A.; Shi, W.; Tarlinton, D.M.; Nutt, S.L. Environmental sensing by mature B cells is controlled by the transcription factors PU.1 and SpiB. *Nat. Commun.* **2017**, *8*, 1426. [CrossRef]
48. Rosales, C. Fcγ Receptor Heterogeneity in Leukocyte Functional Responses. *Front. Immunol.* **2017**, *8*, 280. [CrossRef]
49. Wang, Y.; Jönsson, F. Expression, Role, and Regulation of Neutrophil Fcγ Receptors. *Front. Immunol.* **2019**, *10*, 1958. [CrossRef]
50. Shi, Y.; Yang, C.-Q.; Wang, S.-W.; Li, W.; Li, J.; Wang, S.-M. Characterization of Fc gamma receptor IIb expression within abdominal aortic aneurysm. *Biochem. Biophys. Res. Commun.* **2017**, *485*, 295–300. [CrossRef]
51. Ben Mkaddem, S.; Benhamou, M.; Monteiro, R.C. Understanding Fc Receptor Involvement in Inflammatory Diseases: From Mechanisms to New Therapeutic Tools. *Front. Immunol.* **2019**, *10*, 811. [CrossRef]
52. Arthur, J.S.C.; Ley, S.C. Mitogen-activated protein kinases in innate immunity. *Nat. Rev. Immunol.* **2013**, *13*, 679–692. [CrossRef]
53. Ghosh, A.; DiMusto, P.D.; Ehrlichman, L.K.; Sadiq, O.; McEvoy, B.; Futchko, J.S.; Henke, P.K.; Eliason, J.L.; Upchurch, G.R. The role of extracellular signal-related kinase during abdominal aortic aneurysm formation. *J. Am. Coll. Surg.* **2012**, *215*, 668–680.e1. [CrossRef] [PubMed]
54. Beurel, E.; Michalek, S.M.; Jope, R.S. Innate and adaptive immune responses regulated by glycogen synthase kinase-3 (GSK3). *Trends Immunol.* **2010**, *31*, 24–31. [CrossRef] [PubMed]
55. Neels, J.G.; Hassen-Khodja, R.; Chinetti, G. Nuclear receptors in abdominal aortic aneurysms. *Atherosclerosis* **2020**, *297*, 87–95. [CrossRef] [PubMed]
56. Takeda, K.; Ichiki, T.; Funakoshi, Y.; Ito, K.; Takeshita, A. Downregulation of angiotensin II type 1 receptor by all-trans retinoic acid in vascular smooth muscle cells. *Hypertension* **2000**, *35*, 297–302. [CrossRef] [PubMed]
57. Núñez, V.; Alameda, D.; Rico, D.; Mota, R.; Gonzalo, P.; Cedenilla, M.; Fischer, T.; Boscá, L.; Glass, C.K.; Arroyo, A.G.; et al. Retinoid X receptor α controls innate inflammatory responses through the up-regulation of chemokine expression. *Proc. Natl. Acad. Sci. USA* **2010**, *107*, 10626–10631. [CrossRef]
58. Galán, M.; Varona, S.; Orriols, M.; Rodríguez, J.A.; Aguiló, S.; Dilmé, J.; Camacho, M.; Martínez-González, J.; Rodriguez, C. Induction of histone deacetylases (HDACs) in human abdominal aortic aneurysm: Therapeutic potential of HDAC inhibitors. *Dis. Model. Mech.* **2016**, *9*, 541–552. [CrossRef]
59. Akimova, T.; Beier, U.H.; Liu, Y.; Wang, L.; Hancock, W.W. Histone/protein deacetylases and T-cell immune responses. *Blood* **2012**, *119*, 2443–2451. [CrossRef]
60. Iwasaki, A.; Medzhitov, R. Control of adaptive immunity by the innate immune system. *Nat. Immunol.* **2015**, *16*, 343–353. [CrossRef]
61. Kim, H.W.; de Chantemèle, E.J.B.; Weintraub, N.L. Perivascular Adipocytes in Vascular Disease. *Arterioscler. Thromb. Vasc. Biol.* **2019**, *39*, 2220–2227. [CrossRef]
62. Huh, J.Y.; Park, Y.J.; Ham, M.; Kim, J.B. Crosstalk between Adipocytes and Immune Cells in Adipose Tissue Inflammation and Metabolic Dysregulation in Obesity. *Mol. Cells* **2014**, *37*, 365–371. [CrossRef]
63. Wang, S.K.; Murphy, M.P. Immune Modulation as a Treatment for Abdominal Aortic Aneurysms. *Circ. Res.* **2018**, *122*, 925–927. [CrossRef] [PubMed]
64. Chang, T.W.; Gracon, A.S.A.; Murphy, M.P.; Wilkes, D.S. Exploring autoimmunity in the pathogenesis of abdominal aortic aneurysms. *Am. J. Physiol. Heart Circ. Physiol.* **2015**, *309*, H719–H727. [CrossRef] [PubMed]
65. Bluestone, J.A.; Bour-Jordan, H. Current and future immunomodulation strategies to restore tolerance in autoimmune diseases. *Cold Spring Harb. Perspect. Biol.* **2012**, *4*, a007542. [CrossRef] [PubMed]

66. Sagan, A.; Mikolajczyk, T.P.; Mrowiecki, W.; MacRitchie, N.; Daly, K.; Meldrum, A.; Migliarino, S.; Delles, C.; Urbanski, K.; Filip, G.; et al. T Cells Are Dominant Population in Human Abdominal Aortic Aneurysms and Their Infiltration in the Perivascular Tissue Correlates With Disease Severity. *Front. Immunol.* **2019**, *10*, 1979. [CrossRef] [PubMed]
67. Pinard, A.; Jones, G.T.; Milewicz, D.M. Genetics of Thoracic and Abdominal Aortic Diseases. *Circ. Res.* **2019**, *124*, 588–606. [CrossRef]

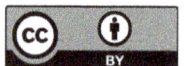

© 2020 by the authors. Licensee MDPI, Basel, Switzerland. This article is an open access article distributed under the terms and conditions of the Creative Commons Attribution (CC BY) license (http://creativecommons.org/licenses/by/4.0/).

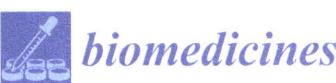

Article

A Systematic Review and Meta-Analysis of the Effect of Pentagalloyl Glucose Administration on Aortic Expansion in Animal Models

Jonathan Golledge [1,2,3,*,†], Shivshankar Thanigaimani [1,3,†] and James Phie [1,3]

1. Queensland Research Centre for Peripheral Vascular Disease, College of Medicine and Dentistry, James Cook University, Townsville, QLD 4810, Australia; shiv.thanigaimani@jcu.edu.au (S.T.); james.phie@jcu.edu.au (J.P.)
2. The Department of Vascular and Endovascular Surgery, The Townsville Hospital, Townsville, QLD 4810, Australia
3. The Australian Institute of Tropical Health and Medicine, James Cook University, Townsville, QLD 4810, Australia
* Correspondence: jonathan.golledge@jcu.edu.au; Tel.: +61-7-4796-1417; Fax: +61-7-4796-1401
† These authors contributed equally and are considered equal first authors.

Abstract: Background: The aim of this systematic review was to pool evidence from studies testing if pentagalloyl glucose (PGG) limited aortic expansion in animal models of abdominal aortic aneurysm (AAA). Methods: The review was conducted according to the PRISMA guidelines and registered with PROSPERO. The primary outcome was aortic expansion assessed by direct measurement. Secondary outcomes included aortic expansion measured by ultrasound and aortic diameter at study completion. Sub analyses examined the effect of PGG delivery in specific forms (nanoparticles, periadventitial or intraluminal), and at different times (from the start of AAA induction or when AAA was established), and tested in different animals (pigs, rats and mice) and AAA models (calcium chloride, periadventitial, intraluminal elastase or angiotensin II). Meta-analyses were performed using Mantel-Haenszel's methods with random effect models and reported as mean difference (MD) and 95% confidence intervals (CIs). Risk of bias was assessed with a customized tool. Results: Eleven studies reported in eight publications involving 214 animals were included. PGG significantly reduced aortic expansion measured by direct observation (MD: −66.35%; 95% CI: −108.44, −24.27; $p = 0.002$) but not ultrasound (MD: −32.91%; 95% CI: −75.16, 9.33; $p = 0.127$). PGG delivered intravenously within nanoparticles significantly reduced aortic expansion, measured by both direct observation (MD: −116.41%; 95% CI: −132.20, −100.62; $p < 0.001$) and ultrasound (MD: −98.40%; 95% CI: −113.99, −82.81; $p < 0.001$). In studies measuring aortic expansion by direct observation, PGG administered topically to the adventitia of the aorta (MD: −28.41%; 95% CI: −46.57, −10.25; $p = 0.002$), studied in rats (MD: −56.61%; 95% CI: −101.76, −11.46; $p = 0.014$), within the calcium chloride model (MD: −56.61%; 95% CI: −101.76, −11.46; $p = 0.014$) and tested in established AAAs (MD: −90.36; 95% CI: −135.82, −44.89; $p < 0.001$), significantly reduced aortic expansion. The findings of other analyses were not significant. The risk of bias of all studies was high. Conclusion: There is inconsistent low-quality evidence that PGG inhibits aortic expansion in animal models.

Keywords: pentagalloyl glucose; abdominal aortic aneurysm; aortic aneurysm

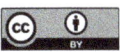

1. Introduction

Abdominal aortic aneurysm (AAA) rupture is estimated to be responsible for approximately 200,000 deaths per year worldwide [1]. The only current treatments for AAA are open or endovascular surgical repair [2,3]. Randomized controlled trials have suggested that the surgical repair of small AAAs (<55 mm) does not reduce mortality [4]. Clinical guidelines recommend that small asymptomatic AAAs are treated conservatively [2,3]; however, up to 70% of non-surgically treated AAAs continue to grow in size, thereby increasing the risk of rupture [5]. A drug therapy for small AAAs would be of great clinical value.

Past preclinical and clinical AAA research has focused on testing drugs that reduce aortic inflammation, inhibit extracellular matrix degradation or lower blood pressure [6–8]. Despite hundreds of preclinical studies and multiple clinical trials, none of these drugs have come into routine clinical practice for treating AAA [6,7]. Pentagalloyl glucose (PGG) is a polyphenolic derivate of tannic acid that is currently under investigation as a treatment to stabilize AAA [9]. PGG has been proposed to reduce the turnover of collagen and elastin by cross-linking these key extracellular matrix proteins [9]. A growing number of studies have examined the effect of PGG administration on aortic expansion in animal models of AAA. Many of these studies have reported reduced aortic expansion [10–13]. However, a recent study reported no effect in two rodent models [14].

Given the conflicting findings of these animal studies and since PGG is now being tested as a treatment for small AAA in patients, a critical review of the past preclinical evidence is needed. The aim of this study was to undertake a systematic review and meta-analysis by pooling data from studies testing the effect of PGG on aortic expansion in animal models of AAA.

2. Methods

2.1. Search Strategy and Eligibility Criteria

This systematic review was conducted according to the Preferred Reporting Items for Systematic Reviews and Meta-Analyses (PRISMA) statement and was registered in the PROSPERO database (Registration number: CRD42021275777) [15]. The PubMed and Web of Science (via ISI Web of Knowledge; 1965) databases were searched from inception to 14 September 2021. The search string ((("Pentagalloyl"[All Fields] AND ("glucose"[MeSH Terms] OR "glucose"[All Fields] OR "glucoses"[All Fields] OR "glucose s"[All Fields])) OR "PGG"[All Fields]) AND ("AAA"[All Fields] OR ("aneurysm"[MeSH Terms] OR "aneurysm"[All Fields] OR "aneurysms"[All Fields] OR "aneurysm s"[All Fields] OR "aneurysmal"[All Fields] OR "aneurysmally"[All Fields] OR "aneurysmic"[All Fields]))) was used. No language or date restrictions were used. Reference lists of the studies identified were also searched. Eligibility criteria for inclusion were: an animal study involving any AAA model testing the effect of PGG on aortic diameter increase; aortic diameter reported at a minimum of one time point after PGG administration; and inclusion of a control group not receiving PGG but otherwise receiving similar care. Studies including animals receiving PGG but not reporting aortic diameter, or where this could not be extracted or obtained from the authors, were excluded. In vitro or ex vivo studies were also excluded.

2.2. Data Extraction

The primary outcome was relative increase in the maximum diameter of the aorta after PGG administration, as compared to controls not receiving PGG, reported as percentage. This was required to be measured by direct observation by analysis of the in situ aortas at laparotomy, or the excised aortas using calipers or pictures. Secondary outcomes were aortic expansion measured by ultrasound, final maximum AAA diameter reported in millimeters, and AAA incidence and aortic rupture reported as numbers and percentage in mice allocated to PGG compared to controls. Other data extracted included: the types of AAA models; animal age, sex and strain; sample sizes; method of aortic diameter measurement; definition of AAA incidence; days after AAA induction that PGG or control were first administered; duration over which aortic expansion was studied; PGG form, dose and route of administration; and the findings of histological, biochemical and biomechanical studies. Data were extracted by three authors separately and inconsistencies were resolved through discussion. In studies where aortic diameters were reported only in graphs, they were extracted using ImageJ 64-bit version 1.8.0_172 (National Institute of Health, Bethesda, MD, USA).

2.3. Risk of Bias

A risk of bias tool was developed by combining the Systematic Review Centre for Laboratory Animal Experimentation (SYRCLE) and a previously developed risk of bias tool for AAA model research [16,17]. This incorporated the first nine questions of the SYRCLE tool and four questions from the AAA model risk of bias tool. These additional questions were focused on: the justification of the dose of PGG used; sample size estimation; whether aortic diameter was reported at first allocation to PGG or control and at study completion; and the reproducibility of aortic diameter measurement. Risk of bias was assessed by three authors and differences were resolved by discussion. The scores of the finally agreed upon risk of bias assessment were summed and reported as a percentage. The studies were rated as high (<50%), medium (51–70%) or low (71–100%) risk of bias.

2.4. Data Analysis

Meta-analyses were planned to be performed for any of the primary and secondary outcomes if data were reported in at least two studies. Sub analyses were also planned, and limited to studies using similar modes of PGG administration (nanoparticle incorporated, aortic periadventitial, or intraluminal); separating treatment starting at the time AAA induction commenced (i.e., testing effect on AAA development) versus starting after AAA had been established for at least one day (i.e., testing effect on AAA growth); performed in the same animals species (e.g., pigs, mice and rats), or AAA model types (calcium chloride, periadventitial, intraluminal elastase or angiotensin II); and excluding studies deemed to be at high risk of bias [18]. A leave-one-out-sensitivity analysis was performed to assess the contribution of each study to the pooled estimates of the primary outcome by excluding individual studies one at a time and recalculating the pooled estimates [19]. All meta-analyses were performed using Mantel-Haenszel's statistical methods and random effect models anticipating substantial heterogeneity [20]. The results were reported as mean differences (MDs), with 95% confidence intervals (CIs), for aortic diameter increase and relative risk (RR) and 95% CIs for AAA incidence and rupture. All statistical tests were two-sided and p-values < 0.05 were considered significant. Statistical heterogeneity was assessed using the I^2 statistic and interpreted as low (0 to 49%), moderate (50 to 74%) or high (75 to 100%) [21]. Publication bias was assessed by funnel plots comparing the summary estimate of each study and its precision (1/standard error) [19]. A minimum of ten studies were required to develop funnel plots to analyze publication bias [19]. Meta-analyses were conducted using 'meta' package, and the sensitivity analysis was performed using the 'dmetar' package of R program version 4.0.3.

3. Results

3.1. Included Studies

From 139 unique publications identified by the search, eight publications met the inclusion criteria and provided a total of 11 unique studies (Figure 1). Three publications included two different eligible studies [10,13,22], while the other five publications included one eligible study each [11,12,23–25]. Six studies used rats, four used mice and one used pigs (see Table 1). Overall, a total of 214 animals were included, with total sample sizes in individual studies varying from 12 to 30 (Table 1). The AAA models used included periadventitial infrarenal aortic calcium chloride application in five studies, intraluminal infrarenal aortic elastase in three studies (including the addition of aortic balloon dilatation and juxta-renal stenosing cuffs in the pig study) [25], periadventitial infrarenal aortic elastase application in two studies and subcutaneous angiotensin II infusion in one study (Table 1). In six studies, PGG and the control interventions were initiated at the time when AAA induction was commenced, whereas in the other five studies, PGG and the control interventions commenced between 10 and 42 days after AAA induction (see Table 2). Animals were monitored for between 14 and 42 days after the PGG and control interventions commenced (Table 2). The routes, forms and doses of the PGG administered varied (see Table 2). Four studies tested the intravenous delivery of PGG incorporated in nanoparticles, another four studies tested PGG applied topically to the adventitia of the aorta and three studies tested PGG infused into the lumen of the aorta (in one case, this was delivered by a drug-eluting balloon). Nine studies included a vehicle control and no intervention was given to the controls in two studies (see Table 2). All eleven studies reported percentage increases in aortic diameter for both the interventional and the control groups. Measurements were performed by direct observation alone in five studies, ultrasound alone in four studies and both measurement methods in two studies (Table 2). Six studies reported the actual aortic diameter at the end of the study. Measurements were performed by direct observation alone in two studies, ultrasound alone in three studies and both measurement methods in one study (Table 2). Only two studies reported AAA incidence [13,24]. Aortic rupture is not a feature of the models used in most studies, with only one study reporting this outcome [10].

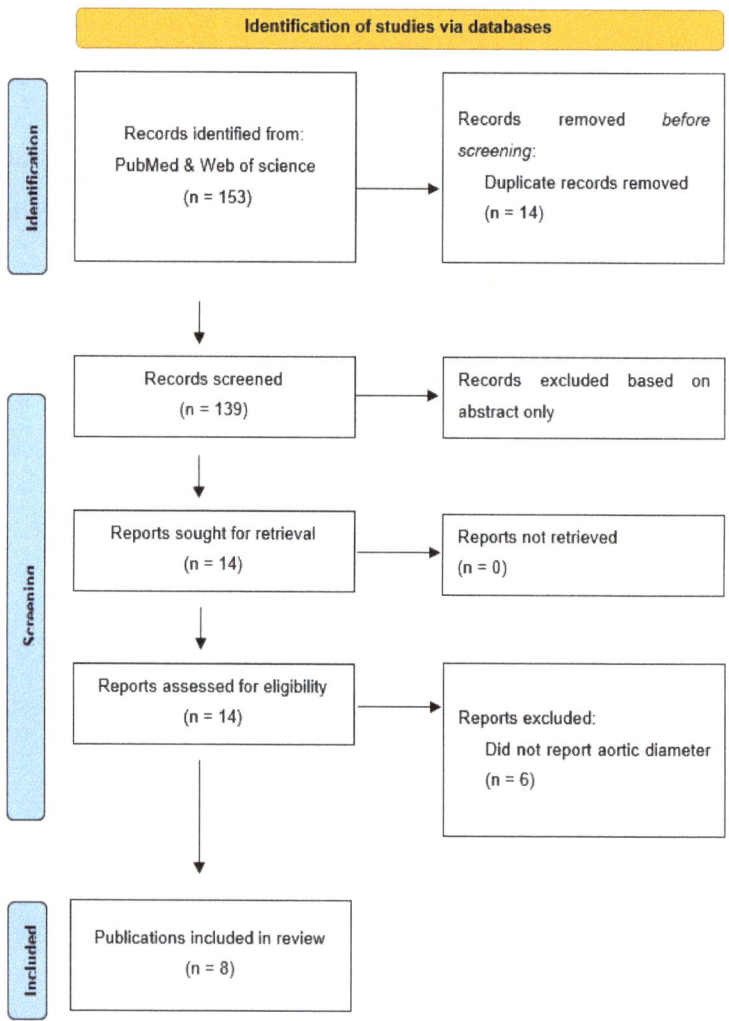

Figure 1. Preferred Reporting Items for Systematic Reviews and Meta-Analyses flow diagram. A total of 153 publications were screened and, after exclusion of irrelevant studies, 8 publications were included.

Table 1. Characteristics of included studies and animals.

Model	Animals	Age (Months)	Sex	Sample Size †	Sample Size ‡	Modality *	Aortic Diameter Measurement Protocol	Reference
Periadventitial infrarenal aortic elastase	C57BL/6 mice	NR	M	10	10	Ultrasound Photographs of excised aortas (end) and in situ measurements at laparotomy (start)	Systolic maximum inner to inner diameter Maximum outer to outer diameter	[11]
Angiotensin II infusion sub-cutaneously	LDLR$^{-/-}$ mice	2	M	12	12	Ultrasound	Inner to inner aortic diameter	[23]
Intraluminal infrarenal aortic elastase	Sprague-Dawley rats	NR	M	9	10	Photographs of in situ aortas	Maximum outer to outer diameter	[10]a
Intraluminal infrarenal aortic elastase	Sprague-Dawley rats	NR	M	15 **	15 **	Ultrasound Photographs of in situ aortas	Maximum inner to inner anterior posterior aortic diameter Maximum outer to outer diameter	[10]b
Periadventitial infrarenal aortic calcium chloride	Sprague-Dawley rats	1	M	6	6	Photographs of aortas	Maximum outer to outer diameter	[24]
Periadventitial infrarenal aortic calcium chloride	Sprague-Dawley rats	1	M	6	6	Photographs of in situ aortas	Maximum outer to outer diameter	[12]
Periadventitial infrarenal aortic calcium chloride	Sprague-Dawley rats	NR	F	11	12	Photographs of in situ aortas	Maximum outer to outer diameter	[13]a
Periadventitial infrarenal aortic calcium chloride	Sprague-Dawley rats	NR	F	11	12	Photographs of in situ aortas	Maximum outer to outer diameter	[13]b
Intraluminal infrarenal aortic elastase following balloon dilatation and juxtarenal stenosing cuff	Danish Landrace pigs	NR	F	10	10	Ultrasound	Maximum outer to outer anterior posterior aortic diameter measured in transverse and longitudinal plane	[25]
Periadventitial infrarenal aortic elastase	C57BL/6 mice	2–3.5	NR	8	9	Ultrasound	Inner to inner diameter during systole	[14]a
Periadventitial infrarenal aortic calcium chloride	C57BL/6 mice	2–3.5	NR	8	6	Ultrasound	Inner to inner diameter during systole	[14]b

NR = Not reported; M = Male; F = Female; LDLR$^{-/-}$ = Low-density lipoprotein-receptor-deficient mice maintained on a high fat diet. a/b: Three of the publications included two separate studies that were considered independently; * Represents imaging modality performed at end point; ** One rat was reported to die during the experiment, but outcomes were reported on 15 rats; † Sample size for intervention group; ‡ Sample size for control group.

Table 2. Pentagalloyl glucose interventions, controls and outcomes.

Group	Dose	Mode of Delivery	Intervention Commenced †	Duration of Follow-Up ‡	Direct Aortic Percentage	p	Direct Aortic Diameter †	p	Ultrasound Aortic Percentage	p	Ultrasound Aortic Diameter †	p Value	AAA Development, n (%)	Reference
Intervention	3 mg PCG in 10 mg/kg nanoparticle (on day 14 and 21)	Intravenous	14	14	24.78 ± 15.62 *	<0.0001	NR		9.69 ± 5.24 *	<0.0001	NR		NR	[11]
Control	No administration	NA	NA	14	144.27 ± 28.18 *		NR		110.54 ± 20.37 *		NR		NR	
Intervention	PCG in 10 mg/kg nanoparticles (on day 28 and 42)	Intravenous	28	28	NR		NR		97.75 ± 49.77	<0.05	NR		NR	[23]
Control	Blank in 10 mg/kg nanoparticles (on day 28 and 42)	Intravenous	28	28	NR		NR		182.44 ± 46.55		NR		NR	
Intervention	0.6 mg/mL PCG for 15 min (Once on day 0)	Direct intraluminal delivery	0	28	71.40 ± 46.00	<0.01	3.48 ± 0.91	<0.01	NR		NR		NR	[10]a
Control	2% ethanol, 2.5% DMSO in isotonic saline (Once on day 0)	Direct intraluminal delivery	0	28	159.00 ± 77.50		5.24 ± 1.61		NR		NR		NR	
Intervention	0.6 mg/mL PCG for 15 min (Once on day 0)	Intraluminal delivery via eluting balloon	0	28	183.00 ± 59.10	NS	6.13 ± 1.01	NS	143.00 ± 91.50	NS	5.22 ± 1.06	NS	NR	[10]b
Control	2% ethanol, 2.5% DMSO in isotonic saline (Once on day 0)	Intraluminal delivery via eluting balloon	0	28	149.00 ± 104.00		5.15 ± 1.96		129.20 ± 97.30		4.75 ± 1.91		NR	
Intervention	PCG in 10 mg/kg nanoparticles (on day 42 and 56)	Intravenous	42	42	66.00 ± 21.00	<0.05	NR		NR		NR		6 (100%)	[24]
Control	Blank in 10 mg/kg nanoparticles (on day 42 and 56)	Intravenous	42	42	185.00 ± 25.00		NR		NR		NR		6 (100%)	

Table 2. Cont.

Group	Dose	Mode of Delivery	Intervention Commenced †	Duration of Follow-Up ‡	Direct Aortic Percentage	p	Direct Aortic Diameter ¶	p	Ultrasound Aortic Percentage	p	Ultrasound Aortic Diameter §	p Value	AAA Development, n (%)	Reference
Intervention	PGG in 10 mg/kg nanoparticles conjugated with elastin antibody (Once every two weeks from day 10)	Intravenous	10	28	57.00 ± 22.00	<0.05	NR		NR		NR		NR	[12]
Control	Blank in 10 mg/kg nanoparticles (Once every two weeks from day 10)	Intravenous	10	28	158.00 ± 43.00		NR		NR		NR		NR	
Intervention	0.03% w/w PGG in saline for 15 min (Once on day 0)	Periadventitial application for 15 min	0	28	8.00 ± 7.00	<0.05	1.60 ± 0.09	NR	NR		NR		8 (66.7%) (p = NR)	[13]a
Control	Saline (Once on day 0)	Periadventitial application for 15 min	0	28	42.00 ± 10.00		1.90 ± 0.10		NR		NR		2 (18.2%) (p = NR)	
Intervention	0.03% w/w PGG in saline for 15 min (Once on day 28)	Periadventitial application for 15 min	28	28	25.00 ± 7.00	<0.05	NR		NR		NR		NR	[13]b
Control	Saline (Once on day 28)	Periadventitial application for 15 min	28	28	47.10 ± 11.00		NR		NR		NR		NR	
Intervention	25 or 50 mg PGG	Intraluminal delivery	0	28	NR		NR		18.41 ± 2.11	<0.001	12.17 ± 0.13	<0.001	NR	[25]
Control	No administration	Intraluminal delivery	0	28	NR		NR		57.03 ± 10.17		16.26 ± 0.93		NR	
Intervention	0.3% w/w PGG in saline for 15 min (Once on day 0)	Periadventitial	0	14	NR		NR		137.65 ± 11.98 *	NS	0.85 ± 0.15	NS	NR	[14]a
Control	Saline (Once on day 0)	Periadventitial	0	14	NR		NR		148.98 ± 15.71 *		0.97 ± 0.18		NR	
Intervention	0.3% w/w PGG in saline for 15 min (Once on day 0)	Periadventitial	0	28	NR		NR		114.48 ± 6.98 *	NS	0.73 ± 0.09	NS	NR	[14]b
Control	Saline (Once on day 0)	Periadventitial	0	28	NR		NR		106.84 ± 3.50 *		0.68 ± 0.07		NR	

NR = Not reported; NA = Not applicable; NS = Not significant; PGG = Pentagalloyl glucose; * Data extracted from graphs or calculated from reported data; † Days after AAA induction was initiated; ‡ Days after intervention commenced; ¶ Represents increase in aortic diameter using ex vivo measurement; § Represents increase in aortic diameter using ultrasound measurement; *† Represents primarily ex vivo, and ultrasound measurement if ex vivo was not reported. a/b: Three of the publications included two separate studies that were considered independently.

3.2. Risk of Bias of Included Studies

All 11 studies were considered to have a high risk of bias with overall scores on the 13 item quality assessment tool ranging between 8% and 31% (see Table 3). Common risks of bias identified were failure to randomize animals to the intervention and control group, failure to blind investigators and outcome assessors, failure to justify PGG dose, absence of sample size rationales and not reporting the reproducibility of aortic diameter measurement (Table 3).

Table 3. Quality assessment of included studies using a modified SYRCLE's tool for assessing risk of bias.

Quality Criteria \ Reference	[11]	[23]	[10]a	[10]b	[24]	[12]	[13]a	[13]b	[25]	[14]a	[14]b
Was the allocation sequence adequately generated and applied?	0	0	0	0	0	0	0	0	0	0	0
Were the groups similar at baseline or were they adjusted for confounders in the analysis?	1	1	1	1	1	0	1	1	1	1	1
Was the allocation adequately concealed?	0	0	0	0	0	0	0	0	0	0	0
Were the animals randomly housed during the experiment?	0	0	0	0	0	0	0	0	0	0	0
Were the caregivers and/or investigators blinded from knowledge of which intervention each animal received during the experiment?	0	0	0	0	0	0	0	0	0	0	0
Were animals selected at random for outcome assessment?	0	0	0	0	0	0	0	0	0	0	0
Was the outcome assessor blinded?	0	0	0	1	0	0	0	0	0	0	0
Were incomplete outcome data adequately addressed?	0	0	1	0	1	1	0	0	1	0	0
Are reports of the study free of selective outcome reporting?	0	0	1	0	1	1	0	0	1	0	0
Was the dose of intervention (PGG) justified?	0	0	0	0	0	0	0	0	0	0	0
Was the sample size estimation performed?	0	0	0	0	1	0	0	0	0	0	0
Was the aortic diameter reported within 1 day prior to first allocation to PGG or control and at study completion?	0	1	1	1	0	0	1	1	1	1	1
Was the reproducibility of aortic diameter measurement reported?	0	0	1	1	0	0	0	0	0	0	0
Total Score	1	2	5	4	4	2	2	2	4	2	2
Percentage of possible score	7.69	15.38	38.46	30.77	30.77	15.38	15.38	15.38	30.77	15.38	15.38
Risk of bias	High	High	High	High	High	High	High	High	High	High	High

a/b: Three of the publications included two separate studies that were considered independently.

3.3. Effect of PGG on Aortic Expansion

PGG was reported to significantly reduce the percentage increase in aortic diameter in six of the seven studies where this was measured by direct observation, and three of the six studies that measured aortic diameter percentage increase by ultrasound (see Table 2). A meta-analysis suggested that PGG significantly reduced aortic expansion when measured by direct observation (MD: −66.35%; 95% CI: −108.44, −24.27; $p = 0.002$), but not ultrasound (MD: −32.91%; 95% CI: −75.16, 9.33; $p = 0.127$), compared to the controls (Figures 2 and 3). In studies measuring aortic expansion by direct observation, PGG administered intravenously through nanoparticles (MD: −116.41%; 95% CI: −132.20, −100.62; $p < 0.001$), topically to the adventitia of the aorta (MD: −28.41%; 95% CI: −46.57, −10.25; $p = 0.002$), studied in rats (MD: −56.61%; 95% CI: −101.76, −11.46; $p = 0.014$), in the calcium chloride model (MD: −68.17%; 95% CI: −115.12, −21.22; $p = 0.004$), and where PGG treatment was initiated after model development on days ranging between 10 and 42 (MD: −90.36; 95% CI: −135.82, −44.89; $p < 0.001$), significantly reduced aortic expansion (Figure 2). A sensitivity analysis of the studies reporting aortic expansion by direct measurement found that the individual removal of any single study did not change the significance of the findings (Supplementary Table S1). In studies measuring aortic expansion by ultrasound measurement, PGG administered intravenously using nanoparticles significantly reduced aortic expansion (MD: −98.40%; 95% CI: −113.99, −82.81; $p < 0.001$) (Figure 3). The findings of other sub analyses were not significant (Figure 3). Funnel plots were not performed, due to data not being available from a minimum number of 10 studies.

3.4. Effect of PGG on Final AAA Diameter

One of three studies reported that PGG significantly reduced AAA diameter measured by direct observation at study completion (Table 2). One of four studies reported that PGG significantly reduced AAA diameter measured by ultrasound at study completion (Table 2). Meta-analyses suggested that PGG did not significantly reduce aortic diameter assessed by both direct measurement (MD: −0.35 mm; 95% CI −1.82, 1.12; $p = 0.642$) and ultrasound (MD −0.93 mm; 95% CI −3.00, 1.15; $p = 0.381$) (Figure 4). The findings of other sub analyses were not significant (Figure 4).

3.5. Effect of PGG on AAA Incidence

Two studies reported the incidence of AAA (see Table 2), but only one study initiated PGG treatment on the day of AAA induction, with 66.7% of rats in the control group developing AAA, compared to 18.2% of the rats receiving periadventitial aortic PGG at study completion [13]. Another study found that 100% of rats receiving PGG-loaded nanoparticles delivered intravenously 42 days after AAA induction developed AAA similar to the control group [24]. A meta-analysis of the two studies suggested that AAA incidence was not significantly different between rats receiving PGG and the controls, with large CIs (RR: 0.62; 95% CI: 0.00, 1751.32; $p = 0.588$, Supplementary Figure S1).

3.6. Findings from Histological and Molecular Biology Analyses

Histology findings from some studies found that animals receiving PGG had less aortic media elastic fiber degradation, more desmosine content and decreased macrophage infiltration (See Table 4). PGG was also reported to significantly reduce aortic matrix metalloproteinase (MMP) activity in three studies and increase lysyl oxidase (LOX) activity in two studies (Table 4). One study reported no significant effect of PGG on MMP-2 and MMP-9 [13]. Another two studies reported no significant effect of PGG on LOX or the markers of aortic macrophage infiltration [10].

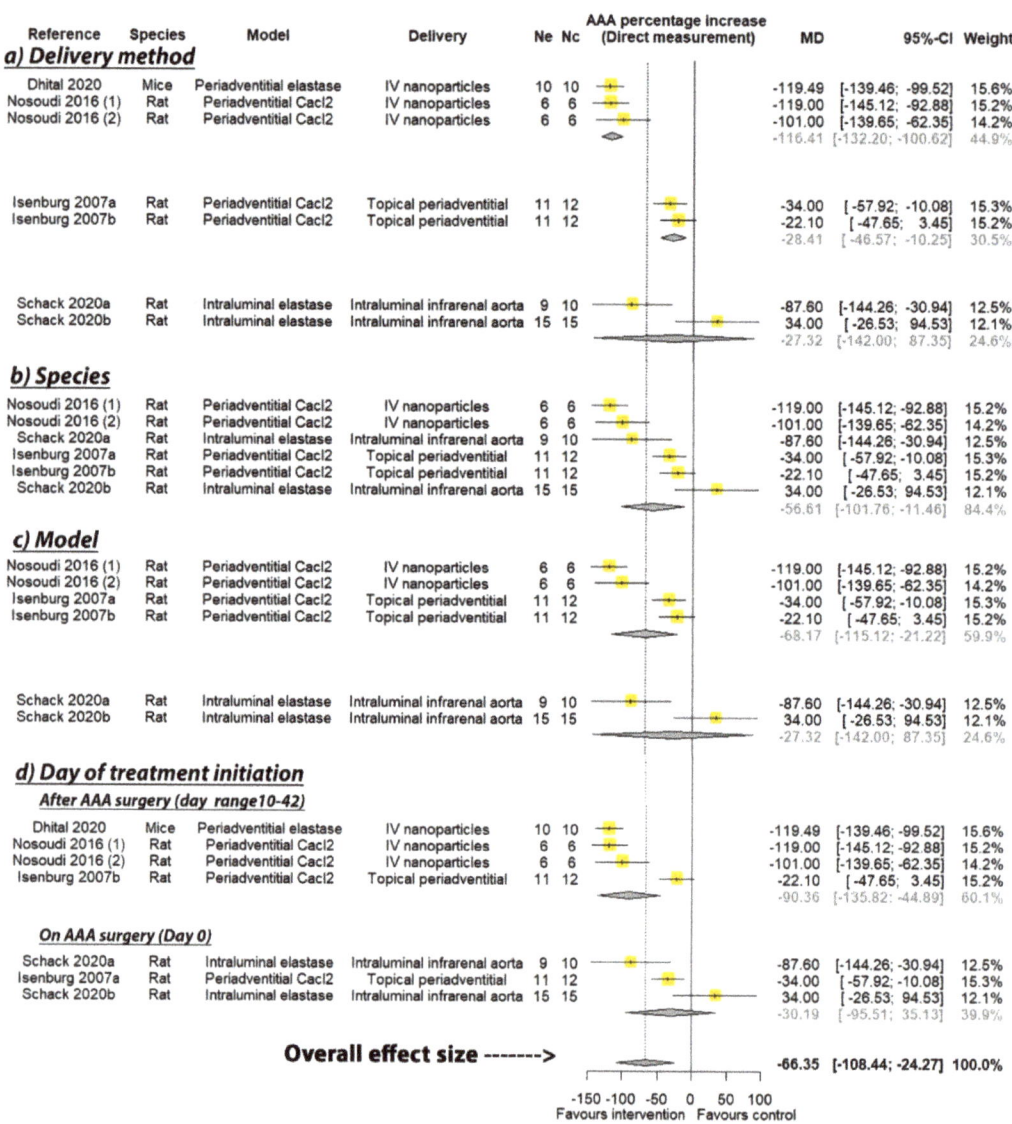

Figure 2. Meta-analysis of studies testing the effect of pentagalloyl glucose on aortic expansion measured by direct observation. MD = Mean difference; Ne = Number of animals in experimental group; Nc = Number of animals in control group; CI = Confidence interval. a/b: Three of the publications included two separate studies that were considered independently.

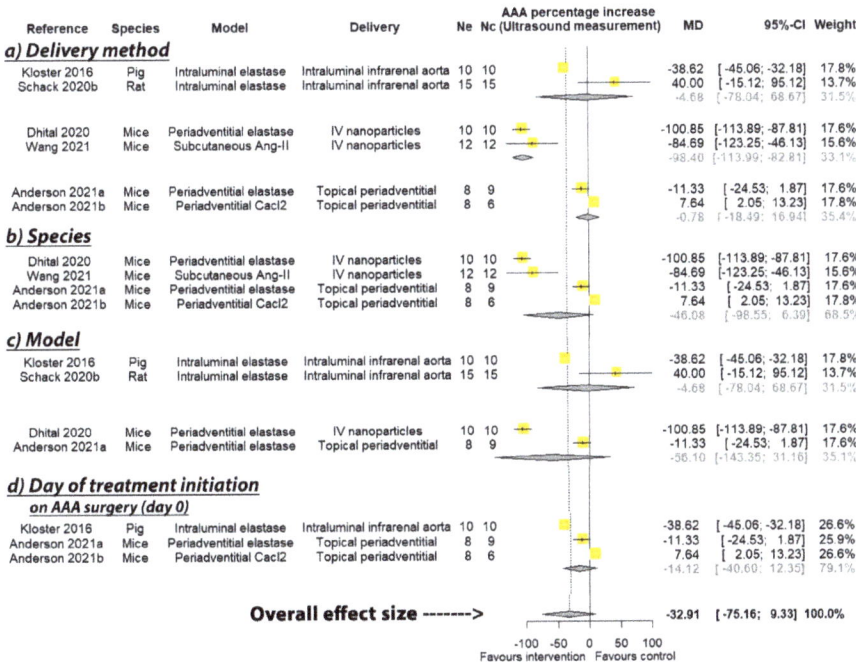

Figure 3. Meta-analysis of studies testing the effect of pentagalloyl glucose on aortic expansion measured by ultrasound. MD = Mean difference; Ne = Number of animals in experimental group; Nc = Number of animals in control group; CI = Confidence interval. a/b: Three of the publications included two separate studies that were considered independently.

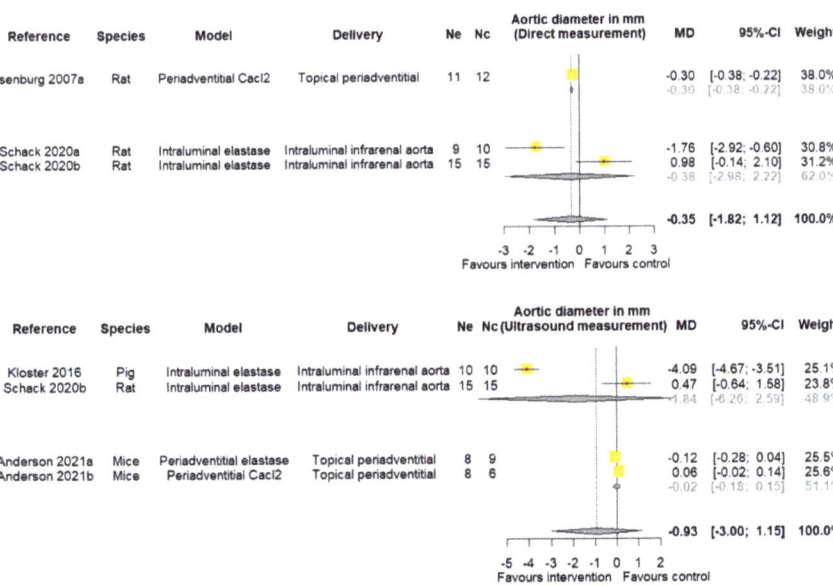

Figure 4. Meta-analysis of studies testing the effect of pentagalloyl glucose on final aortic diameter in animal models of abdominal aortic aneurysm. MD = Mean difference; Ne = Number of animals in experimental group; Nc = Number of animals in control group; CI = Confidence interval. a/b: Three of the publications included two separate studies that were considered independently.

Table 4. Reported effects of PGG on aortic histology and molecular biology findings.

Histology Findings	Molecular Biology Findings	Reference
Suggested aortic elastic fibers were restored in the medial layer (no quantitation); Significantly decreased CD68 positive aortic macrophages ($p < 0.05$)	Suggested decreased MMP-2 (p = NR), MMP-9 (p = NR) and TGF-b1 (p = NR)	[11]
Repaired aortic elastic laminae, improved morphology, and minimal cell infiltration.	Significantly reduced aortic MMP-2 ($p < 0.05$) activity and increased TIMP-1 and -2 ($p < 0.05$). Significantly reduced serum IFN-y and spleen CD68 positive cells ($p < 0.05$)	[23]
Controls had significantly more degraded aortic medial elastic fibers than the PGG-administered group ($p < 0.01$)	mRNA levels of LOX and macrophage marker F4/80 not significantly different between groups	[10]a
NR	mRNA levels of LOX, LOXL1 and macrophage marker F4/80 not significantly different between groups	[10]b
Reduced aortic collagen deposition in PGG-administered compared to controls (not quantitated)	Significant suppression of aortic MMP ($p < 0.05$) and increased LOX ($p < 0.05$) activity compared to controls	[24]
Reduced elastin degradation, calcification, macrophage staining in the adventitial layers (not quantitated)	Significant suppression of aortic MMP ($p < 0.05$) and increased LOX ($p < 0.05$) activity and desmosine content ($p < 0.05$) compared to controls	[12]
Minimal decrease in elastin content and preserved elastic laminar integrity and waviness visually; Significantly greater aortic desmosine ($p < 0.05$)	No significant difference in MMP-2, 9 and TIMP-2. Macrophages and lymphocytes were unaffected (All $p > 0.05$).	[13]a
Improved preservation of elastic laminar integrity and waviness and overall preserved tissue architecture. Aorta media thickness was significantly reduced ($p < 0.05$).	NR	[13]b
Integrity of elastic lamellae was preserved. Light to moderate irregular scattered focal muscle atrophy in the tunica media	NR	[25]
Unchanged levels of calcium and elastin content. Did not exhibit inflammatory characteristic seen in controls.	NR	[14]a
Calcium content was found to be significantly lower in the PGG-treated cohort ($p = 0.036$). No change in elastin content. The extracellular microarchitecture was well preserved (p = NR).	NR	[14]b

NR = Not reported; MMP = Matrix metalloproteinase; TIMP = Tissue inhibitor of MMP; CD68 = Cluster of Differentiation 68; LOX = Lysyl oxidase; LOXL1 = Lysyloxidase-like protein 1; IFN-y = Interferon gamma; TGF-b1 = Transforming growth factor beta-1; PGG = Pentagalloyl glucose. a/b: Three of the publications included two separate studies that were considered independently.

4. Discussion

This systematic review of past studies found that the administration of PGG reduced aortic expansion within AAA animal models when measured by direct observation. The findings were not consistent when measured by ultrasound. PGG administered within intravenously injected nanoparticles significantly reduced aortic expansion in studies consistently, whether measured by direct observation or ultrasound. Surprisingly, when PGG treatment was initiated later than when AAA induction commenced (range from 10 to 42 days), it significantly reduced aortic expansion. This was, however, not the case when PGG treatment was started at the time of AAA induction. The findings of other analyses were inconsistent, depending on the method used to measure aortic expansion. A number of important limitations of these prior studies should be noted. Firstly, all studies had a high risk of bias. None of the studies included methods typically thought to be critical in human clinical trials, such as randomization and blinding. Only one study included a sample size calculation [24]. All studies were small and there has been concern that findings from animal models do not translate to AAA patients. This has been particularly reported in relation to doxycycline, but also for fenofibrate, an angiotensin receptor blocker and an angiotensin-converting enzyme inhibitor, which have all been reported to limit aortic expansion in animal models but have not been found to limit AAA growth in clinical trials [7,8,26–28].

In addition to the animal experiments reported in this study, there have been other experimental studies reporting the beneficial effects of PGG. In vitro studies have suggested that PGG reduces oxidative stress and MMP secretion and improves the elastic properties of a myoblast cell line [22]. Ex vivo studies of the carotid arteries of mice suggest that PGG protected against elastase-induced artery destruction and limited the mechanical failure of the artery by repairing the elastic lamellae and limiting changes in the mechanical properties of the tissue [29]. A similar ex vivo study using pig aortic samples reported that PGG partially protected against elastase- and collagenase-induced biomechanical changes [30].

One of the key challenges to the use of PGG as a clinical treatment is clarity on the most appropriate route of delivery. None of the animal studies used oral administration, which would be the most straightforward way to administer a medical treatment for AAA. The pharmacokinetics of oral PGG administration are poorly understood, as summarized in detail in a recent review [9]. Low and variable bioavailability of PGG has been reported after oral administration [9]. As illustrated in the included animal studies, a wide range of other routes of administration have been proposed, such as nanoparticles and periadventitial routes, but all are not ideal. Given the low risk (approximately 1% per year) of rupture of small AAAs, any treatment needs to have a good safety profile and, ideally, should be minimally invasive [7].

Despite the limitations of the past animal studies, the positive findings of some studies have encouraged the investigation of PGG as an AAA treatment in patients. In a recent presentation at Aortic Asia, it was announced that PGG delivery via an endovascularly placed balloon to the lumen of the infrarenal aorta is being tested as a treatment of small AAA within a clinical trial. Whether this route of administration, given its relatively invasive nature, is appropriate and feasible to use on a wider scale needs further consideration. Most AAAs contain large volumes of intraluminal thrombus that may interfere with PGG delivery to the aortic wall, and also be at risk of embolization during balloon inflation [31]. Further information on the safety and efficacy of intraluminal PGG is thus required. It is possible that, if this initial clinical trial is encouraging, there could be scope to combine PGG treatment with the endovascular repair of large AAA. A recent systematic review reported a long-term reintervention rate of 18% following endovascular aneurysm repair due to the continued expansion of the AAA sac [32]. The combination of an effective drug and surgical treatment could be a valuable addition to the clinical care of patients with large AAAs. This would need widescale testing to ensure that it is an effective and durable treatment.

A number of limitations of this systematic review should be noted. Firstly, the included studies were small and at high risk of bias. There was insufficient investigation or reporting of aortic rupture to assess this outcome. Finally, and most importantly, since all the current evidence is from animal, ex vivo, or in vitro studies, the clinical relevance of these findings remains unclear. The failure to translate past findings from these types of experiments is again emphasized.

In conclusion, this systematic review suggests inconsistent and low-quality evidence from animal studies that PGG may represent a treatment to restore aortic structure in patients with early-stage AAA. Whether this can translate into a clinically useful treatment is currently unclear, but under investigation by at least one company.

Supplementary Materials: The following are available online at https://www.mdpi.com/article/10.3390/biomedicines9101442/s1, Figure S1: Meta-analysis of studies testing the effect of pentagalloyl glucose on AAA incidence. RR = Relative risk; Ne = Number of animals in experimental group; Nc = Number of animals in control group; CI = Confidence interval, Table S1: Leave-one-out sensitivity analysis of studies reporting aortic expansion through direct measurement.

Author Contributions: Conceptualization, J.G.; methodology, J.G., S.T. and J.P.; software, S.T.; validation, S.T., J.P. and J.G.; formal analysis, S.T.; investigation, J.G. and S.T.; resources, S.T. and J.P.; data curation, S.T. and J.P.; writing—original draft preparation, J.G.; writing—review and editing, J.G., S.T. and J.P.; visualization, S.T., J.P. and J.G.; supervision, J.G.; project administration, J.G.; funding acquisition, J.G. All authors have read and agreed to the published version of the manuscript.

Funding: This research was supported by grants from the National Health and Medical Research Council (1180736), Townsville Hospital and Health Service Study, Education and Research Trust Fund, and the Queensland Government. JG holds a Practitioner Fellowship from the National Health and Medical Research Council (1117601), and a Senior Clinical Research Fellowship from the Queensland Government.

Institutional Review Board Statement: Not applicable.

Informed Consent Statement: Not applicable.

Data Availability Statement: Not applicable.

Conflicts of Interest: The authors declare no conflict of interest.

References

1. Abubakar, I.; Tillmann, T.; Banerjee, A. Global, regional, and national age-sex specific all-cause and cause-specific mortality for 240 causes of death, 1990–2013: A systematic analysis for the Global Burden of Disease Study 2013. *Lancet* **2015**, *385*, 117–171.
2. Chaikof, E.L.; Dalman, R.L.; Eskandari, M.K.; Jackson, B.M.; Lee, W.A.; Mansour, M.A.; Mastracci, T.M.; Mell, M.; Murad, M.H.; Nguyen, L.L. The Society for Vascular Surgery practice guidelines on the care of patients with an abdominal aortic aneurysm. *J. Vasc. Surg.* **2018**, *67*, 2–77.e2. [CrossRef]
3. Wanhainen, A.; Verzini, F.; Van Herzeele, I.; Allaire, E.; Bown, M.; Cohnert, T.; Dick, F.; van Herwaarden, J.; Karkos, C.; Koelemay, M. Editor's choice–European society for vascular surgery (ESVS) 2019 clinical practice guidelines on the management of abdominal aorto-iliac artery aneurysms. *Eur. J. Vasc. Endovasc. Surg.* **2019**, *57*, 8–93. [CrossRef] [PubMed]
4. Filardo, G.; Powell, J.T.; Martinez, M.A.M.; Ballard, D.J. Surgery for small asymptomatic abdominal aortic aneurysms. *Cochrane Database Syst. Rev.* **2015**. [CrossRef] [PubMed]
5. Lederle, F.A.; Johnson, G.R.; Wilson, S.E.; Ballard, D.J.; Jordan, W.D., Jr.; Blebea, J.; Littooy, F.N.; Freischlag, J.A.; Bandyk, D.; Rapp, J.H. Rupture rate of large abdominal aortic aneurysms in patients refusing or unfit for elective repair. *JAMA* **2002**, *287*, 2968–2972. [CrossRef] [PubMed]
6. Golledge, J.; Moxon, J.V.; Singh, T.P.; Bown, M.J.; Mani, K.; Wanhainen, A. Lack of an effective drug therapy for abdominal aortic aneurysm. *J. Intern. Med.* **2020**, *288*, 6–22. [CrossRef] [PubMed]
7. Golledge, J. Abdominal aortic aneurysm: Update on pathogenesis and medical treatments. *Nat. Rev. Cardiol.* **2019**, *16*, 225–242. [CrossRef] [PubMed]
8. Golledge, J.; Singh, T.P. Effect of blood pressure lowering drugs and antibiotics on abdominal aortic aneurysm growth: A systematic review and meta-analysis. *Heart* **2021**, *107*, 1465–1471. [CrossRef] [PubMed]
9. Patnaik, S.S.; Simionescu, D.T.; Goergen, C.J.; Hoyt, K.; Sirsi, S.; Finol, E.A. Pentagalloyl Glucose and Its Functional Role in Vascular Health: Biomechanics and Drug-Delivery Characteristics. *Ann. Biomed. Eng.* **2019**, *47*, 39–59. [CrossRef] [PubMed]
10. Schack, A.S.; Stubbe, J.; Steffensen, L.B.; Mahmoud, H.; Laursen, M.S.; Lindholt, J.S. Intraluminal infusion of Penta-Galloyl Glucose reduces abdominal aortic aneurysm development in the elastase rat model. *PLoS ONE* **2020**, *15*, e0234409. [CrossRef]
11. Dhital, S.; Vyavahare, N.R. Nanoparticle-based targeted delivery of pentagalloyl glucose reverses elastase-induced abdominal aortic aneurysm and restores aorta to the healthy state in mice. *PLoS ONE* **2020**, *15*, e0227165. [CrossRef] [PubMed]
12. Nosoudi, N.; Chowdhury, A.; Siclari, S.; Parasaram, V.; Karamched, S.; Vyavahare, N. Systemic Delivery of Nanoparticles Loaded with Pentagalloyl Glucose Protects Elastic Lamina and Prevents Abdominal Aortic Aneurysm in Rats. *J. Cardiovasc. Transl. Res.* **2016**, *9*, 445–455. [CrossRef] [PubMed]
13. Isenburg, J.C.; Simionescu, D.T.; Starcher, B.C.; Vyavahare, N.R. Elastin stabilization for treatment of abdominal aortic aneurysms. *Circulation* **2007**, *115*, 1729–1737. [CrossRef] [PubMed]
14. Anderson, J.L.; Niedert, E.E.; Patnaik, S.S.; Tang, R.; Holloway, R.L.; Osteguin, V.; Finol, E.A.; Goergen, C.J. Animal Model Dependent Response to Pentagalloyl Glucose in Murine Abdominal Aortic Injury. *J. Clin. Med.* **2021**, *10*, 219. [CrossRef] [PubMed]
15. Page, M.J.; McKenzie, J.E.; Bossuyt, P.M.; Boutron, I.; Hoffmann, T.C.; Mulrow, C.D.; Shamseer, L.; Tetzlaff, J.M.; Akl, E.A.; Brennan, S.E.; et al. The PRISMA 2020 statement: An updated guideline for reporting systematic reviews. *BMJ* **2021**, *372*, n71. [CrossRef]
16. Hooijmans, C.R.; Rovers, M.M.; de Vries, R.B.; Leenaars, M.; Ritskes-Hoitinga, M.; Langendam, M.W. SYRCLE's risk of bias tool for animal studies. *BMC Med. Res. Methodol.* **2014**, *14*, 43. [CrossRef] [PubMed]

17. Phie, J.; Thanigaimani, S.; Golledge, J. Systematic Review and Meta-Analysis of Interventions to Slow Progression of Abdominal Aortic Aneurysm in Mouse Models. *Arter. Thromb. Vasc. Biol.* **2021**, *41*, 1504–1517. [CrossRef] [PubMed]
18. Sterne, J.A.C.; Savovic, J.; Page, M.J.; Elbers, R.G.; Blencowe, N.S.; Boutron, I.; Cates, C.J.; Cheng, H.Y.; Corbett, M.S.; Eldridge, S.M.; et al. RoB 2: A revised tool for assessing risk of bias in randomised trials. *BMJ* **2019**, *366*, l4898. [CrossRef]
19. Sterne, J.A.; Gavaghan, D.; Egger, M. Publication and related bias in meta-analysis: Power of statistical tests and prevalence in the literature. *J. Clin. Epidemiol.* **2000**, *53*, 1119–1129. [CrossRef]
20. Kulinskaya, E.; Morgenthaler, S.; Staudte, R.G. Combining Statistical Evidence. *Int. Stat. Rev.* **2014**, *82*, 214–242. [CrossRef]
21. Higgins, J.P.; Thompson, S.G.; Deeks, J.J.; Altman, D.G. Measuring inconsistency in meta-analyses. *BMJ* **2003**, *327*, 557–560. [CrossRef]
22. Arnold, F.; Muzzio, N.; Patnaik, S.S.; Finol, E.A.; Romero, G. Pentagalloyl Glucose-Laden Poly(lactide-co-glycolide) Nanoparticles for the Biomechanical Extracellular Matrix Stabilization of an In Vitro Abdominal Aortic Aneurysm Model. *ACS Appl. Mater. Interfaces* **2021**, *13*, 25771–25782. [CrossRef] [PubMed]
23. Wang, X.; Parasaram, V.; Dhital, S.; Nosoudi, N.; Hasanain, S.; Lane, B.A.; Lessner, S.M.; Eberth, J.F.; Vyavahare, N.R. Systemic delivery of targeted nanotherapeutic reverses angiotensin II-induced abdominal aortic aneurysms in mice. *Sci. Rep.* **2021**, *11*, 8584. [CrossRef] [PubMed]
24. Nosoudi, N.; Chowdhury, A.; Siclari, S.; Karamched, S.; Parasaram, V.; Parrish, J.; Gerard, P.; Vyavahare, N. Reversal of Vascular Calcification and Aneurysms in a Rat Model Using Dual Targeted Therapy with EDTA- and PGG-Loaded Nanoparticles. *Theranostics* **2016**, *6*, 1975–1987. [CrossRef]
25. Kloster, B.O.; Lund, L.; Lindholt, J.S. Inhibition of early AAA formation by aortic intraluminal pentagalloyl glucose (PGG) infusion in a novel porcine AAA model. *Ann. Med. Surg.* **2016**, *7*, 65–70. [CrossRef] [PubMed]
26. Golledge, J.; Pinchbeck, J.; Tomee, S.M.; Rowbotham, S.E.; Singh, T.P.; Moxon, J.V.; Jenkins, J.S.; Lindeman, J.H.; Dalman, R.L.; McDonnell, L.; et al. Randomised-controlled trial testing the efficacy of telmisartan to slow growth of small abdominal aortic aneurysms. *JAMA Cardiol.* **2020**, *5*, 1374–1381. [CrossRef]
27. Moxon, J.V.; Rowbotham, S.E.; Pinchbeck, J.L.; Lazzaroni, S.M.; Morton, S.K.; Moran, C.S.; Quigley, F.; Jenkins, J.S.; Reid, C.M.; Cavaye, D.; et al. A Randomised Controlled Trial Assessing the Effects of Peri-operative Fenofibrate Administration on Abdominal Aortic Aneurysm Pathology: Outcomes From the FAME Trial. *Eur. J. Vasc. Endovasc. Surg.* **2020**, *60*, 452–460. [CrossRef]
28. Pinchbeck, J.L.; Moxon, J.V.; Rowbotham, S.E.; Bourke, M.; Lazzaroni, S.; Morton, S.K.; Matthews, E.O.; Hendy, K.; Jones, R.E.; Bourke, B.; et al. Randomized Placebo-Controlled Trial Assessing the Effect of 24-Week Fenofibrate Therapy on Circulating Markers of Abdominal Aortic Aneurysm: Outcomes From the FAME-2 Trial. *J. Am. Heart Assoc.* **2018**, *7*, e009866. [CrossRef]
29. Pavey, S.N.; Cocciolone, A.J.; Marty, A.G.; Ismail, H.N.; Hawes, J.Z.; Wagenseil, J.E. Pentagalloyl glucose (PGG) partially prevents arterial mechanical changes due to elastin degradation. *Exp. Mech.* **2021**, *61*, 41–51. [CrossRef]
30. Patnaik, S.S.; Piskin, S.; Pillalamarri, N.R.; Romero, G.; Escobar, G.P.; Sprague, E.; Finol, E.A. Biomechanical Restoration Potential of Pentagalloyl Glucose after Arterial Extracellular Matrix Degeneration. *Bioengineering* **2019**, *6*, 58. [CrossRef]
31. Golledge, J.; Wolanski, P.; Parr, A.; Buttner, P. Measurement and determinants of infrarenal aortic thrombus volume. *Eur. Radiol.* **2008**, *18*, 1987–1994. [CrossRef] [PubMed]
32. Li, B.; Khan, S.; Salata, K.; Hussain, M.A.; de Mestral, C.; Greco, E.; Aljabri, B.A.; Forbes, T.L.; Verma, S.; Al-Omran, M. A systematic review and meta-analysis of the long-term outcomes of endovascular versus open repair of abdominal aortic aneurysm. *J. Vasc. Surg.* **2019**, *70*, 954–969.e30. [CrossRef] [PubMed]

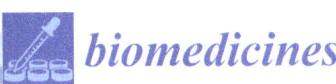

Article

Cycloastragenol Inhibits Experimental Abdominal Aortic Aneurysm Progression

Leander Gaarde Melin [1,2,3], Julie Husted Dall [1,2,3], Jes S. Lindholt [1,2], Lasse B. Steffensen [3], Hans Christian Beck [1,4], Sophie L. Elkrog [3], Pernille D. Clausen [3], Lars Melholt Rasmussen [1,4] and Jane Stubbe [1,3,*]

1. Centre for Individualized Medicine in Arterial Diseases (CIMA), Odense University Hospital (OUH), 5000 Odense, Denmark; leander.gaarde@rsyd.dk (L.G.M.); julie.husted.dall@regionh.dk (J.H.D.); jes.sanddal.lindholt@rsyd.dk (J.S.L.); hans.christian.beck@rsyd.dk (H.C.B.); lars.melholt.rasmussen@rsyd.dk (L.M.R.)
2. Department of Cardiothoracic and Vascular Surgery, Odense University Hospital, 5000 Odense, Denmark
3. Cardiovascular and Renal Research Unit, Institute for Molecular Medicine, University of Southern Denmark, 5000 Odense, Denmark; lsteffensen@health.sdu.dk (L.B.S.); soelk17@student.sdu.dk (S.L.E.); pecla17@student.sdu.dk (P.D.C.)
4. Department of Clinical Biochemistry and Pharmacology, Odense University Hospital, 5000 Odense, Denmark
* Correspondence: jstubbe@health.sdu.dk; Tel.: +45-6550-3709

Abstract: The pathogenesis of abdominal aortic aneurysm involves vascular inflammation and elastin degradation. *Astragalus radix* contains cycloastragenol, which is known to be anti-inflammatory and to protect against elastin degradation. We hypothesized that cycloastragenol supplementation inhibits abdominal aortic aneurysm progression. Abdominal aortic aneurysm was induced in male rats by intraluminal elastase infusion in the infrarenal aorta and treated daily with cycloastragenol (125 mg/kg/day). Aortic expansion was followed weekly by ultrasound for 28 days. Changes in aneurysmal wall composition were analyzed by mRNA levels, histology, zymography and explorative proteomic analyses. At day 28, mean aneurysm diameter was 37% lower in the cycloastragenol group ($p < 0.0001$). In aneurysm cross sections, elastin content was insignificantly higher in the cycloastragenol group (10.5% ± 5.9% vs. 19.9% ± 16.8%, $p = 0.20$), with more preserved elastin lamellae structures ($p = 0.0003$) and without microcalcifications. Aneurysmal matrix metalloprotease-2 activity was reduced by the treatment ($p = 0.022$). Messenger RNA levels of inflammatory- and anti-oxidative markers did not differ between groups. Explorative proteomic analysis showed no difference in protein levels when adjusting for multiple testing. Among proteins displaying nominal regulation were fibulin-5 ($p = 0.02$), aquaporin-1 ($p = 0.02$) and prostacyclin synthase ($p = 0.007$). Cycloastragenol inhibits experimental abdominal aortic aneurysm progression. The suggested underlying mechanisms involve decreased matrix metalloprotease-2 activity and preservation of elastin and reduced calcification, thus, cycloastragenol could be considered for trial in abdominal aortic aneurysm patients.

Keywords: aortic aneurysm; pathogenesis; pharmacological therapy; experimental model; drug delivery

1. Introduction

Abdominal aortic aneurysm (AAA) is a localized enlargement of the aorta exceeding 3 cm in diameter and is potentially life-threatening [1]. Globally, AAA rupture is a major cause of mortality in elderly men, being responsible for the death of 1% of men above 65 years [1,2]. Today, patients with known AAAs are carefully monitored and offered surgical repair when the AAA possesses a diameter above 5–6 cm. Thus, an urgent unmet clinical need of medical therapies for small AAAs exists, to prevent progressive dilatation, acute or elective surgical repair, rupture, and death [3–5].

Chronic inflammation, due to persistent infiltration of inflammatory cells into the aortic wall and degradation of elastin, seems to fundamentally characterize the pathology

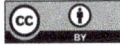

of AAAs [6]. Elastin in the medial layer of the aortic wall is degraded when the aneurysm is formed. This loss of elastin is partly compensated by the continuous formation of collagen and elastin by vascular smooth muscle cells along with expression of structural proteins such as tropoelastin and fibrillin 1, which is cross-linked by lysyl oxidase (LOX) and fibulin-5 to form elastic fibers [6–8]. This process is diminished by inflammation when elastin-degrading enzymes, such as matrix metalloproteases (MMPs), are released from macrophages, monocytes, neutrophils and activated vascular smooth muscle cells [6,7]. Especially the M1 proinflammatory macrophages, which produce proinflammatory cytokines and MMPs, augment AAA progression [9]. Moreover, reactive oxygen species (ROS) contribute to AAA expansion by enhancing MMP activity, which further degrades the extracellular matrix (ECM) and weakens the aneurysm wall [6,10–13].

A promising dietary supplement in the fight against AAA progression is cycloastragenol (CAG). It is a crystalline solid triterpenoid saponin compound and a hydrolyzed product of the main active ingredient in the Chinese herb *Astragalus membranaceus*. CAG has been used in traditional Chinese medicine for over 2000 years with no commonly known side effects [14]. Recent literature describes various anti-inflammatory effects of CAG in heart, vascular, liver and skin tissue including inhibition of lymphocyte activation. CAG also reduces MMP-2 and MMP-9 expression and activity, thereby preserving extracellular matrix (ECM) integrity [15–19]. CAG supplement has recently been proven to attenuate AAA expansion in mice using an elastase wrapping model and in angiotensin-II induced AAA in Apolipoprotein E (ApoE)$^{-/-}$ mice [19]. However, the model can be criticized for not producing human-like-AAA in contrast to the elastase perfusion model in rats, which uses porcine pancreatic elastase (PPE) applied intraluminally in the infrarenal aortic segment through laparotomy and atherectomy [20]. This imitates human AAA well, as it displays various pathological similarities, such as inflammation, elastin degradation, thrombus formation and calcification [21]. Thus, the growing base of evidence describing the anti-inflammatory properties of CAG illustrates its potential as a possible future medical treatment against AAA expansion in humans.

In this study, we hypothesize that CAG inhibits the progressive dilatation of AAA in the rat PPE aneurysm-model by its anti-inflammatory and anti-oxidative effects leading to reduced protease activity and, thereby, preserving elastin integrity.

2. Materials and Methods

2.1. Study Design

The rats were randomly allocated to either CAG treatment (125 mg/kg/day) or controls, starting on the first postoperative day, by an external investigator, not participating in any of the experimental procedures. Therefore, rats were housed independent of treatment, and daily caretakers were blinded to treatment.

2.2. Outcomes

The primary outcome was peak-systolic infrarenal aortic anterior to posterior inner-to-inner diameter. Secondary explanatory outcome were: AAA wall content of elastin, its structure and LOX mRNA levels. Determine the effect of CAG on matrix-dependent MMP-2, -9 and -12 mRNA levels and MMP activity. Measure mRNA levels of leukocyte marker CD45 mRNA, macrophage marker F4/80 mRNA and IL-6 and -10 mRNA levels together with the pro-inflammatory M1 macrophage marker iNOS, the antioxidative markers Nrf2 and HO-1 in the aneurysms. Furthermore, perform histological assessments of cluster of differentiation (CD)68 and CD206 and the presence of calcification in the aneurysm wall. Finally, identify potential new targets of CAG treatment in aneurysm wall by discovery proteomic analysis.

Potential harm outcomes were weight of liver, spleen, heart, and kidneys, as well as morphology of the inferior right liver lobe.

2.3. Sample Size Calculation

We have, in previous experiments with the rat model, observed a mean diameter increase of 158.75% ± 77.5 SD. To detect a 50% difference, which is considered clinically relevant, by a *t*-test using 5% significance level and 80% power, 24 rats are needed (12 in each group). This sample size estimation is conservative, as two-way repeated measure ANOVA tests were used to determine the correlation of the aortic diameters between the groups over time.

2.4. Experimental Animals, Ethical Statement, Housing and Husbandry

Male Sprague-Dawley rats purchased from Janvier Laboratories, Le Genest-Saint-Isle, France, were housed in cages of up to 4 rats per cage under twelve-hours light/dark cycle, room temperature of 20 °C, air humidity of 55% with free access to standard chow and tap water at the Biomedical Laboratory at the University of Southern Denmark. Rats were acclimatized for at least one week after delivery before entering the experimental protocol.

All animal experiments were conducted in accordance with a protocol ethically approved by the Danish Animal Experiments Inspectorate (license nr. 2016−15−0201−01046), and in accordance with arrive guidelines [22]. As females are generally protected against AAA formation [1,2,23,24], we only used males in this study.

2.5. Induction of Abdominal Aortic Aneurysm by Perfusion of Pancreatic Porcine Elastase (PPE) in the Infrarenal Region of the Aorta

On the day of surgery, male Sprague-Dawley rats (260–435 g corresponding to age 7–10 weeks) were given 0.2 mg temgesic (buprenorphine, Indivior, North Chesterfield, VA, USA) administered in 1 g of nut paste (Nutella) for pain management [25]. Then, the rats were anesthetized by a subcutaneous injection of a mixture of fentanyl (236 µg/kg), fluanisone (7.5 mg/kg, Skanderborg Apotek, Skanderborg, Denmark) and midazolam (3.75 mg/kg, Hameln Pharma, Hamelin, Germany) and underwent AAA induction by intraluminal PPE infusion of the infrarenal region by the procedure previously described by Shack et al. [26]. The only variation was that pancreatic porcine elastase concentration was increased to 12 units/mL for 30 min and post-surgical pain management was provided with additional 0.2 mg temgesic in nut paste (Nutella) [25]. The surgical procedure lasted between 60–70 min. If needed rats were supplemented with 20% of the initial dose of anesthesia by subcutaneous injection during the operation. Representative pictures of the surgical steps and post-surgery day 28 are shown in Figure 1. All rats were observed post-surgery until they were fully awake from anesthesia. They were housed in individual cages in a heated cabinet until next morning, where treatment of the rats was initiated, and the rats were housed together throughout the rest of the experimental period. Rats were treated daily from day 1 post-surgery with CAG (125 mg/kg, Chengdu King-tiger Pharmchem. Tech. Co., Ltd., Chengdu, China, n = 12) or vehicle (deionized reverse osmosis water containing 0.05% methylcellulose (*w/v*, Merck), 2% tween 80 (*v/v*, Merck), n = 12) by oral gavage using Soft Flex feeding tubes (Vetagree, Oslo, Norway) for 28 consecutive days; AAA expansion was monitored weekly by ultrasound measurements, as described below. Four rats were excluded; two vehicle controls died due to surgical and post-surgical complications and two did not consistently receive CAG due to difficulties with oral gavage.

2.6. Ultrasound Measurement of Aneurysm Progression

The abdominal aorta was video recorded from the renal artery to the bifurcation using ultrasound (LogiQ e ultrasound machine and a L10-22-RS transducer, GE Healthcare, Brøndby, Denmark) on the day of AAA induction, day 0 prior to surgery and, thereafter, on days 7, 14, 21 and 28 during treatment using 4% isoflurane inhalation anesthesia (Sigma-Aldrich, Søborg, Denmark). All ultrasound scans were performed by the same investigator, as our pilot study of 76 ultrasound recordings from 16 rats displayed a 6.9% variance between two investigators and stored for later analysis. Measurements of maximal vertical anterior to posterior diameter of the aorta spanning from internal edges during peak systolic blood pressure were performed blinded to the treatment group by two independent investigators using standard software on the LogiQ e Ultrasound machine. Inter-observer variation of the measured diameters was determined to be 3.7% based on the 76 pilot study ultrasound recordings. Values for the relative increase were obtained by adjusting to the diameter on day 0.

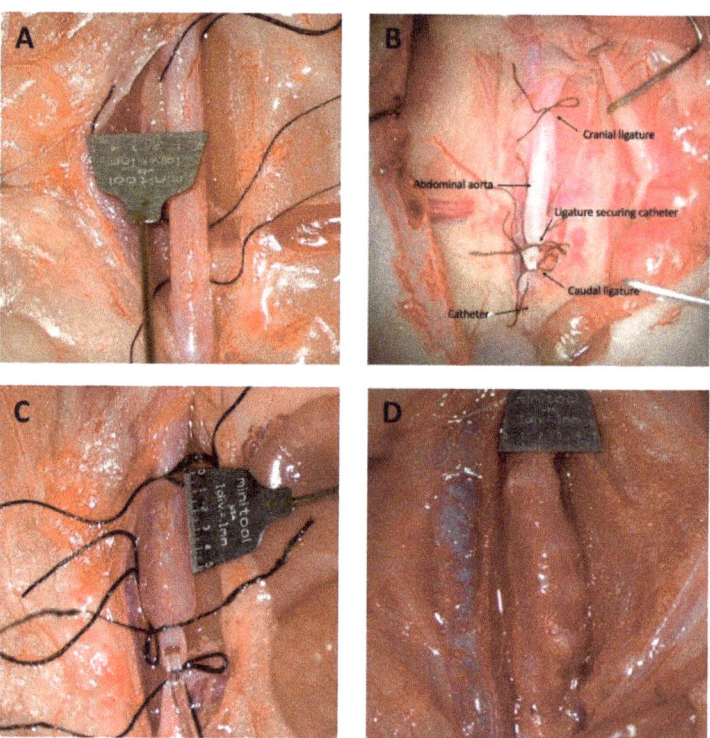

Figure 1. Induction of the surgical steps. (**A**) Isolated infrarenal aorta, (**B**) placing catheter in the infrarenal aorta, (**C**) intraluminal porcine pancreatic elastase infusion, (**D**) isolated AAA on day 28 post surgery.

2.7. At Termination

All rats were euthanized by exsanguination 28 days after AAA induction, resulting in 10 rats in each group. Liver, spleen, heart, and kidneys were collected and weighed. Subsequently, a specimen from the inferior right liver lobe was fixed as described below for morphological analysis.

The aneurysm specimens were isolated and divided into two pieces; the cranial piece was fixed in a 10% normal formalin buffer (Hounisen Laboratorie udstyr A/S, Skanderborg, Denmark) over night at 4 °C, then placed in phosphate-buffered saline (PBS) (Thermo Fisher, Slangerup, Denmark) with 0.05% azide (Sigma-Adrich, Søborg, Denmark) and subsequently embedded in paraffin for morphological analysis. Two samples from the vehicle-group and three from the CAG-group, were unfortunately damaged in the embedding process. The caudal piece was immediately snap frozen in liquid nitrogen and kept at −80 °C until RNA and protein isolation.

2.8. Miller's Elastin and Calcium Von Kossa's Staining

Five μm cross-sections of paraffin embedded aneurysm specimens were sectioned, deparaffinized and hydrated. For identification of elastin fibers, Miller's elastin stain kit

(Atom Scientific, Hyde, UK) was used according to the manufacturer's instructions. In brief, sections were stained for 3 h in Miller's elastin stain, subsequently washed and counterstained with Van Gieson's stain.

Micro-calcium deposits in the aneurysm wall were detected by the silverplating kit according to Von Kossa's stain instructions (Merck, Søborg, Denmark). Calcium deposits were visualized using a 20-watt energy-saving lamp (Quantification method, described below). One additional sample from the vehicle group was damaged during the Von Kossa staining process.

2.9. Immunohistochemistry

Aneurysm cross-sections were deparaffinized and hydrated, followed by antigen retrieval by heating to 100 °C for 15 min in a citrate buffer (10 mM; pH 6, Merck, Søborg, Denmark) for CD206, MMP2or in a TEG-buffer (10 mM TrisBase; 0.5 mM EGTA; pH 9, Sigma Aldrich, Søborg, Denmark) for CD68.

Sections were subsequently blocked for endogenous peroxide activity using, respectively, a 3% and a 1.5% hydrogen peroxide (Merck, Søborg, Denmark) in tris-buffered saline (TBS, Sigma Aldrich, Søborg, Denmark) solution for, respectively, 10 and 30 min. This was followed by one hour blocking in a 5% milk/1× TBS/0.05% Tween-20 (TBST) solution for CD68 and α-actin 3% BSA-TBST solution for CD206 and MMP2.

After washing in TBST, the aneurysm sections were incubated overnight at 4 °C with primary anti-CD68 (Abcam, Cambridge, UK) 1:500 and α-actin (Sigma Aldrich, Søborg, Denmark) 1:500 in 5% milk/TBST and anti-CD206 (Abcam, Cambridge, UK) 1:1000 and MMP2 (Abcam, Cambridge, UK) 1:500, both in 3% BSA/TBST. The next day sections were washed in TBST and incubated with horseradish peroxidase (HRP) conjugated goat-anti-rabbit (DAKO, Glostrup, Denmark) 1:1000 or HRP conjugated anti mouse (DAKO, Glostrup, Denmark) 1:1000 in 5% milk/TBST or 3% BSA/TBST. Positive staining was visualized with 3,3'-Diaminobenzidine tetrahydrochloride hydrate (DAB, Merck, Søborg, Denmark) and sections were counterstained in Mayer's hematoxylin (Merck, Søborg, Denmark) and rinsed in tap water. As negative controls rabbit immunoglobulin IgG corresponding to the primary antibody concentration was applied (DAKO, Glostrup, Denmark). All staining was analyzed in an Olympus Bx51 microscope and micrographs were captured using an Olympus DP26 camera. After analysis, whole frame micrographs were adjusted for brightness and contrast using Photoshop (ver. 9, San Jose, CA, USA).

2.10. Elastin Content Analysis and Immunohistochemical Cell Count

For the assessment of elastin percentage in the medial layer, Image J software (ImageJ 1.53a Wayne Rasband, National Institutes of Health, Bethesda, MD, USA) was used. The external edge of the medial layer was defined as the transition site from disrupted or concentric rings of elastin to connective tissue in the adventitial layer. To quantify the percentage of elastin, the color threshold tool was used. For the scoring of aneurysmal wall disruption, each micrograph was divided into 8 areas, and each field was scored from 1–4, 4 being severe wall disruption and 1 minimal wall disruption. All assessments of elastin content were performed by two investigators blinded to treatment. The interobserver variation was 2.2% and the average score was used for statistical calculations.

Thereafter, elastin lamellae externa was used to identify the border between the medial layer and adventitial layer when identifying the adventitial area with CD68 and CD206 positive cell count per mm^2. The total area of adventitial layer was divided by the number of positive labeled cells to determine positive cells per mm^2. One investigator blinded to treatment determined numbers of positive CD68 and CD206 cells per adventitial area.

2.11. Zymography

Aneurysm samples were homogenized in protein extraction buffer (0.3 M sucrose; 25 mM Imidazole, 1 mM EDTA, pH 7.2 complete protease inhibitor cocktail 2 and 3, Sigma

Aldrich, Søborg, Denmark). Samples were centrifuged for 10 min at 6000× g at 4 °C. Protein concentration was determined by Bicinchoninic Acid Kit for Protein Determination (Sigma Aldrich, Søborg, Denmark) using bovine serum albumin as the standard. A total of 12 µg protein samples and 1.25 µL recombinant MMP-2 (Sigma Aldrich, Søborg, Denmark) were mixed with an equal amount of 2× tris-glycine SDS sample buffer (Thermo Fischer) loaded onto a Novex zymogram gel containing 10% gelatin (Thermo Fisher, Slangerup, Denmark) and proteins were separated by gel electrophoresis at 125 V for 90 min. Proteins were then allowed to refold 30 min in renaturation buffer (Thermo Fisher, Slangerup, Denmark) followed by 24 h at 37 °C in developing buffer (Thermo Fischer, Slangerup, Denmark). Finally, undigested proteins in the gel were stained with simple blue stain (Thermo Fisher) for 30 min. White bands were inverted and quantified in Molecular Imager Image Lab (ChemiDoc WRS+, Biorad, Copenhagen, Denmark).

2.12. Proteomic Analysis

Preparation of AAA tissue for mass spectrometry was performed as previously described [27]. In brief, snap frozen tissue was homogenized in a lysis buffer, then denatured, alkylated, and digested with trypsin overnight. Tryptic peptides were purified on custom-made Poros R2/R3 (Thermo Fisher Scientific, Slangerup, Denmark) columns, and peptide concentration was normalized across samples. Samples (4 µg tryptic peptides per sample) were randomly labelled with 10-plex tandem mass tags (TMT, Thermo Scientific, Waltham, MA, USA); mass tag 126 was a pool of all AAA samples and served as internal control. Proteome data are protein abundances relative to the internal control. Mixed peptide samples were high-pH fractionated and analyzed by nano-LC–MS/MS virtually, as previously described [28]. All Eclipse raw data files were processed and quantified using Proteome Discoverer version 2.4 (Thermo Scientific, Waltham, MA, USA) as previously described [28].

2.13. Quantitative Polymerase Chain Reaction Measurements (qPCR)

The methods of total RNA isolation, cDNA synthesis and qPCR quantification have been described previously by Wintmo et al. [29]. Addition of 1 µL glycoblue (Thermo Fisher, Slangerup, Denmark) as a carrier for enhancement of RNA precipitation was the only modification. Primers used for determining mRNA levels are shown in Table 1.

Table 1. Primer sequences for qPCR analyses. The coefficient of correlation obtained for the standard curve expressed as R^2-value is stated for each PCR product.

Target	Forward Primer (5'-3')	Reverse Primer (5'-3')	R^2-Value
Lysyl oxidase (LOX)	ACCTGGTACCCGATCCCTAC	AGTCTCTGACATCCGCCCTA	0.99
Inducible nitric oxidase synthase (iNOS)	AGGCAAGCCCTCACCTACTT	GATGGGAACTCTTCCAGCAC	0.98
Mature macrophages (F4/80)	TTTTGGCTGCTCCTCTTCTG	TGGCATAAGCTGGACAAGTG	0.98
Interleukin-6 (IL-6)	CAGAGTCATTCAGAGCAATAC	CTTTCAAGATGACTTGGATGG	0.98
Interleukin-10 (IL-10)	TCTCCCCTGTGAGAATAAAA	TAGACACCTTTGTCTTGGAG	0.96
Matrix Metalloprotease 2 (MMP-2)	GATCTTCTTCCTTCAAGGATCG	TACACGGCATCAATCTTTTC	0.99
Matrix Metalloprotease 9 (MMP-9)	TACTTTGGAAACGCAAATGG	GTGTAGGATTCTACTGGG	0.99
Matrix Metalloprotease 12 (MMP-12)	CAATATTGGAGGTACGATGTG	GTCATATTCCAATTGGTAGGC	0.90
Cluster of differentiation 45 (CD45)	GCTATAAAAGACCCCTTCAG	CATTAGGCAAATAGAGACACTG	0.99
Heme oxygenase 1 (HO-1)	ACAGAAGAGGCTAAGACCG	CAGGCATCTCCTTCCATT	0.99
Nuclear factor erythroid-2-related factor (Nrf2)	CCATTTGTAGATGACCATGAG	CTATTAAGACACTGTAACTCGG	0.95
Ribsomal Protein L41 (RPL41)	TGGCGGAAGAAGAGAATGC	TGGACCTCTGCCTCATCTTT	0.99

Messenger RNA (mRNA) levels of genes of interest and five standards (10-fold dilutions) were run in duplicate using SYBR green (Biorad, Copenhagen, Denmark) as the detector system. RNase-free water and RNA samples without reverse transcriptase were used as negative controls. All samples were loaded on 96 Aria Max well plates (Agilent Technologies, Santa Clara, CA, USA), and the PCR amplification was done using three steps (initial 3 min at 95 °C, followed by 40 cycles: 95 °C 20 s; 60 °C 20 s, 72 °C 15 s) followed by a melting curve for the determination of PCR-product selectivity. RNA yield in one sample from each group was low; therefore, these samples were only included in RPL41, LOX, F4/80 and iNOS. Each mRNA expression level of the gene of interest was normalized to the complimentary expression level of the housekeeping gene ribosomal protein L41 (RPL41) that we first tested and did not change significantly between vehicle- and CAG-treated aneurysms.

2.14. Statistical Methods

D'Angostino and Pearson test was used for normality testing. A two-way repeated measures ANOVA adjusted for weight at entry with a Greenhouse-Geisser correction, due to the violation of the assumption of sphericity (Mauchly's test), was used to analyze difference in relative aneurysm diameter between groups, calculated in SPSS (IBM SPSS Statistics, IBM Corporation, Endicott, NY, USA, 1989, 2020). Sidak's multiple comparison test was subsequently applied in Graphpad Prism (ver. 8, San Diego, CA, USA) for each time point.

For the secondary explanatory data, two-tailed unpaired Student's t-test was used to analyze normally distributed data. Values are presented as mean ± standard deviation (SD). Welch's correction was used if F-test for variance was significant. A non-parametric Mann–Whitney test was used if data failed normality testing by the D'Angostino and Pearson test. Values are then presented as median ± interquartile range (IQR). Chi-square test was used for categorial outcome variables.

Explorative proteomics data were analyzed by Student's t-test for each protein and subsequent false discovery rate (FDR) correction for multiple testing and GO enrichment analysis was performed using default settings of the DAVID Bioinformatics Resources [30,31]. The p-values < 0.05 were considered significant.

3. Results

All rats tolerated daily treatment well, except for the two CAG rats excluded due to difficulties with the daily gavage. Treatment did, however, seem to affect liver, spleen, and heart to body weight ratios with a higher ratio among CAG treated rats (Supplementary Figure S1A–C), while kidney to body weight ratio was unaffected (Supplementary Figure S1D). Microscopic analysis of HE-stained liver lobes displayed no obvious differences as evaluated by investigators. As mentioned, a total of four rats were excluded causing an unintendedly higher non-significant mean initial body weight in the vehicle treated rats when compared to the CAG-treated group. Furthermore, there was a large variation in body weight within groups (vehicle: 351.8 g ± 52.2 g vs. CAG: 332.0 g ± 50.1 g, p = 0.33, n = 10/10). To make sure initial body weight did not influence AAA expansion, the statistical analysis was adjusted for body weight. Body weight increase during the experimental period was similar in both groups (Supplementary Figure S1E, 35.6% ± 11.3% vs. 36.78% ± 11.2%; p = 0.83, n = 10/10).

3.1. CAG Treatment Inhibited AAA Expansion

The relative increase in aortic aneurysm diameter at the widest point during peak systolic blood pressure, adjusted for weight at entry, increased gradually in both groups during the experimental period of 28 days (Figure 2). CAG treatment led to significantly smaller aneurysms on days 7, 14, 21 and 28 compared to vehicle treatment (Figure 2). Aneurysm growth was most pronounced during the first 14 days after induction and reached maximal enlargement after 21 days with a mean relative increase of 124% ± 10% and 88% ± 10% for vehicle and CAG groups, respectively (Figure 2). No further change in aneurysm growth was observed at day 28 in either group.

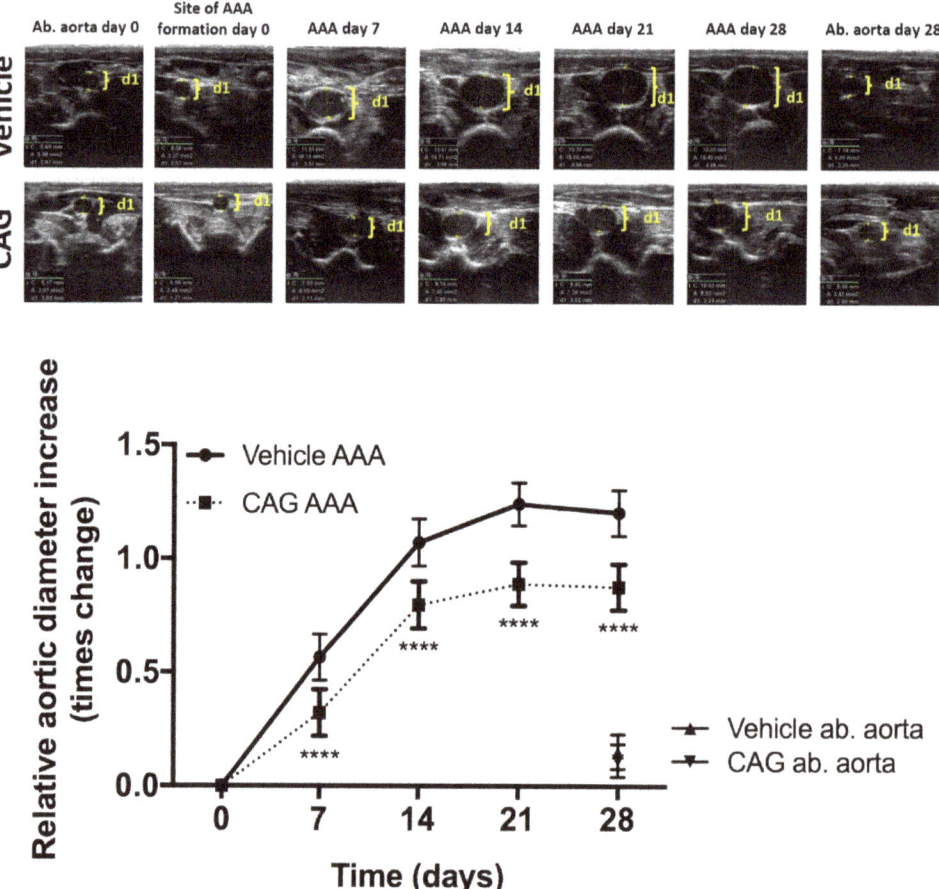

Figure 2. The effect of CAG on AAA growth. Upper panel shows representative ultrasound recordings at baseline and post-surgery days 7, 14, 21, 28 for both vehicle and CAG treated rats. The abdominal aorta (Ab. Aorta) just distal from the left renal artery was used as a reference point for developmental aortic expansion in the experimental period (day 0 and post-surgery day 28). D1: shows aortic diameter. Below, the relative increase in maximal aortic aneurysm diameter adjusted for weight at entry from day 0–28 measured by ultrasound in CAG treated group and vehicle treated group (n = 10/10). Values are mean ± standard deviation. **** indicates $p < 0.0001$.

3.2. CAG Treatment Affects Elastin Integrity

Comparing cross sections of aneurysms at day 28 from both groups to unaffected abdominal aortas proximal to the aneurysm, revealed significant degradation and disruption of elastin lamellae in the medial layer (Figure 3A). Assessing the elastin content in the medial layer in both the vehicle and CAG treated AAA sections showed the mean percentage of elastin content was nearly doubled in the CAG treated group compared to the vehicle treated group, though not significantly (Figure 3B, $p = 0.20$). Elastin degradation and disruption was not affected uniformly in the aneurysm cross sections. Scoring 8 areas on each cross-section showed that areas more prone to rupture (grade 4) were significantly more pronounced in the vehicle-treated group, while larger areas in the CAG-treated group were minimally affected, with large areas scoring grade 1 (Figure 3C, $p = 0.0003$), indicating less wall thinning and destruction, thus, less potential for rupture. This protective effect on elastin was most likely not caused by augmented synthesis of elastin, as the mRNA levels of lysyl oxidase (LOX), an enzyme involved in elastin synthesis and cross-linking [7], was similar in both groups (Figure 3D, $p = 0.57$).

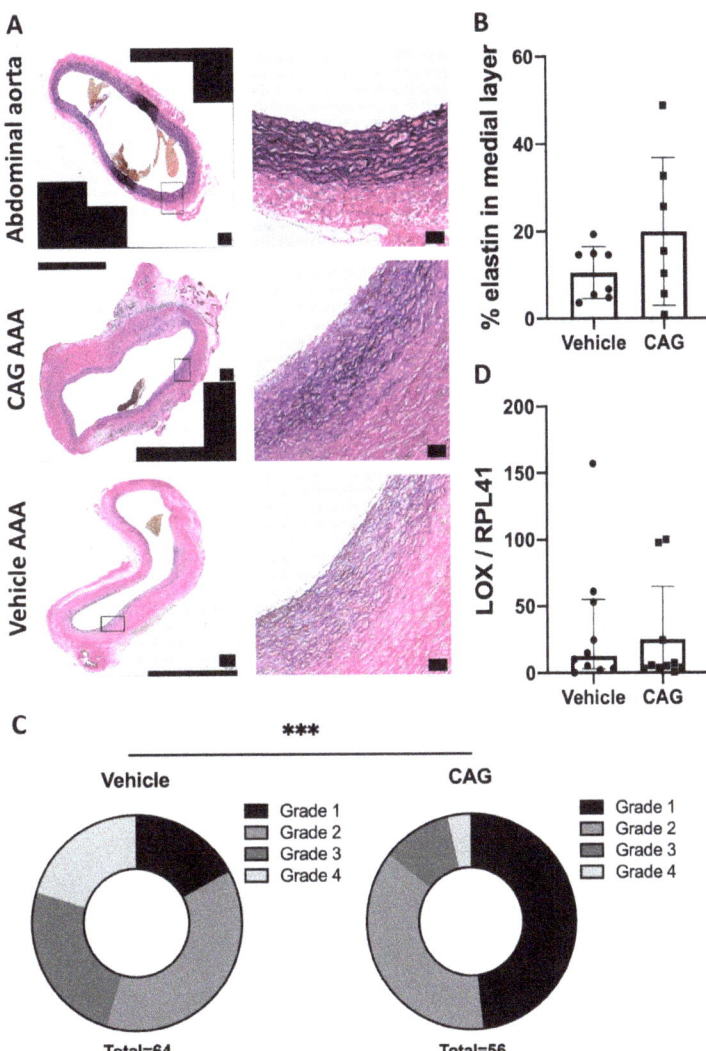

Figure 3. Elastin assessment in abdominal aortic aneurysms (AAA) (**A**) Representative micrographs of Miller's elastin stain (black) from abdominal aorta, vehicle AAA and CAG AAA at day 28 (enlargements correspond to black square on the left image). Scale bar (black box) in micrographs to the left: 100 μm and micrographs to the right: 50 μm (**B**) Percentage of elastin in medial layer in vehicle and CAG group AAA at day 28 (n = 8/7). (**C**) Scoring of aneurysmal wall elastin disruption in vehicle and CAG group 1–4, 4 being severe wall disruption and 1 minimal wall disruption (n = 8/7; $p = 0.0003$). (**D**) Elastin related mRNA coding for LOX gene (n = 10/10) normalized to RPL41 mRNA levels. Values are median ± inter quartile range. *** Indicates $p < 0.001$.

To investigate whether CAG protects against elastin degradation, mRNA levels of MMPs known to play a major role in AAA development [32] were determined. Neither mRNA levels of MMP-2 ($p = 0.22$), MMP-9 ($p = 0.24$) nor MMP-12 ($p = 0.60$) were affected by CAG treatment (Figure 4A–C). In contrast, MMP-2 activity measured by zymography was significantly decreased in the CAG-treated group (Figure 4D), suggesting CAG treatment partly prevents elastin degradation and AAA growth by dampening MMP-2 activity. MMP-2 was associated with a subset of vascular smooth muscle cells in the aneurysm wall, where weak labeling of MMP-2 was detected in the medial layer. There was no apparent difference between the two groups (Figure 4E).

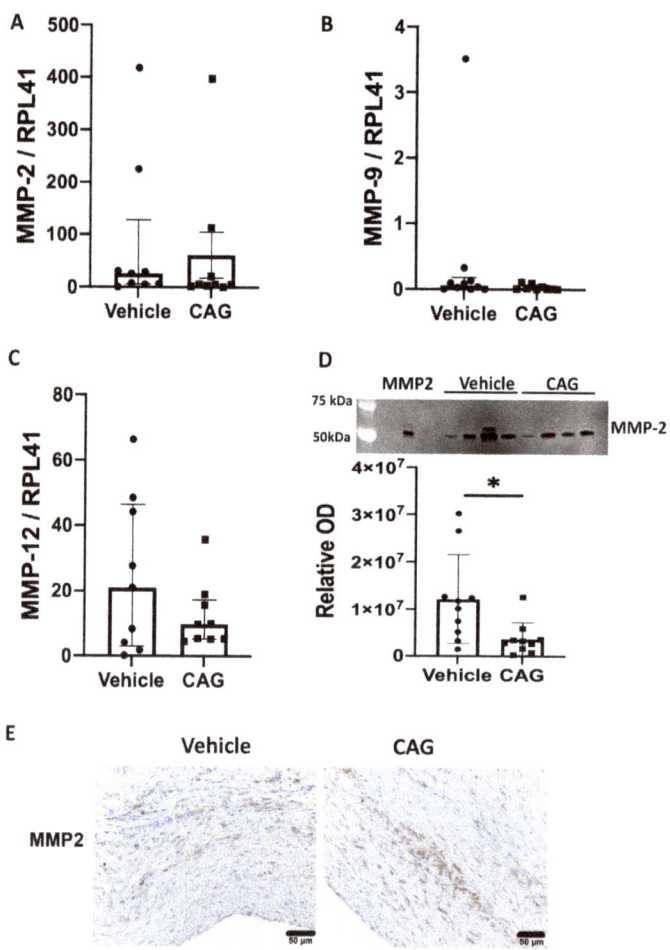

Figure 4. Quantity and activity of matrix metalloproteinases (MMPs) in AAAs. Assessment of messenger RNA (mRNA) from aneurysmal wall samples from vehicle and CAG group coding for (**A**) MMP-2 (n = 9/9), (**B**) MMP-9 (n = 9/9), and (**C**) MMP-12 (n = 9/9). (**D**) Zymography and quantification of zymography showing significantly increased activity of MMP-2 in vehicle compared to CAG group (n = 10/10; $p = 0.02$). (**E**) Displays weak MMP-2 labeling in a subset of vascular smooth muscle cells of the aneurysm wall from both vehicle- and CAG-treated rats (n = 8/7), scalebar = 50 μm. Values in (**A–C**) are median ± interquartile range and normalized to RPL41 mRNA levels. Values in (**D**) are mean ± SD, * indicates $p = 0.02$.

3.3. The Effect of CAG on Infiltration of Inflammatory Cells into the Aneurysm Wall

Next, we determined the suggested anti-inflammatory properties of CAG by determining infiltration of immune cells into the aneurysm wall. The mRNA levels of the common lymphocyte marker CD45 (Figure 5A, $p = 0.63$) and the monocyte/macrophage marker F4/80 (Figure 5B, $p = 0.44$) were not affected in the CAG treated aneurysms.

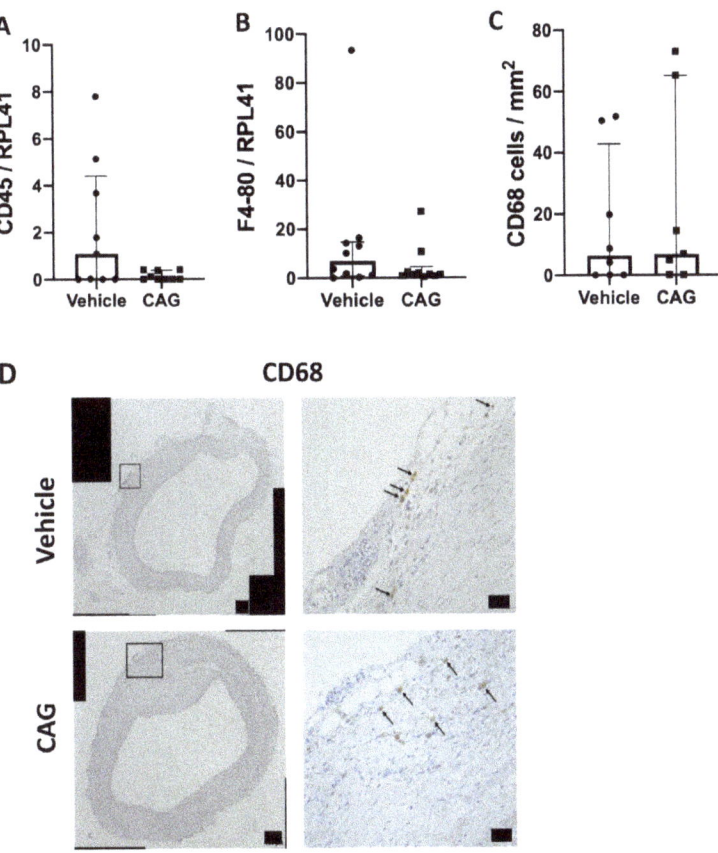

Figure 5. Immune cells in abdominal aortic aneurysms. (**A**) Relative mRNA levels from aneurysmal wall samples from vehicle and CAG treated group of common lymphocyte marker CD45 (n = 9/9), and (**B**) macrophage/monocyte marker F4-80 (n = 10/10). All RNA data were normalized to RPL41 mRNA levels. (**C**) Semi-quantification of aneurysmal CD68 positive cells in AAA of each group per mm^2 in the adventitial layer (n = 8/7). (**D**) Representative micrographs of CD68 positive cells in vehicle and CAG AAAs on day 28 (enlargement represents black square on the left image). Arrows mark positive cells (n = 8/7). Scale bar (black box) in micrographs to the left: 100 µm and in micrographs to the left: 50 µm. Values are median ± interquartile range.

The number of infiltrating macrophages identified as CD68 positive cells, localized to the adventitial layer of the aneurysms, did not show any difference between groups (Figure 5C, D, $p = 0.56$).

As the balance between pro-inflammatory M1 macrophages and tissue repairing M2 macrophages has previously been shown to be important for AAA expansion [9], the M2 macrophages identified as CD206 positive cells were determined in the aneurysm wall (Figure 6A). CD206 positive cells were limited to the adventitial layer, and there were no differences in the number of CD206 positive cells per mm^2 between the two groups

(Figure 6B, $p = 0.99$). In agreement, there were no difference in the aneurysmal mRNA levels of the anti-inflammatory cytokine IL-10 between groups (Figure 6C, $p = 0.114$). Moreover, levels of iNOS mRNA, another marker for M1 macrophages, did not differ between the vehicle and CAG treated groups (Figure 6D, $p = 0.684$) and there was no difference in aneurysmal mRNA levels of the pro-inflammatory cytokine IL-6 between groups (Figure 6E, $p = 0.340$). Thus, the inflammatory response seemed not to be affected by CAG treatment.

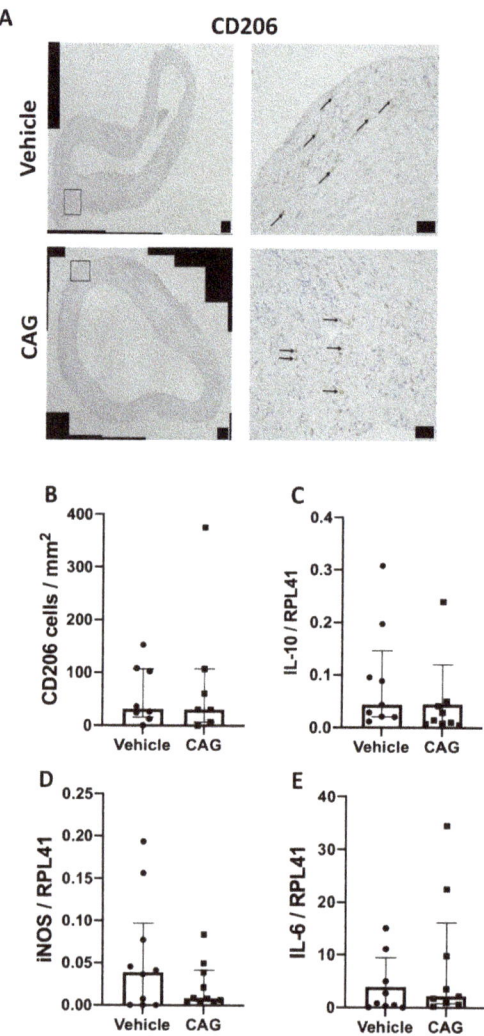

Figure 6. Markers for M1 and M2 macrophages and cytokine expression in the aneurysm wall after 28 days on vehicle or CAG treatment. (A) Representative micrographs of CD206 positive staining from vehicle and CAG AAAs at day 28 (enlargement represent black square on the left image). Arrows mark positive cells (n = 8/7). Scale bar (black box) in micrographs to the left: 100 μm and in micrographs to the right: 50 μm. (B) Semi-quantification of CD206 positive cells in each group per mm^2 in adventitia. (C) Relative mRNA levels of IL-10 (n = 10/10), (D) inducible NO synthase (iNOS) (n = 10/10), and (E) IL-6 (n = 9/9) in the aneurysm tissue. All RNA data is normalized to RPL41 mRNA levels. All values are median ± interquartile range.

3.4. The Effect of CAG on Oxidative Stress and Calcification of the Aneurysm Wall

To determine if CAG dampens AAA progression by reducing oxidative stress, the levels of antioxidative marker Nrf2 mRNA and its downstream target HO-1 were determined in the aneurysms. Neither Nrf2 nor HO-1 mRNA levels differed between treatment groups (Figure 7A,B; $p = 0.171$ and $p = 0.489$, respectively).

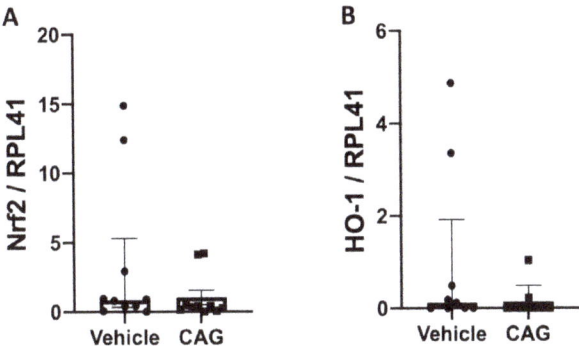

Figure 7. Effect of CAG on aneurysmal oxidative stress. (**A**) Relative mRNA levels of nuclear factor erythroid 2–related factor (Nrf2) (n = 9/9) and (**B**) relative mRNA levels of Heme oxygenase (HO)-1 (n = 9/9) in the aneurysm tissue. All values are median ± interquartile range. All RNA data is normalized to RPL41 mRNA levels.

In more advanced AAAs, calcifications become significant [33]; therefore, the effect of CAG on calcifications was examined by Von Kossa's calcium deposit staining. Calcifications were present in 4 out of 7 AAA samples in the vehicle treated group, while no calcifications were detected in 7 out of 7 in the CAG-treated group (Figure 8A,B, $p = 0.018$).

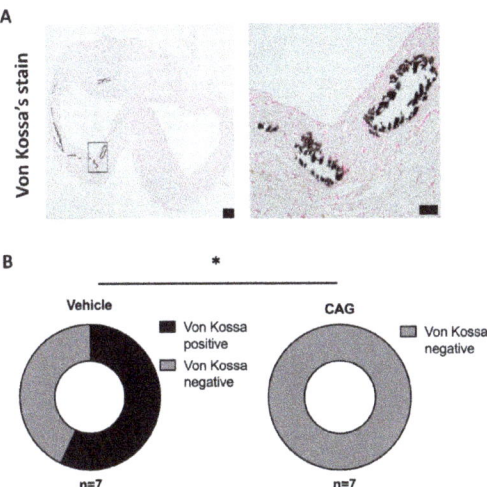

Figure 8. The effect of CAG treatment on aneurysm calcification. (**A**) Representative micrographs of calcium deposits (Black) in the aneurysm wall visualized by Von Kossa's staining (enlargement represent black square on the left image). Scale bar (black box) in micrograph to the left: 100 μm and in micrograph to the right: 50 μm. (n = 7/7). (**B**) Donut plot of percentage of Von Kossa's positive aneurysm sections in CAG and vehicle treated groups (n = 7/7; $p = 0.018$). All values are median ± interquartile range. All RNA data is normalized to RPL41 mRNA levels. * Indicates $p < 0.05$.

3.5. The Effect of CAG AAA Protein Composition Using Explorative Proteomics

To identify new mechanisms of CAG in limiting aneurysm progression, protein samples of the aneurysms were analyzed by liquid chromatography mass spectrometry (LC-MS/MS). We identified 2011 unique proteins (minimum n = 3/3), of which 57% were detected across all samples (n = 10/10) (Supplementary Table S1). No significant differences were found between CAG-treated and vehicle-treated aneurysms when correcting for multiple testing (Supplementary Figure S2); thus, one should bear in mind that some unadjusted de-regulated proteins might be false positive.

The top 20 de-regulated proteins in the aneurysm wall are shown in Table 2. The proteins identified in the aneurysm wall include the structural fibulin-5 involved in elastin assembly [8], the anti-aggregatory and vasodilatory PGI_2-producing enzyme prostacyclin synthase [34], and the water channel aquaporin-1 (AQP1). Table 2: Top 20 hits of proteins deregulated in CAG treated AAA tissue compared to vehicle treated AAA by explorative proteomics (n = 10/10). In this table, data is not adjusted for multiple testing. FC: fold change.

Table 2. Top Deregulated Proteins in CAG Treated AAA vs. Vehicle Treated AAA.

Accession	Description	Fold Change	p-Value
O08658	Nuclear pore complex protein	1.17	0.001
Q9Z1X1	Extended synaptotagmin-1	1.15	0.003
P61227	Ras-related protein Rap-2b	0.77	0.003
P20171	GTPase HRas OS = Rattus norvegicus	0.79	0.004
P53534	Glycogen phosphorylase, brain form (Fragment)	1.14	0.004
P21263	Nestin	1.71	0.005
Q62969	Prostacyclin synthase	1.25	0.007
O35353	Guanine nucleotide-binding protein subunit beta-4	1.22	0.010
Q4V8H8	EH domain-containing protein 2	1.16	0.012
P09414	Nuclear factor 1 A-type	1.39	0.014
O89043	DNA polymerase alpha subunit B	1.19	0.014
Q8CF97	Deubiquitinating protein VCIP135	0.80	0.014
P63029	Translationally-controlled tumor protein	0.90	0.014
P29975	Aquaporin-1	1.25	0.016
Q62745	CD81 antigen	1.07	0.016
B2RYW9	Fumarylacetoacetate hydrolase domain-containing protein 2	1.20	0.018
Q7TQ16	Cytochrome b-c1 complex subunit 8	1.18	0.018
P60892	Ribose-phosphate pyrophosphokinase 1	1.14	0.019
Q9JLZ1	Glutaredoxin-3	0.93	0.020
Q9WVH8	Fibulin-5	1.15	0.020

3.6. Effect of CAG on Vascular Smooth Muscle Cells

To determine if vascular smooth muscle cell layers in the aneurysm wall were changed by CAG treatment, the α-actin positive cells were examined in aneurysm cross-sections from the two groups. Intense α-actin labeling was detected in the medial layer of the aneurysms in both groups; there was no difference in the area of positive α-actin staining between vehicle and CAG-treated rats (Figure 9A,B, $p = 0.56$). That no major change in vascular smooth muscle cell layer was observed was further supported by the quantitative proteome analyses of the aneurysm wall showing no change in proteins associated with vascular smooth muscle cells contractile phenotype [35]; myosin 11, α-actin, transgelin/SM22, calponin-1, myosin regulatory light polypeptide 9, and topomyosin β chain (Supplementary Table S2 and Supplementary Figure S2, yellow dots) between vehicle and CAG-treated rats.

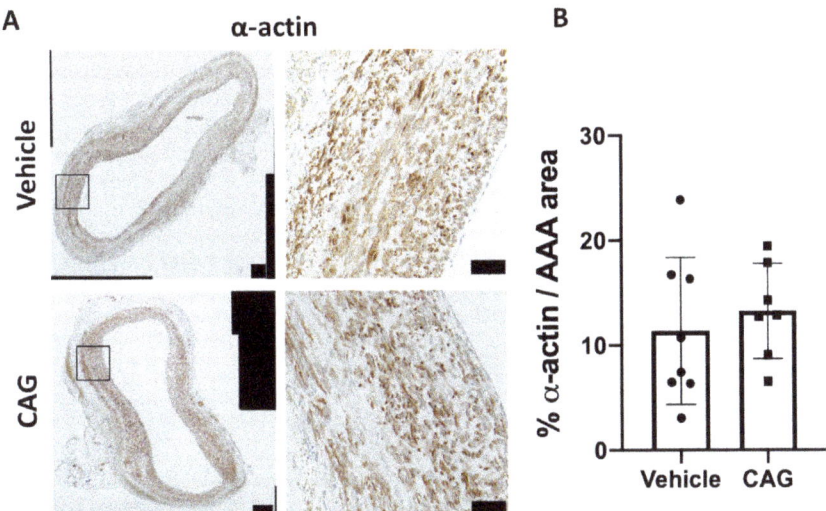

Figure 9. CAG does not affect α-actin positive area in the aneurysm wall. (**A**) Representative micrographs of α-actin staining from vehicle and CAG AAAs at day 28 (enlargement represent black square on the left image, (n = 8/7). Scale bar (black box) in micrographs to the left: 100 μm and in micrographs to the right: 50 μm. (**B**) Semi-quantification of α-actin positive area of total AAA area. Values are mean ± SD.

4. Discussion

In the present study, we aimed to test the proposed protective effects of CAG supplementation on AAA progression. We found that daily administration of CAG significantly attenuated expansion of intraluminal elastase-induced AAA in rats. The aneurysms displayed more preserved elastic lamellae. The underlying mechanism could be linked to diminished aneurysmal MMP-2 activity.

Preservation of elastic lamellae in the CAG treated AAAs could be explained by decreased degradation of elastin or augmented synthesis. Our data suggest that it may not be caused by increased elastin synthesis, as LOX mRNA levels were unchanged. However, we did detect a non-significant upregulation of fibulin-5 by our explorative proteome analysis (FC 1.15 and unadjusted p-value = 0.020). Both LOX and fibulin-5 enable the formation of elastin fibers in the aorta by binding to structural proteins such as tropoelastin and fibrillin-1, thereby facilitating increased elastin assembly in AAAs [8]. Moreover, in cultured rat vascular smooth muscle cells, CAG restored the TNF-mediated reduction in expression of fibulin-5 and -1 [19]. The effect of CAG is, however, more likely caused by decreased MMP-2 activity in the CAG-treated aneurysms produced in vascular smooth muscle cells. This is in line with previous murine studies showing a reduced AAA expansion associated with decreased MMP activity, both in the murine elastase wrapping model and the angiotensin II-induced AAA model in hyperlipidemic ApoE$^{-/-}$ mice [19]. That CAG directly affects vascular smooth muscle cells and, thereby inhibits MMP activity, has been shown in TNF-stimulated cultured primary rat vascular smooth muscle cells; the affected molecular signaling pathway was ascribed to dampening of the ERK/JNK signaling pathway [19].

One of the critical elements in AAA progression includes chronic inflammation associated with continuous infiltration of macrophages and lymphocytes because of degradation of the ECM in the aneurysm wall. The infiltrated immune cells release pro-inflammatory cytokines and proteases that activate VSMCs to phenotypic shift and increased collagen production as a compensatory mechanism for the degradation of elastin fibers. Eventually VSMCs become stressed and undergo apoptosis resulting in high production of RNS and

ROS [36–39]. In murine models, inflammation is the primary driver of AAA progression in the first two weeks of AAA expansion [40,41]; thus, this could explain why we, in this study, did not observe any effect of CAG on the monocyte/macrophage marker F4/80 at the mRNA level, along with no reduction of CD68 positive macrophages in the wall of the CAG treated aneurysms. A reduction in infiltrating CD68 positive cells in the aneurysm wall has previously been observed after CAG treatment in aneurysms in mice induced by local elastase wrapping around the abdominal aorta, and in mice where the component 3,4-benzopyrene (an active ingredient in cigarettes) enhanced angiotensin II AAA two weeks, but also six weeks, after AAA induction [19,42]. The underlying mechanisms were ascribed to reduction in transforming growth factor beta (TGFβ) and nuclear factor kB-induced production of pro-inflammatory cytokines resulting in diminished inflammation. A similar effect of CAG on macrophages was observed in chronic psoriatic skin lesions in mice, where CAG administration reduced infiltration of macrophages and decreased mRNA levels of the pro-inflammatory cytokines IL-1β, TNF, and IL-6 in the inflamed skin and in LPS stimulated bone marrow-derived macrophages in vitro. The effect of CAG was shown to dampen inflammation by preventing NRLP3 inflammasome activation in bone marrow derived macrophages [18].

As there is consensus that CAG seems to inhibit macrophage infiltration and expression of pro-inflammatory cytokines, we would have expected to detect lower mRNA expression levels of IL-6 in the CAG-treated aneurysms. IL-6 is believed to act as a chemoattractant for immune cells in aneurysms. However, it has not been proven to individually affect progression or expansion of AAAs in mice [43]. Our findings of no difference in IL-6 expression between groups contradicts the existing literature [19]. IL-6 belongs to one of the early inflammatory response genes in inflamed tissue [44]. However, we examined the aneurysmal tissue after 28 days, a phase that, in rats, is more regenerative [40]; macrophages shift to favor the anti-inflammatory and tissue repairing phenotype [12,45], which could be why we did not detect any difference in IL-6 levels.

The balance between M1 and M2 macrophages is important for tissue homeostasis [12]. Dale et al. demonstrated that favoring M1 macrophages augmented AAA expansion, while favoring M2 macrophages dampened AAA progression [9]. Thus, we expected that CAG administration would favor the M2 phenotype. We did not find any difference between groups in our semi-quantifications of CD206 positive cells in aneurysm wall cross-sections. In addition, the mRNA levels of the anti-inflammatory cytokine IL-10 in the aneurysms were not significantly different, nor were mRNA levels of iNOS used as an indicator of M1 macrophages in the aneurysms. Thus, in our study, CAG did not seem to favor a shift from M1 to M2 macrophages. No change in inflammatory status was observed in the aneurysm wall. This corresponds with the absence of changes in the media layer of α-actin positive cells and the fact that we did not detect any difference in quantitative proteins associated with vascular smooth muscle cell contractile phenotype.

As previously described, ROS contribute significantly to AAA progression in both human and murine models [46,47] as ROS promote macrophages to release pro-inflammatory cytokines such as IL-6. Astragaloside IV (AST) obtained from *Astragalus membranaceus* is easily converted by intestinal microbes to CAG by deglycosylation [48]. In murine models of AAA, both AST and CAG reduced ROS and, thereby, dampened the release of pro-inflammatory cytokines IL-6, TNF and MMPs from macrophages [19,42]. The underlying mechanism relates to augmented Nrf2 and HO-1 signaling pathways. Nrf2 is a transcription factor that controls the expression of antioxidant genes [10]. Thus, upregulation of Nrf2 will diminish ROS and, thereby, ROS-mediated inflammation [46]. HMOX1 is a cellular stress response gene regulated by Nrf2 that produces HO-1. HO-1 is responsible for the oxidative cleavage of heme groups released from damaged erythrocytes in the vascular wall, leading to the generation of biliverdin with antioxidant properties, thereby scavenging ROS, carbon monoxide with vasodilatory properties, and release of ferrous iron. Thus, HO-1 has important antioxidant, anti-inflammatory, and cytoprotective effects in vascular cells. Thus, the presence of HO-1 protects vascular smooth muscle cells and endothelial cells from further damage in response to injury. Furthermore, HO-1 deficiency in mice augments AAA progression [49]. Moreover, in humans, polymorphisms in the promoter region of the HMOX1 gene, resulting in decreased expression of HO-1, are associated with increased risk of developing AAA [50]. In our experiments, neither Nrf2 nor HO-1 mRNA levels changed after CAG treatment, suggesting that, in our setting, CAG did not influence ROS or exert antioxidative effects at the examined time point. Perhaps, this could be explained by species difference or the dose of CAG used. The studies showing that CAG or AST reduced the expression of Nrf2 and HO-1 were performed in mice using two different models: the elastase wrapping model and the angiotensin II and 3,4 benzopyrene-induced AAA model in 8–10 months old C57BL/6 mice. As in our experiments, CAG was given orally. In the angiotensin II and 3.4-benzopyrene model, they used daily doses of 20 mg/kg and 80 mg/kg for 6 weeks [42], while CAG, in the elastase wrapping model, was given in a low dose 62.5 mg/kg or high dose 125 mg/kg daily for 14 or 28 days perorally, starting at the day of experiment or at 14 days (high dose only) after AAA induction [19]. We initiated our CAG administration the day after surgery to prevent pre-priming of the aortic wall prior to elastase treatment. The high dose in our experiment was chosen based on the daily dose of CAG on an oral no-observed-adverse-effect-level (NOAEL) > 150 mg/day in rats, achieved by oral administration of 150 mg CAG/kg/day for 91 consecutive days [51] and corresponded to the dose used in Wang et al. [19], though there might be species difference.

To find new potential mechanisms that CAG might affect to dampen AAA progression, we used an explorative proteome approach. We did not find any deregulated proteins in the aneurysm wall in comparing the two groups, when adjustment for multiple testing was done. This might reflect the highly heterogenous tissue that requires numerous samples to detect differences. Amongst the unadjusted regulated genes with a p-value below 0.02 was prostacyclin synthase (PGIS) (FC 1.27, unadjusted p-value = 0.006). PGIS produces prostacyclin with known vasodilatory, anti-inflammatory, and anti-thrombotic properties counteracting the prothrombotic thromboxane [34,52,53]. The water channel AQP1 was also upregulated (FC 1.26, unadjusted p-value = 0.01). We have previously shown that loss of AQP1 accelerates angiotensin II-induced atherosclerosis in hyperlipidemic mice [29]. The underlying mechanism was not identified; however, AQP1 channels in the endothelial cells could, perhaps, contribute to washing out substances, such as LDL, trapped in the subendothelial intimal layer in areas of endothelial dysfunction.

The protective effect of CAG could also be mediated by lowering arterial blood pressure. We did not measure blood pressure in our study, but we did observe a difference in heart to body weight ratios, with a higher ratio among CAG-treated rats that could suggest an elevated blood pressure. However, we believe that the elevated heart to body ratio more likely relates to the relatively lower body weights within the CAG-treated rats, as liver and spleen to body ratios were also slightly elevated. Others have reported that the compound astragaloside IV, which is converted by intestinal microbes to CAG [54], did not affect arterial blood pressure in pregnant rats [55]. They did, however, observe a dose-dependent (20–80 mg/kg) blood pressure lowering effect in preeclampsia-induced pregnant rats, as well as a reduction in preeclampsia-induced oxidative stress [55], suggesting that CAG in our model could potentially have a minor blood pressure lowering effect rather than elevating blood pressure. In comparison, we treated our rats with a higher dose of CAG that seemed to be well tolerated; the rats had a similar weight gain as the vehicle treated controls, in line with the existing literature [19,51].

There are some limitations to the study. Our primary end point was progressive aneurysm dilatation. Therefore, we chose the PPE AAA model in rats, as it is, to our knowledge, the model that presents most of the features of the human disease [20,40,41]. All models are short term, while human AAA develops over years [1,6]. The length of the experimental protocol is, in most studies, either 14 days or 28 days. The first 14 days of AAA expansion is fastest and involves inflammation and oxidative stress as drivers [56]. While, in the last 14 days, AAA expansion declines and reaches a plateau, reflecting tissue-repairing mechanisms with extensive elastin production. To get the full effect of CAG on

AAA expansion, we chose to end the experiment after 28 days, when AAA size and elastin integrity could be analyzed, while proinflammatory responses may be less pronounced. Although the reduction in MMP-2 activity seen at day 28 in the aneurysm wall may reflect reduced inflammation and/or oxidative stress at an earlier timepoint.

The effect of CAG in already established AAA has yet to be evaluated. This would be clinically relevant. Although, in our experiments, CAG treatment was provided after induction of AAA by elastase infusion. Thus, we did not affect the aortic wall by initiating CAG treatment prior to AAA induction, which suggests that CAG could likely be beneficial in existing AAA and is supported by findings in mice [19].

5. Conclusions

In conclusion, CAG reduced experimental AAA progression. Our data suggest that underlying mechanisms might be mediated by reduced MMP-2 activity and by preserving elastin and reduced calcification. Based on these findings, CAG should be considered as a possible candidate for future dietary supplementation that may dampen AAA expansion in humans.

Supplementary Materials: The following supporting information can be downloaded at: https://www.mdpi.com/article/10.3390/biomedicines10020359/s1, Figure S1: Body weight changes and tissue weights after 28 days of CAG treatment. Figure S2: Volcano plot showing changes in aneurysmal protein levels between CAG treated and vehicle treated groups using proteomic analyses. Table S1:All identified proteins in CAG vs. vehicle treated AAAs. Table S2: CAG treatment does not affect aneurysm protein levels related to VSMC contractile phenotype compared to vehicle treated rats.

Author Contributions: Conceptualization and methodology: L.G.M., J.H.D., J.S.L. and J.S.; software, validation, formal analysis, resources, data curation and visualization: L.G.M., J.H.D., L.B.S., S.L.E., P.D.C., H.C.B., J.S.L. and J.S.; writing—original draft preparation: L.G.M., L.B.S., J.S.L. and J.S.; writing—review and editing: L.G.M., L.B.S., J.H.D., J.S.L., H.C.B., S.L.E., P.D.C., L.M.R. and J.S.; supervision and project administration: J.S., J.S.L. and L.G.M.; Funding acquisition: J.S.L., L.G.M. and J.S. All authors have read and agreed to the published version of the manuscript.

Funding: The research was funded by The Region of Southern Denmark (19/25225), A. P. Moeller Foundation (19-L-0069) and Novo Nordisk Foundation (NNF19OC0058959).

Institutional Review Board Statement: Not applicable. All animal experiments were as described in the method section conducted as according to an animal protocol approved by the Danish Animal Experiments Inspectorate (license nr. 2016−15−0201−01046).

Informed Consent Statement: Not applicable.

Data Availability Statement: The mass spectrometry proteomics data have been deposited to the ProteomeXchange Consortium via the PRIDE [57] partner repository with the dataset identifier PXD030441.

Acknowledgments: We would like to thank our skillful technicians Lene Bundgaard Andersen, Amalie Kamstrup Mogensen, Kenneth Kjærsgaard, Inger Nissen, Bianca Jørgensen, Anne Mette Durand, and Maja Friis Waltersdorff for their excellent technical assistance. We thank Anthony M. Carter for linguistic correction.

Conflicts of Interest: The authors have no conflict of interest. The funders had no role in the design of the study; in the collection, analyses, or interpretation of data; in the writing of the manuscript; or in the decision to publish the results.

References

1. Kuivaniemi, H.; Ryer, E.J.; Elmore, J.R.; Tromp, G. Understanding the pathogenesis of abdominal aortic aneurysms. *Expert Rev. Cardiovasc. Ther.* **2015**, *13*, 975–987. [CrossRef] [PubMed]
2. Howard, D.P.; Banerjee, A.; Fairhead, J.F.; Handa, A.; Silver, L.E.; Rothwell, P.M. Population-Based Study of Incidence of Acute Abdominal Aortic Aneurysms With Projected Impact of Screening Strategy. *J. Am. Heart Assoc.* **2015**, *4*, e001926. [CrossRef] [PubMed]
3. Filardo, G.; Powell, J.T.; Martinez, M.A.; Ballard, D.J. Surgery for small asymptomatic abdominal aortic aneurysms. *Cochrane Database Syst Rev.* **2015**, *2015*, Cd001835. [CrossRef] [PubMed]

4. Kent, K.C. Clinical practice. Abdominal aortic aneurysms. *N. Engl. J. Med.* **2014**, *371*, 2101–2108. [CrossRef] [PubMed]
5. Moll, F.L.; Powell, J.T.; Fraedrich, G.; Verzini, F.; Haulon, S.; Waltham, M.; van Herwaarden, J.A.; Holt, P.J.; van Keulen, J.W.; Rantner, B.; et al. Management of abdominal aortic aneurysms clinical practice guidelines of the European society for vascular surgery. *Eur. J. Vasc. Endovasc. Surg.* **2011**, *41* (Suppl. 1), S1–S58. [CrossRef] [PubMed]
6. Ailawadi, G.; Eliason, J.L.; Upchurch, G.R., Jr. Current concepts in the pathogenesis of abdominal aortic aneurysm. *J. Vasc. Surg.* **2003**, *38*, 584–588. [CrossRef]
7. Campa, J.S.; Greenhalgh, R.M.; Powell, J.T. Elastin degradation in abdominal aortic aneurysms. *Atherosclerosis* **1987**, *65*, 13–21. [CrossRef]
8. Yanagisawa, H.; Schluterman, M.K.; Brekken, R.A. Fibulin-5, an integrin-binding matricellular protein: Its function in development and disease. *J. Cell Commun. Signal.* **2009**, *3*, 337–347. [CrossRef]
9. Dale, M.A.; Xiong, W.; Carson, J.S.; Suh, M.K.; Karpisek, A.D.; Meisinger, T.M.; Casale, G.P.; Baxter, B.T. Elastin-Derived Peptides Promote Abdominal Aortic Aneurysm Formation by Modulating M1/M2 Macrophage Polarization. *J. Immunol.* **2016**, *196*, 4536–4543. [CrossRef]
10. Kovac, S.; Angelova, P.R.; Holmström, K.M.; Zhang, Y.; Dinkova-Kostova, A.T.; Abramov, A.Y. Nrf2 regulates ROS production by mitochondria and NADPH oxidase. *Biochim. Biophys. Acta* **2015**, *1850*, 794–801. [CrossRef]
11. Chen, Q.; Wang, Q.; Zhu, J.; Xiao, Q.; Zhang, L. Reactive oxygen species: Key regulators in vascular health and diseases. *Br. J. Pharmacol.* **2018**, *175*, 1279–1292. [CrossRef] [PubMed]
12. Dale, M.A.; Ruhlman, M.K.; Baxter, B.T. Inflammatory cell phenotypes in AAAs: Their role and potential as targets for therapy. *Arterioscler. Thromb. Vasc. Biol.* **2015**, *35*, 1746–1755. [CrossRef] [PubMed]
13. McCormick, M.L.; Gavrila, D.; Weintraub, N.L. Role of oxidative stress in the pathogenesis of abdominal aortic aneurysms. *Arterioscler. Thromb. Vasc. Biol.* **2007**, *27*, 461–469. [CrossRef] [PubMed]
14. Yu, Y.; Zhou, L.; Yang, Y.; Liu, Y. Cycloastragenol: An exciting novel candidate for age-associated diseases. *Exp. Ther. Med.* **2018**, *16*, 2175–2182. [CrossRef]
15. Sun, C.; Jiang, M.; Zhang, L.; Yang, J.; Zhang, G.; Du, B.; Ren, Y.; Li, X.; Yao, J. Cycloastragenol mediates activation and proliferation suppression in concanavalin A-induced mouse lymphocyte pan-activation model. *Immunopharmacol. Immunotoxicol.* **2017**, *39*, 131–139. [CrossRef]
16. Wang, J.; Wu, M.L.; Cao, S.P.; Cai, H.; Zhao, Z.M.; Song, Y.H. Cycloastragenol ameliorates experimental heart damage in rats by promoting myocardial autophagy via inhibition of AKT1-RPS6KB1 signaling. *Biomed. Pharmacother.* **2018**, *107*, 1074–1081. [CrossRef]
17. Gu, M.; Zhang, S.; Zhao, Y.; Huang, J.; Wang, Y.; Li, Y.; Fan, S.; Yang, L.; Ji, G.; Tong, Q.; et al. Cycloastragenol improves hepatic steatosis by activating farnesoid X receptor signalling. *Pharmacol. Res.* **2017**, *121*, 22–32. [CrossRef]
18. Deng, G.; Chen, W.; Wang, P.; Zhan, T.; Zheng, W.; Gu, Z.; Wang, X.; Ji, X.; Sun, Y. Inhibition of NLRP3 inflammasome-mediated pyroptosis in macrophage by cycloastragenol contributes to amelioration of imiquimod-induced psoriasis-like skin inflammation in mice. *Int. Immunopharmacol.* **2019**, *74*, 105682. [CrossRef]
19. Wang, Y.; Chen, C.; Wang, Q.; Cao, Y.; Xu, L.; Qi, R. Inhibitory effects of cycloastragenol on abdominal aortic aneurysm and its related mechanisms. *Br. J. Pharmacol.* **2019**, *176*, 282–296. [CrossRef]
20. Anidjar, S.; Salzmann, J.L.; Gentric, D.; Lagneau, P.; Camilleri, J.P.; Michel, J.B. Elastase-induced experimental aneurysms in rats. *Circulation* **1990**, *82*, 973–981. [CrossRef]
21. Lysgaard Poulsen, J.; Stubbe, J.; Lindholt, J.S. Animal Models Used to Explore Abdominal Aortic Aneurysms: A Systematic Review. *Eur. J. Vasc. Endovasc. Surg.* **2016**, *52*, 487–499. [CrossRef] [PubMed]
22. Kilkenny, C.; Browne, W.; Cuthill, I.C.; Emerson, M.; Altman, D.G.; Group NCRRGW. Animal research: Reporting in vivo experiments: The ARRIVE guidelines. *Br. J. Pharmacol.* **2010**, *160*, 1577–1579. [CrossRef] [PubMed]
23. Johnston, W.F.; Salmon, M.; Su, G.; Lu, G.; Ailawadi, G.; Upchurch, G.R., Jr. Aromatase is required for female abdominal aortic aneurysm protection. *J. Vasc. Surg.* **2015**, *61*, 1565–1574.e4. [CrossRef] [PubMed]
24. Ailawadi, G.; Eliason, J.L.; Roelofs, K.J.; Sinha, I.; Hannawa, K.K.; Kaldjian, E.P.; Lu, G.; Henke, P.K.; Stanley, J.C.; Weiss, S.J.; et al. Gender differences in experimental aortic aneurysm formation. *Arterioscler. Thromb. Vasc. Biol.* **2004**, *24*, 2116–2122. [CrossRef]
25. Abelson, K.S.; Jacobsen, K.R.; Sundbom, R.; Kalliokoski, O.; Hau, J. Voluntary ingestion of nut paste for administration of buprenorphine in rats and mice. *Lab. Anim.* **2012**, *46*, 349–351. [CrossRef]
26. Schack, A.S.; Stubbe, J.; Steffensen, L.B.; Mahmoud, H.; Laursen, M.S.; Lindholt, J.S. Intraluminal infusion of Penta-Galloyl Glucose reduces abdominal aortic aneurysm development in the elastase rat model. *PLoS ONE* **2020**, *15*, e0234409. [CrossRef]
27. Steffensen, L.B.; Stubbe, J.; Lindholt, J.S.; Beck, H.C.; Overgaard, M.; Bloksgaard, M.; Genovese, F.; Nielsen, S.H.; Tha, M.L.T.; Bang-Moeller, S.K.; et al. Basement membrane collagen IV deficiency promotes abdominal aortic aneurysm formation. *Sci. Rep.* **2021**, *11*, 12903. [CrossRef]
28. Mulorz, J.; Spin, J.M.; Beck, H.C.; Tha Thi, M.L.; Wagenhäuser, M.U.; Rasmussen, L.M.; Lindholt, J.S.; Tsao, P.S.C.; Steffensen, L.B. Hyperlipidemia does not affect development of elastase-induced abdominal aortic aneurysm in mice. *Atherosclerosis* **2020**, *311*, 73–83. [CrossRef]
29. Wintmo, P.; Johansen, S.H.; Hansen, P.B.L.; Lindholt, J.S.; Urbonavicius, S.; Rasmussen, L.M.; Bie, P.; Jensen, B.L.; Stubbe, J. The water channel AQP1 is expressed in human atherosclerotic vascular lesions and AQP1 deficiency augments angiotensin II-induced atherosclerosis in mice. *Acta Physiol.* **2017**, *220*, 446–460. [CrossRef]

30. Huang da, W.; Sherman, B.T.; Lempicki, R.A. Systematic and integrative analysis of large gene lists using DAVID bioinformatics resources. *Nat. Protoc.* **2009**, *4*, 44–57. [CrossRef]
31. Huang da, W.; Sherman, B.T.; Lempicki, R.A. Bioinformatics enrichment tools: Paths toward the comprehensive functional analysis of large gene lists. *Nucleic Acids Res.* **2009**, *37*, 1–13. [CrossRef] [PubMed]
32. Rabkin, S.W. The Role Matrix Metalloproteinases in the Production of Aortic Aneurysm. *Prog. Mol. Biol. Transl. Sci.* **2017**, *147*, 239–265. [PubMed]
33. Buijs, R.V.; Willems, T.P.; Tio, R.A.; Boersma, H.H.; Tielliu, I.F.; Slart, R.H.; Zeebregts, C.J. Calcification as a risk factor for rupture of abdominal aortic aneurysm. *Eur. J. Vasc. Endovasc. Surg.* **2013**, *46*, 542–548. [CrossRef] [PubMed]
34. Moncada, S.; Vane, J.R. The role of prostacyclin in vascular tissue. *Fed. Proc.* **1979**, *38*, 66–71.
35. Wirka, R.C.; Wagh, D.; Paik, D.T.; Pjanic, M.; Nguyen, T.; Miller, C.L.; Kundu, R.; Nagao, M.; Coller, J.; Koyano, T.K.; et al. Atheroprotective roles of smooth muscle cell phenotypic modulation and the TCF21 disease gene as revealed by singlecell analysis. *Nat. Med.* **2019**, *25*, 1280–1289. [CrossRef]
36. Li, P.F.; Dietz, R.; von Harsdorf, R. Reactive oxygen species induce apoptosis of vascular smooth muscle cell. *FEBS Lett.* **1997**, *404*, 249–252. [CrossRef]
37. Morimoto, K.; Hasegawa, T.; Tanaka, A.; Wulan, B.; Yu, J.; Morimoto, N.; Okita, Y.; Okada, K. Free-radical scavenger edaravone inhibits both formation and development of abdominal aortic aneurysm in rats. *J. Vasc. Surg.* **2012**, *55*, 1749–1758. [CrossRef]
38. Peppin, G.J.; Weiss, S.J. Activation of the endogenous metalloproteinase, gelatinase, by triggered human neutrophils. *Proc. Natl. Acad. Sci. USA* **1986**, *83*, 4322–4326. [CrossRef]
39. Rajagopalan, S.; Meng, X.P.; Ramasamy, S.; Harrison, D.G.; Galis, Z.S. Reactive oxygen species produced by macrophage-derived foam cells regulate the activity of vascular matrix metalloproteinases in vitro. Implications for atherosclerotic plaque stability. *J. Clin. Investig.* **1996**, *98*, 2572–2579. [CrossRef]
40. Sénémaud, J.; Caligiuri, G.; Etienne, H.; Delbosc, S.; Michel, J.B.; Coscas, R. Translational Relevance and Recent Advances of Animal Models of Abdominal Aortic Aneurysm. *Arterioscler. Thromb. Vasc. Biol.* **2017**, *37*, 401–410. [CrossRef]
41. Pyo, R.; Lee, J.K.; Shipley, J.M.; Curci, J.A.; Mao, D.; Ziporin, S.J.; Ennis, T.L.; Shapiro, S.D.; Senior, R.M.; Thompson, R.W. Targeted gene disruption of matrix metalloproteinase-9 (gelatinase B) suppresses development of experimental abdominal aortic aneurysms. *J. Clin. Investig.* **2000**, *105*, 1641–1649. [CrossRef] [PubMed]
42. Wang, J.; Zhou, Y.; Wu, S.; Huang, K.; Thapa, S.; Tao, L.; Wang, J.; Shen, Y.; Wang, J.; Xue, Y.; et al. Astragaloside IV Attenuated 3,4-Benzopyrene-Induced Abdominal Aortic Aneurysm by Ameliorating Macrophage-Mediated Inflammation. *Front. Pharmacol.* **2018**, *9*, 496. [CrossRef] [PubMed]
43. Nishihara, M.; Aoki, H.; Ohno, S.; Furusho, A.; Hirakata, S.; Nishida, N.; Ito, S.; Hayashi, M.; Imaizumi, T.; Fukumoto, Y. The role of IL-6 in pathogenesis of abdominal aortic aneurysm in mice. *PLoS ONE* **2017**, *12*, e0185923. [CrossRef] [PubMed]
44. Tanaka, T.; Narazaki, M.; Kishimoto, T. IL-6 in inflammation, immunity, and disease. *Cold Spring Harb. Perspect. Biol.* **2014**, *6*, a016295. [CrossRef] [PubMed]
45. Cheng, Z.; Zhou, Y.Z.; Wu, Y.; Wu, Q.Y.; Liao, X.B.; Fu, X.M.; Zhou, X.M. Diverse roles of macrophage polarization in aortic aneurysm: Destruction and repair. *J. Transl. Med.* **2018**, *16*, 354. [CrossRef] [PubMed]
46. Emeto, T.I.; Moxon, J.V.; Au, M.; Golledge, J. Oxidative stress and abdominal aortic aneurysm: Potential treatment targets. *Clin. Sci.* **2016**, *130*, 301–315. [CrossRef] [PubMed]
47. Usui, F.; Shirasuna, K.; Kimura, H.; Tatsumi, K.; Kawashima, A.; Karasawa, T.; Yoshimura, K.; Aoki, H.; Tsutsui, H.; Noda, T.; et al. Inflammasome activation by mitochondrial oxidative stress in macrophages leads to the development of angiotensin II-induced aortic aneurysm. *Arterioscler. Thromb. Vasc. Biol.* **2015**, *35*, 127–136. [CrossRef]
48. Ran, R.; Zhang, C.; Li, R.; Chen, B.; Zhang, W.; Zhao, Z.; Fu, Z.; Du, Z.; Du, X.; Yang, X.; et al. Evaluation and Comparison of the Inhibition Effect of Astragaloside IV and Aglycone Cycloastragenol on Various UDP-Glucuronosyltransferase (UGT) Isoforms. *Molecules* **2016**, *21*, 1616. [CrossRef]
49. Azuma, J.; Wong, R.J.; Morisawa, T.; Hsu, M.; Maegdefessel, L.; Zhao, H.; Kalish, F.; Kayama, Y.; Wallenstein, M.B.; Deng, A.C.; et al. Heme Oxygenase-1 Expression Affects Murine Abdominal Aortic Aneurysm Progression. *PLoS ONE* **2016**, *11*, e0149288. [CrossRef]
50. Schillinger, M.; Exner, M.; Mlekusch, W.; Domanovits, H.; Huber, K.; Mannhalter, C.; Wagner, O.; Minar, E. Heme oxygenase-1 gene promoter polymorphism is associated with abdominal aortic aneurysm. *Thromb. Res.* **2002**, *106*, 131–136. [CrossRef]
51. Szabo, N.J. Dietary safety of cycloastragenol from Astragalus spp.: Subchronic toxicity and genotoxicity studies. *Food Chem. Toxicol.* **2014**, *64*, 322–334. [CrossRef] [PubMed]
52. Canaud, B.; Mion, C.; Arujo, A.; N'Guyen, Q.V.; Paleyrac, G.; Hemmendinger, S.; Cazenave, J.P. Prostacyclin (epoprostenol) as the sole antithrombotic agent in postdilutional hemofiltration. *Nephron* **1988**, *48*, 206–212. [CrossRef] [PubMed]
53. Stitham, J.; Midgett, C.; Martin, K.A.; Hwa, J. Prostacyclin: An inflammatory paradox. *Front. Pharmacol.* **2011**, *2*, 24. [CrossRef] [PubMed]
54. Zhao, Y.; Li, Q.; Zhao, W.; Li, J.; Sun, Y.; Liu, K.; Liu, B.; Zhang, N. Astragaloside IV and cycloastragenol are equally effective in inhibition of endoplasmic reticulum stress-associated TXNIP/NLRP3 inflammasome activation in the endothelium. *J. Ethnopharmacol.* **2015**, *169*, 210–218. [CrossRef] [PubMed]
55. Yang, S.; Zhang, R.; Xing, B.; Zhou, L.; Zhang, P.; Song, L. Astragaloside IV ameliorates preeclampsia-induced oxidative stress through the Nrf2/HO-1 pathway in a rat model. *Am. J. Physiol. Endocrinol. Metab.* **2020**, *319*, E904–E911. [CrossRef] [PubMed]

56. Carsten, C.G., 3rd; Calton, W.C.; Johanning, J.M.; Armstrong, P.J.; Franklin, D.P.; Carey, D.J.; Elmore, J.R. Elastase is not sufficient to induce experimental abdominal aortic aneurysms. *J. Vasc. Surg.* **2001**, *33*, 1255–1262. [CrossRef] [PubMed]
57. Perez-Riverol, Y.; Csordas, A.; Bai, J.; Bernal-Llinares, M.; Hewapathirana, S.; Kundu, D.J.; Inuganti, A.; Griss, J.; Mayer, G.; Eisenacher, M.; et al. The PRIDE database and related tools and resources in 2019: Improving support for quantification data. *Nucleic Acids Res.* **2019**, *47*, D442–D450. [CrossRef]

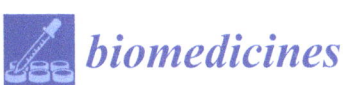

Article

Intra-Operative Video-Based Measurement of Biaxial Strains of the Ascending Thoracic Aorta

Shaiv Parikh [1], Berta Ganizada [2], Gijs Debeij [2], Ehsan Natour [2], Jos Maessen [2], Bart Spronck [1], Leon Schurgers [3], Tammo Delhaas [1], Wouter Huberts [1,†], Elham Bidar [2,†] and Koen Reesink [1,*,†]

1. Department of Biomedical Engineering, CARIM School for Cardiovascular Diseases, Maastricht University, 6229 ER Maastricht, The Netherlands; s.parikh@maastrichtuniversity.nl (S.P.); b.spronck@maastrichtuniversity.nl (B.S.); tammo.delhaas@maastrichtuniversity.nl (T.D.); wouter.huberts@maastrichtuniversity.nl (W.H.)
2. Department of Cardiothoracic Surgery, Heart & Vascular Centre, Maastricht University Medical Centre, 6229 HX Maastricht, The Netherlands; berta.ganizada@mumc.nl (B.G.); gijs.debeij@mumc.nl (G.D.); ehsan.natour@mumc.nl (E.N.); j.g.maessen@mumc.nl (J.M.); elham.bidar@mumc.nl (E.B.)
3. Department of Biochemistry, CARIM School for Cardiovascular Diseases, Maastricht University, 6229 ER Maastricht, The Netherlands; l.schurgers@maastrichtuniversity.nl
* Correspondence: k.reesink@maastrichtuniversity.nl; Tel.: +31-6-4216-1888
† These authors have contributed equally to this work.

Abstract: Local biaxial deformation measurements are essential for the in-depth investigation of tissue properties and remodeling of the ascending thoracic aorta, particularly in aneurysm formation. Current clinical imaging modalities pose limitations around the resolution and tracking of anatomical markers. We evaluated a new intra-operative video-based method to assess local biaxial strains of the ascending thoracic aorta. In 30 patients undergoing open-chest surgery, we obtained repeated biaxial strain measurements, at low- and high-pressure conditions. Precision was very acceptable, with coefficients of variation for biaxial strains remaining below 20%. With our four-marker arrangement, we were able to detect significant local differences in the longitudinal strain as well as in circumferential strain. Overall, the magnitude of strains we obtained (range: 0.02–0.05) was in line with previous reports using other modalities. The proposed method enables the assessment of local aortic biaxial strains and may enable new, clinically informed mechanistic studies using biomechanical modeling as well as mechanobiological profiling.

Keywords: aortic aneurysm; vascular biomechanics and mechanobiology; tissue deformation; image feature tracking

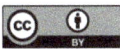

1. Introduction

Ascending thoracic aortic aneurysm formation is potentially lethal, with an annual incidence of approximately 6–10 cases/100,000 patient-years [1]. In current practice, the decision for surgical intervention considers the maximum diameter (≥5.5 cm) and/or growth rate (>1 cm/year) of the aneurysm [2–5]. However, treatment guidance based on these indicators still results in unexpected dissections in 60% of cases [4], as well as ruptures in 0.3% of cases for diameters < 4 cm and in 1.7% of cases for diameters < 5 cm [6]. In up to 95% of aortic dissections, aortic dimensions did not meet the guideline criteria prior to the event [7]. Additionally, recently introduced anatomical criteria such as aortic elongation have so far shown a limited predictive value [7]. Clearly, these current clinical metrics do not fully capture aortic wall integrity [4]. Aortic wall deformations as induced by the pulsating blood pressure could provide more insight into degenerative changes taking place in the aortic wall [4].

Many studies consider pulsatile changes in the aortic lumen area in response to changes in transmural pressure (i.e., distensibility) to estimate the structural stiffness of the aorta [8,9], and consider only circumferential stress [4]. However, these approaches for vessel stiffness and wall stress assessment ignore longitudinal deformations, which have been shown to be significant [10]. Moreover, accurate wall stress calculations in both healthy and aneurysmatic aorta are dependent on the biaxial mechanical behavior of the vessel wall, which is determined by the structural arrangement and properties of the extracellular matrix [11,12]. Taken together, the assessment of biaxial deformations appears highly important for understanding ascending thoracic aortic wall mechanics, material properties, and aneurysm formation.

Existing methods to capture the biaxial deformations of ascending aorta are based on non-invasive magnetic resonance (MR), computed tomography (CT), and ultrasound (US) imaging [8–10,13]. However, for the assessment of local biaxial mechanics of the ascending thoracic aorta, these imaging modalities are hampered by a more global region of interest definition (from the aortic root to brachiocephalic bifurcation) [8–10], as well as by a limited number of anatomical features that can be used to track deformations [9].

Considering the above, we developed an intra-operative video-tracking technique to assess local biaxial strains of the ascending thoracic aorta. Such an approach also enables investigation of the correlations between biaxial strain, tissue histology, as well as cell biology profiles in patients in whom tissue is resected [14,15]. Additionally, the strain measurements may serve as inputs to mathematical modeling studies [16]. In the present paper, we introduce and evaluate our method in patients undergoing open thorax surgery.

2. Materials and Methods

2.1. Study Population

Thirty-two consecutive patients undergoing open-chest cardiac surgery at Maastricht University Medical Centre were included. Prior to enrolment, patients gave written informed consent. The study was approved by the Maastricht University medical ethics committee (protocol METC2019-1235).

2.2. Video-Based Biaxial Strain Method Description

Figure 1 illustrates the key elements of the presented method. The biaxial strain method includes video recording, marker tracking, displacement measurements, filtering, and strain assessments, which are further detailed below.

2.2.1. Intra-Operative Set-Up and Video Recording Settings

A camera (HERO7, GoPro Inc., San Mateo, CA, USA) with a mounting arm (GoPro stick, GoPro Inc., San Mateo, CA, USA) was secured to the surgical table at the head end (Figure 1A) during the routine clinical preparations for open-chest surgery. The arm consisted of a commercial action-cam extension arm (GoPro stick, GoPro Inc., San Mateo, CA, USA) and a custom mounting bracket adapted to the bed. The rigidity of the arm made sure that the camera position with respect to the opened chest was maintained during table tilting. To prevent manual artifacts during the starting and stopping of the recording, remote control was obtained by pairing a smartphone with the camera. The camera used was a commercial action cam (HERO7, GoPro Inc., San Mateo, CA, USA), with the following settings: 2.7k video resolution (screen resolution in pixels: 2704 × 1520; pixel size about ~0.08 mm), at 50 frames per second, and with a linear field of view.

After sternotomy and exposure of the ascending aortic region, four sterile surgical pledgets (BARD PTFE Felt Pledgets, Bard Peripheral Vascular, Inc., Tempe, AZ, USA) were sutured to the adventitial surface of the aorta (Figure 1B) cranial to the sinotubular junction. The two pledgets of a pair were placed as diametrically opposite as possible (Figure 1B). For all cases, the (axial) distance between the two pairs of markers was kept between 0.5 to 1 times the diametrical distance, as exemplified in Figure 1B.

Just prior to recordings, the camera was manually positioned to ensure that its focal plane was parallel to the imaging plane as defined by the four markers. The distance between the camera and imaging plane was about 40 cm (Figure 1A). For calibration, a sterile steel or paper ruler was placed in the imaging plane.

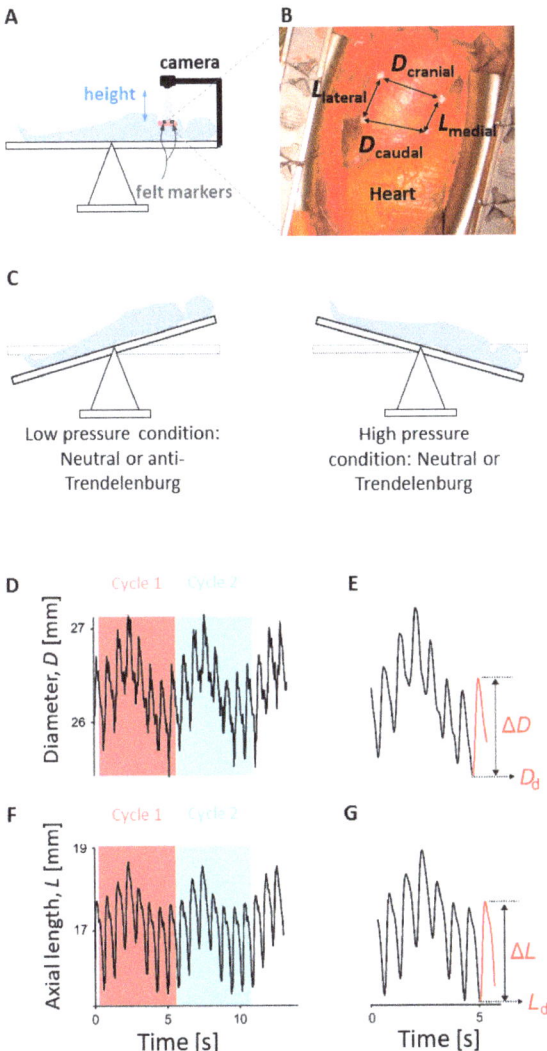

Figure 1. Key elements of the intra-operative, video-based strain measurement method. (**A**): Intra-operative set-up. The remote-controlled camera mounted on a rigid arm attached to the table was positioned at a height of about 40 cm above the imaging plane, as defined by the markers, with a viewing angle close to zero degrees. (**B**): Single video image showing heart on bottom and markers sutured on the adventitia of an ascending aortic aneurysm. Arrows between markers define the positions at which cranial and caudal (circumferential) strains, and medial and lateral (axial) strains were assessed. (**C**): Low and high transmural pressure conditions were created by tilting the table. Tilted table position for low-pressure condition shown is anti-Trendelenburg, while tilted-table position for high-pressure condition shown is Trendelenburg position. Horizontal position of the table is referred to as neutral position. (**D,F**): Examples of diameter and axial length signals, comprising two ventilatory cycles. (**E,G**): Smoothed signals for diameter and axial length, respectively (single ventilation cycles). The variables D_d and L_d represent magnitudes of diameter and axial length corresponding to diastolic pressure, while ΔD and ΔL are deformations of diameter and axial length caused by the change in pressure from diastole to systole (i.e., pulse pressure).

2.2.2. Blood Pressure Conditions and Recording Protocol

Systolic and diastolic blood pressure (BP) were measured using a regular arterial pressure catheter (Edward Lifesciences, Irvine, CA, USA) placed in the (left) radial artery. Subsequently, pressure catheter readings were taken from the clinical routine hemodynamics monitor (stored in a case report form) just prior to and directly after video recordings. Videos were made during both 'low' and 'high' pressure conditions that were induced by table-tilting (Figure 1C).

The first video recording was obtained with the patient in either supine (neutral), anti-Trendelenburg, or Trendelenburg position. The second video recording was then obtained at a different pressure level after tilting the table. The initial table position determined whether the second measurement was made with an increased or decreased BP condition, utilizing the expected BP differences between positioning: Trendelenburg BP > supine BP > anti-Trendelenburg BP. This means that a low-pressure condition was induced by either a neutral or anti-Trendelenburg position, with a corresponding high-pressure condition achieved by Trendelenburg or neutral position, respectively (Figure 1C). The sequence (low-then-high or high-then-low) was arbitrary and determined by the surgeon, who merely targeted a mean arterial pressure (MAP) difference of about 10 mmHg between positions, for which positioning sequence was not relevant. It should be noted that the aim was to measure strains at a distinctly different transmural pressure without invoking pharmacological side-effects.

Video recording duration was 12 s to capture at least two ventilation cycles, enabling assessment of (ventilation) cycle-to-cycle reproducibility. The video recordings and pressure readings did not span more than 2 min, after which the surgical procedure continued.

In the aneurysm-repair cases, the resected tissue was further sectioned and stored in vials for genetic and tissue characterization. These data are not included in the analysis as they are beyond the scope of the present paper. After the procedure, all video files (.mp4 format) and blood-pressure case report forms were stored on a secure local server for further processing.

2.2.3. Video Processing and Strain Calculations

To determine diameters and axial lengths from acquired videos, markers on the ascending aorta were tracked across all video frames (Figure 1B), using a proprietary program written in MATLAB (MATLAB R2018a; The MathWorks, Natick, MA, USA). In the first step, the region of aorta with markers and ruler from the first frame was selected manually using the MATLAB Image Processing Toolbox function imrect. The same imrect box was used to crop all other frames in the video. Subsequently, small regions around the markers were manually assigned to obtain sub-images used for correlation-based tracking across the video frames. A normalized cross-correlation matrix was used and implemented by the function normxcorr2. Sub-image displacements between frames were defined as those at which the normalized cross-correlation coefficient was maximum. Using the obtained positions of the markers in all video frames, dimensions of the line segments connecting the markers were determined as a function of time, yielding diameter (D) and axial length (L) signals (illustrated in Figure 1D,F).

To calibrate the measured distances to physical distances (in mm), a known reference distance visible on the ruler in a video frame was used. Note that this calibration is relevant only for the diastolic diameter (D_d) and length (L_d) estimates but not for the strain estimates (see calculations below).

The D and L signals were subjected to Fourier analysis to identify the lowest frequency (about 0.2 Hz in our subjects) resulting from the ventilation cycle (Figure 1D,F). Ventilation cycles and individual beats were then segmented manually from the raw D and L signals, with the start and end points selected manually. Subsequently, signals were smoothed, using a zero-phase, 6-point, bi-directional (forward and backward), moving-average filter (filtfilt, MATLAB). Beat-by-beat minimum and maximum points were determined, yielding diastolic values (D_d and L_d) and the corresponding systolic-diastolic changes (ΔD and ΔL).

The circumferential strains and axial strains were then calculated for each beat as the engineering strains $\Delta D/D_d$ and $\Delta L/L_d$, respectively (Figure 1E,G). The diastolic dimensions and strains were averaged over the number of beats (in one full ventilation cycle) by taking the median.

In addition, pulse pressure (ΔP) and circumferential distensibility ($\Delta D/(\Delta P \cdot D_d)$) were calculated. The two ventilatory cycles (Figure 1D,F) present in every recording were considered as repeated measurements ($m = 2$), to assess reproducibility (see Statistical analysis).

2.3. Statistical Analysis

Data are presented as median [25th, 75th percentile], unless noted otherwise. Non-normality of presented measurement data was verified using a Shapiro–Wilk test. For $p < 0.05$, the distribution of measurements was not considered normal.

We tested for statistical differences between low- and high-pressure conditions, and for differences between cranial and caudal strain as well as between lateral and medial strain measurements using paired Wilcoxon Signed-Rank tests.

Based on the two ventilatory cycles in each recording (see above), the intra-measurement standard deviation (σ_{intra}) was determined as the square root of the average of variances of the repeated measurements for each recording:

$$\sigma_{intra} = \sqrt{\frac{1}{n}\sum_{i=1}^{n} s_i^2} \qquad (1)$$

where, $\frac{1}{n}\sum_{i=1}^{n} s_i^2$ is the average of variances for n subjects. We expressed reproducibility using the coefficient of variation (CV), defined as σ_{intra} divided by the corresponding sample mean value $\bar{x}$ of each group times 100%:

$$CV = \frac{\sigma_{intra}}{\bar{x}} \cdot 100\% \qquad (2)$$

Using Bland's estimate of the uncertainty about reproducibility, the σ_{intra} we calculated has an uncertainty of 25%, given the number of repetitions $m = 2$ and $n = 30$ [17].

3. Results

Twenty-seven male and five female patients were included in the present analysis. Videos of patients where tracking of markers was not accomplished—either due to decorrelation ($n = 1$) or loss of visibility of the tracking marker in all frames ($n = 1$)—were excluded. Patient characteristics are mentioned in Table 1. The age of the patient population was 64 ± 12 years (mean ± SD).

Table 1. Patient characteristics.

Type of Surgical Intervention	Aortic Repair	AVR	CABG
Number of patients	17	9	6
Male/female	14/3	7/2	6/-
Age (years)	62 ± 9	59 ± 17	72 ± 5

AVR = aortic valve replacement; CABG = coronary artery bypass grafting; age is presented as mean ± SD.

Table 2 shows the blood pressure (BP) and video-derived measurements. In one subject we did not obtain video results in the high-pressure condition, due to loss of view on one marker (hence $n = 29$ for high pressure). There were two subjects in which the ruler appeared not visible enough. In these cases, marker dimensions (4.8 mm × 6.0 mm) were used for calibration instead of the ruler.

Diastolic and systolic blood pressures (DBP and SBP) changed significantly ($p < 0.001$) from low- to high-pressure conditions (Table 2), with a mean arterial pressure (MAP) difference of 10 mmHg between both conditions. The absolute dimensions (D_d and L_d) and strains ($\Delta D/D_d$ for caudal and cranial, and $\Delta L/L_d$ for lateral) did not vary significantly with the change in transmural pressure. Medial axial strain increased significantly by 0.01 from low- to high-pressure ($p = 0.007$). For most direct measures, the measurement variability was of the order 10%, although for the strains, the CVs tended to be higher but remained below 20% (Table 2).

Table 2. Blood pressure and video-derived measures.

Measurements	Pressure Conditions			CV (%)	
	Low (n = 30)	High (n = 29)	p Value * (-)	Low	High
Blood pressure (mmHg)					
SBP	84 [70, 93]	98 [90, 105]	<0.001	4	3
DBP	47 [36, 52]	54 [47, 62]	<0.001	10	5
ΔP	35 [26, 48]	43 [33, 53]	<0.001	4	7
Diastolic diameter, D_d (mm)					
Caudal	30 [25, 36]	30 [23, 38]	0.97	2	2
Cranial	33 [23, 40]	34 [23, 41]	0.8	2	2
Circumferential strain, $\Delta D/D_d$ (-)					
Caudal	0.03 [0.02, 0.05]	0.03 [0.02, 0.05]	0.19	8	8
Cranial	0.02 [0.01, 0.03]	0.02 [0.01, 0.03]	0.3	19	12
Distensibility (MPa^{-1})					
Caudal	7 [4, 9]	4 [3, 9]	0.078	8	13
Cranial	6 [3, 7]	3 [2, 6]	0.02	22	15
Axial diastolic length, L_d (mm)					
Medial	20 [17, 27]	19 [17, 25]	0.92	2	3
Lateral	24 [20, 30]	24 [19, 29]	0.97	2	1
Axial strain, $\Delta L/L_d$ (-)					
Medial	0.04 [0.02, 0.08]	0.05 [0.02, 0.09]	0.007	10	11
Lateral	0.04 [0.01, 0.05]	0.04 [0.02, 0.06]	0.3	19	12

Values are indicated as median [25th, 75th percentile]; CV = coefficient of variation ((σ_{intra}/mean)·100%); SBP = systolic blood pressure; DBP = diastolic blood pressure; ΔP = pulse pressure; Distensibility = $(\Delta D/(\Delta P \cdot D_d \cdot 133)) \cdot 10^6$; * values compared for low pressure vs. high pressure conditions using paired Wilcoxon Signed-Rank test (performed on 29 subjects); n = number of subjects.

From low- to high-pressure, pulse pressure (ΔP) increased by 8 mmHg ($p < 0.001$) and distensibility showed a trend towards decrease: from 7 MPa^{-1} to 4 MPa^{-1}, $p = 0.078$ for caudal and from 6 MPa^{-1} to 3 MPa^{-1}, $p = 0.020$ for cranial.

Figure 2 summarizes differences between locations. For the high-pressure condition, we detected differences between caudal and cranial circumferential strains (0.03 and 0.02, respectively; $p = 0.005$), as well as between medial and lateral axial strains (0.05 and 0.04, respectively; $p = 0.006$). Interestingly, for the low-pressure condition, we did not observe clear differences between locations.

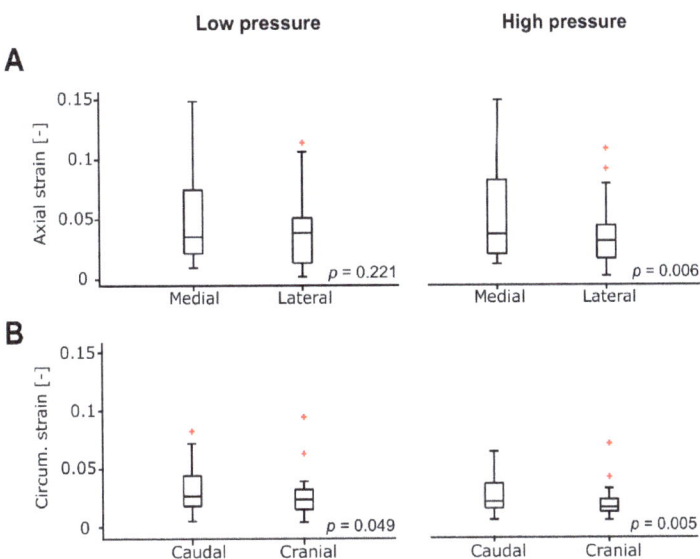

Figure 2. Potential for detecting local strain differences. *p*-values indicate paired Wilcoxon Signed Ranks testing, with *n* = 30 for low and *n* = 29 for high pressure. Boxplots indicate medians [25th, 75th percentile], with whiskers indicating variability beyond the first and the third quartile, while red plus signs are the outliers. (**A**): Lateral axial strains tended to be lower than those captured medially, but only achieving statistical significance in the high-pressure condition. (**B**): Cranial circumferential strains tended to be significantly lower than at the caudal location. Note: one outlier not shown in B (values for caudal and cranial strains > 0.2 for both pressure conditions).

4. Discussion

At present, the assessment of aortic aneurysm progression is limited to monitoring (slow changes in) vessel dimensions [2,3,7]. Current clinical imaging modalities show limitations for assessing dynamic biaxial strains in the ascending thoracic aorta. In the present study, we introduce and evaluate an intra-operative video-based method for measuring biaxial strains in the ascending thoracic aorta. Our findings show the ability–in patients with and without aneurysm–to capture local circumferential as well as axial strains, including changes in response to changes in transmural pressure, with very acceptable reproducibility (CV range 8–19%).

Our approach differs from existing methods reported in previous studies [8,10], where global rather than local longitudinal deformations were quantified. These global approaches consider as a region of interest the entire trajectory between the aortic root at the one end and the brachiocephalic bifurcation at the other end. Our method enables the measurement of local axial strains, and particularly in aneurysmatic regions of the ascending aorta.

Longitudinal strains obtained using global approaches are in the order of 6–9% [8,10] in patients and in the order of 15% in presumably healthy volunteers [10], while our study subjects exhibited local longitudinal strains in the order of 4–5%. The global approaches idealize the entire region of interest for longitudinal strains into a cylindrical geometry, presuming a homogenous distribution of strains [8,10]. However, owing to the bend in the aorta, possible differences in local strains between inner and outer curvature may exist. Our method (with four markers) does enable the assessment of such differences (Figure 2). We expect that the bent form with its complex deformation, even if wall material were assumed homogenous, may lead to differences between the medial and lateral axial strains. Yet, at this point, we do not have a clear concept of how to interpret such differences in local longitudinal strains. Changes in such differences could be instrumental in identifying remodeling processes at the constitutive level.

Circumferential strains reported in the literature [8–10,13,18] range between 3 and 14%, whereas we observed circumferential strains in the order of 2–3%. The strains we found are in the same range as those reported by Morrison et al. [9], who observed substantially decreased circumferential strain at the aortic root and the ascending segment (proximal to the first branch of the brachiocephalic trunk) in older patients (3% strain; mean age of 68 years), as compared to younger patients (10% strain, mean age of 41 years) using cardiac-gated CT image data. Van Disseldorp [18] also estimated ascending aortic circumferential strains in the order of 4–7% in aneurysm patients (age ranging from 44 to 72 years) using 3D transesophageal (TEE) ultrasound. On the other hand, Wittek et al. [13] reported circumferential strains in the order of 11% for healthy young volunteers (median age of 25.5 years) using 3D ultrasound speckle tracking, which inclined more towards the circumferential strain range of 7–14% [8,10] reported by global approaches using magnetic resonance imaging (MRI). In addition, the pressure-dependence of strain measurements must also be considered, as likely caused by the non-linear elastic behavior of the blood vessel wall [16,19]. Our observation of a decrease in distensibility with increasing pressure (Table 1) corroborates this clinically important phenomenon. Taken together, differences in the magnitude of strains may well be attributed to differences between studies pertaining to age [20], disease stage of the study population, imaging modality, as well as hemodynamic conditions.

When considered in more detail, strain differences between our novel method and existing imaging modalities may also be due to differences in temporal and spatial resolution. 3D ultrasound enables imaging of the aorta at a moderate temporal frequency of 11–25 Hz [13] with a voxel size on the order of 0.2–0.7 mm [13,18]. However, access to the whole segment of the aorta is cumbersome, thereby limiting the ability to (keep) focus on the desired region of interest. Additionally, MR and CT rely on the reconstruction of the cardiac cycle from multiple beat snapshots (30 phases per cardiac cycle [8,10]; spatial resolution: 0.5–1.5 mm [8,10]), presuming that consecutive beats are 'identical'. In contrast, our method is able to capture single beats at a 50 Hz frame rate as well as at 10 times better spatial resolution: about 0.08 mm.

Some methods with established imaging modalities use a fixed location in the image to determine circumferential strains [8,10]. Such an approach may lead to errors due to through-plane movement of the aorta, yielding an overestimation in the circumferential strain of up to 50% as reported by Morrison et al. [9]. Identification of fixed anatomical markers in the images avoids this problem, but these are generally limited to bifurcations or valve features. Our approach solves the lack of anatomical markers for a local region of interest by utilizing pledget markers placed at desired locations.

The local differences (between caudal and cranial) in circumferential strain were found to suggest that our method may also detect these regional differences (Figure 2). However, we did not expect to find a trend towards lower cranial strains when compared to the caudal location (Figure 2). Clearly, the relevance and potential of regional differences in tissue properties due to local strain variations (owing to the complex geometry of the aorta) call for future, sufficiently powered studies. In that respect, it is highly relevant to consider the reproducibility of our strain-measurement method. Overall, CVs were less than 20%, and these reproducibility estimates were obtained with an uncertainty of about 25% (see Statistical Analysis). Assuming an expected absolute difference in strain of about 0.01 (e.g., a difference of 0.04 in one group and 0.03) and the 20% reproducibility as the lower limit of variability, the required minimum sample size for a case–control study would be about 11 per group (groups of equal size, power $1 - \beta = 0.8$, type-I error $\alpha = 0.05$).

We deem our method particularly useful for mechanistic studies. For instance, our method may be of interest to investigate the correlation between CT-based atherosclerotic burden (i.e., regional wall thickness abnormalities) and local biaxial strains [21]. Such studies would be very interesting, because the (assumed) changes in stiffness with atherosclerotic burden would depend on, e.g., how and to what extent the intimal disease processes affect medial structure and properties. The 'innate' invasive nature of our method obviously precludes a wider clinical application.

For computational (e.g., finite-element) studies, the availability of high-quality input data is essential [22]. Constitutive models, that capture the elastic properties of the aortic wall under large deformations, rely on reliable estimates of (local) strains and biaxial data. Direct mapping of video marker displacements onto finite element models, using an inverse modeling approach, may enable the estimation of constitutive properties. Besides facilitating realistic computational modeling, well-parameterized constitutive models may provide insight into microstructural changes such as increased cross-linking of collagen and/or elastin degradation, which in turn may help in developing therapeutic approaches in silico [22,23]. Furthermore, computational modeling estimates based on our strain measurements may serve as a benchmark for non-invasive imaging techniques. Moreover, comparative studies correlating our method to MRI or TEE could provide the knowledge base to translate mechanistic insights towards clinical use.

Lastly, reliable strain data accompanied by immunohistochemical and cytochemical assays may allow comprehensive studies on the mechanobiological factors in ascending thoracic aortic aneurysm formation [14,15].

5. Conclusions

The proposed intra-operative, video-based method enables the assessment of regional biaxial strains of the ascending thoracic aorta with very acceptable precision. Our method provides a steppingstone towards clinically informed mechanistic studies using biomechanical modeling as well as mechanobiological profiling.

Author Contributions: Conceptualization, S.P., G.D., E.B. and K.R.; methodology, S.P., B.S., W.H., E.B. and K.R.; data analysis, S.P. and B.G.; resources, J.M., T.D., E.B. and K.R.; data curation, S.P., B.G., G.D., E.N. and E.B.; writing—original draft preparation, S.P. and K.R.; writing—review and editing, S.P., B.G., G.D., E.N., J.M., B.S., L.S., T.D., W.H., E.B. and K.R.; visualization, S.P.; supervision, W.H., E.B. and K.R. All authors have read and agreed to the published version of the manuscript.

Funding: BS was funded by the European Union's Horizon 2020 research and innovation program (No 793805).

Institutional Review Board Statement: The study was conducted according to the guidelines of the Declaration of Helsinki and approved by the Institutional Review Board (or Ethics Committee) of MUMC+ (protocol code METC2019-1235 niet-WMO and 2 October 2019).

Informed Consent Statement: Informed consent was obtained from all subjects involved in the study.

Data Availability Statement: Data are available upon reasonable request addressed to the corresponding author.

Acknowledgments: The authors would like to thank Ciprian Mateescu, Maarten Heusinkveld, and Jeroen Hameleers for their pioneering work on the proposed intra-operative video-based method. Authors are also indebted to the research assistants Karina V. Chaibekava, Willemijn H.J.M. Tunnissen, Colin J. Willems, Inez Cortenraad, Fleur E.C.M. Vande Kerckhove, and Anke M. Merks for their support in recruitment, measurements, and logistics.

Conflicts of Interest: The authors declare no conflict of interest.

References

1. Kuzmik, G.A.; Sang, A.X.; Elefteriades, J.A. Natural history of thoracic aortic aneurysms. *J. Vasc. Surg.* **2012**, *56*, 565–571. [CrossRef]
2. Coady, M.A.; Rizzo, J.A.; Hammond, G.L.; Mandapati, D.; Darr, U.; Kopf, G.S.; Elefteriades, J.A. What is the appropriate size criterion for resection of thoracic aortic aneurysms? *J. Thorac. Cardiovasc. Surg.* **1997**, *113*, 476–491, discussion 489–491. [CrossRef]
3. Davies, R.R.; Goldstein, L.J.; Coady, M.A.; Tittle, S.L.; Rizzo, J.A.; Kopf, G.S.; Elefteriades, J.A. Yearly rupture or dissection rates for thoracic aortic aneurysms: Simple prediction based on size. *Ann. Thorac. Surg.* **2002**, *73*, 17–27, discussion 27–28. [CrossRef]
4. Martufi, G.; Forneris, A.; Appoo, J.J.; Di Martino, E.S. Is There a Role for Biomechanical Engineering in Helping to Elucidate the Risk Profile of the Thoracic Aorta? *Ann. Thorac. Surg.* **2016**, *101*, 390–398. [CrossRef] [PubMed]

5. Wang, T.K.M.; Desai, M.Y. Thoracic aortic aneurysm: Optimal surveillance and treatment. *Cleve. Clin. J. Med.* **2020**, *87*, 557–568. [CrossRef] [PubMed]
6. Elefteriades, J.A. Natural history of thoracic aortic aneurysms: Indications for surgery, and surgical versus nonsurgical risks. *Ann. Thorac. Surg.* **2002**, *74*, S1877–S1880, discussion S1892–S1898. [CrossRef]
7. Heuts, S.; Adriaans, B.; Rylski, B.; Mihl, C.; Bekkers, S.C.A.M.; Olsthoorn, J.R.; Natour, E.; Bouman, H.; Berezowski, M.; Kosiorowska, K.; et al. Evaluating the diagnostic accuracy of maximal aortic diameter, length and volume for prediction of aortic dissection. *Heart* **2020**, *106*, 892–897. [CrossRef]
8. Bell, V.; Mitchell, W.A.; Sigurethsson, S.; Westenberg, J.J.; Gotal, J.D.; Torjesen, A.A.; Aspelund, T.; Launer, L.J.; de Roos, A.; Gudnason, V.; et al. Longitudinal and circumferential strain of the proximal aorta. *J. Am. Heart Assoc.* **2014**, *3*, e001536. [CrossRef]
9. Morrison, T.M.; Choi, G.; Zarins, C.K.; Taylor, C.A. Circumferential and longitudinal cyclic strain of the human thoracic aorta: Age-related changes. *J. Vasc. Surg.* **2009**, *49*, 1029–1036. [CrossRef]
10. Guala, A.; Teixido-Tura, G.; Rodriguez-Palomares, J.; Ruiz-Munoz, A.; Dux-Santoy, L.; Villalva, N.; Granato, C.; Galian, L.; Gutierrez, L.; Gonzalez-Alujas, T.; et al. Proximal aorta longitudinal strain predicts aortic root dilation rate and aortic events in Marfan syndrome. *Eur. Heart J.* **2019**, *40*, 2047–2055. [CrossRef]
11. Duprey, A.; Trabelsi, O.; Vola, M.; Favre, J.P.; Avril, S. Biaxial rupture properties of ascending thoracic aortic aneurysms. *Acta Biomater.* **2016**, *42*, 273–285. [CrossRef]
12. Ferruzzi, J.; Vorp, D.A.; Humphrey, J.D. On constitutive descriptors of the biaxial mechanical behaviour of human abdominal aorta and aneurysms. *J. R. Soc. Interface* **2011**, *8*, 435–450. [CrossRef]
13. Wittek, A.; Karatolios, K.; Fritzen, C.P.; Bereiter-Hahn, J.; Schieffer, B.; Moosdorf, R.; Vogt, S.; Blase, C. Cyclic three-dimensional wall motion of the human ascending and abdominal aorta characterized by time-resolved three-dimensional ultrasound speckle tracking. *Biomech. Model. Mechanobiol.* **2016**, *15*, 1375–1388. [CrossRef] [PubMed]
14. Korneva, A.; Humphrey, J.D. Maladaptive aortic remodeling in hypertension associates with dysfunctional smooth muscle contractility. *Am. J. Physiol. Heart Circ. Physiol.* **2019**, *316*, H265–H278. [CrossRef] [PubMed]
15. Jaminon, A.; Reesink, K.; Kroon, A.; Schurgers, L. The Role of Vascular Smooth Muscle Cells in Arterial Remodeling: Focus on Calcification-Related Processes. *Int. J. Mol. Sci.* **2019**, *20*, 5694. [CrossRef] [PubMed]
16. Reesink, K.D.; Spronck, B. Constitutive interpretation of arterial stiffness in clinical studies: A methodological review. *Am. J. Physiol. Heart Circ. Physiol.* **2019**, *316*, H693–H709. [CrossRef] [PubMed]
17. How Can I Decide the Sample Size for a Repeatability Study? Available online: https://www-users.york.ac.uk/~{}mb55/meas/sizerep.htm (accessed on 1 April 2021).
18. Van Disseldorp, E. Mechanical Analysis of Aortic Aneurysms Using 3D Ultrasound: Towards Patient-Specific Risk Assessment. Ph.D. Thesis, Eindhoven University of Technology, Eindhoven, The Netherlands, 2019.
19. Spronck, B.; Heusinkveld, M.H.; Vanmolkot, F.H.; Roodt, J.O.; Hermeling, E.; Delhaas, T.; Kroon, A.A.; Reesink, K.D. Pressure-dependence of arterial stiffness: Potential clinical implications. *J. Hypertens.* **2015**, *33*, 330–338. [CrossRef]
20. Redheuil, A.; Yu, W.C.; Mousseaux, E.; Harouni, A.A.; Kachenoura, N.; Wu, C.O.; Bluemke, D.; Lima, J.A. Age-related changes in aortic arch geometry: Relationship with proximal aortic function and left ventricular mass and remodeling. *J. Am. Coll. Cardiol.* **2011**, *58*, 1262–1270. [CrossRef] [PubMed]
21. Malayeri, A.A.; Natori, S.; Bahrami, H.; Bertoni, A.G.; Kronmal, R.; Lima, J.A.; Bluemke, D.A. Relation of aortic wall thickness and distensibility to cardiovascular risk factors (from the Multi-Ethnic Study of Atherosclerosis [MESA]). *Am. J. Cardiol.* **2008**, *102*, 491–496. [CrossRef]
22. Stalhand, J. Determination of human arterial wall parameters from clinical data. *Biomech. Model. Mechanobiol.* **2009**, *8*, 141–148. [CrossRef]
23. Heusinkveld, M.H.G.; Quicken, S.; Holtackers, R.J.; Huberts, W.; Reesink, K.D.; Delhaas, T.; Spronck, B. Uncertainty quantification and sensitivity analysis of an arterial wall mechanics model for evaluation of vascular drug therapies. *Biomech. Model. Mechanobiol.* **2018**, *17*, 55–69. [CrossRef] [PubMed]

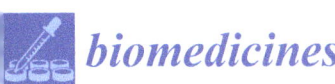

Article

Syndecan-1 Expression Is Increased in the Aortic Wall of Patients with Type 2 Diabetes but Is Unrelated to Elevated Fasting Plasma Glucagon-Like Peptide-1

Stelia Ntika [1,2,*], Linda M. Tracy [1], Anders Franco-Cereceda [2], Hanna M. Björck [3] and Camilla Krizhanovskii [1,2]

1. Department of Research, Södertälje Hospital, Södertälje, 152 86 Stockholm, Sweden; lindamtracy@gmail.com (L.M.T.); camilla.krizhanovskii@sll.se (C.K.)
2. Cardiothoracic Surgery Unit, Department of Molecular Medicine and Surgery, Karolinska Institutet & Karolinska University Hospital, 171 76 Stockholm, Sweden; anders.franco-cereceda@ki.se
3. Cardiovascular Medicine Unit, Center for Molecular Medicine, Department of Medicine, Karolinska Institutet, Karolinska University Hospital, 171 76 Stockholm, Sweden; hanna.bjorck@ki.se
* Correspondence: stelia.ntika@ki.se; Tel.: +46-72-7395762

Abstract: A reduced prevalence of a thoracic aortic aneurysm (thoracic AA) is observed in type 2 diabetes (T2D). Glucagon-like peptide-1 (GLP-1)/GLP-1-based anti-diabetic therapy has indicated protective effects in thoracic AA and regulates the processes controlling the vascular tissue expression of Syndecan-1 (Sdc-1). Sdc-1 expression on macrophages infiltrating the aortic tissue contributes to a counter-regulatory response to thoracic AA formation in animal models through the interplay with inflammation/proteolytic activity. We hypothesized that elevated fasting plasma GLP-1 (fpGLP-1) increases the aortic Sdc-1 expression in T2D, which may contribute to a reduced prevalence of thoracic AA. Consequently, we determined whether T2D/thoracic AA associates with an altered Sdc-1 expression in the aortic tissue and the possible associations with fpGLP-1 and inflammation/proteolytic activity. From a cohort of surgical patients with an aortic valve pathology, we compared different disease groups (T2D/thoracic AA) with the same sub-cohort group of controls (patients without T2D and thoracic AA). The MMP-2 activity and Sdc-1, GLP-1R and CD68 expression were analyzed in the aortic tissue. GLP-1, Sdc-1 and cytokines were analyzed in the plasma. The aortic Sdc-1 expression was increased in T2D patients but did not correlate with fpGLP-1. Thoracic AA was associated with an increased aortic expression of Sdc-1 and the macrophage marker CD68. CD68 was not detected in T2D. In conclusion, an increased aortic Sdc-1 expression may contribute to a reduced prevalence of thoracic AA in T2D.

Keywords: thoracic aortic aneurysm; type 2 diabetes; adventitia; syndecan-1; glucagon-like peptide-1

Citation: Ntika, S.; Tracy, L.M.; Franco-Cereceda, A.; Björck, H.M.; Krizhanovskii, C. Syndecan-1 Expression Is Increased in the Aortic Wall of Patients with Type 2 Diabetes but Is Unrelated to Elevated Fasting Plasma Glucagon-Like Peptide-1. *Biomedicines* 2021, 9, 697. https://doi.org/10.3390/biomedicines9060697

Academic Editor: Elena Kaschina

Received: 13 April 2021
Accepted: 17 June 2021
Published: 20 June 2021

Publisher's Note: MDPI stays neutral with regard to jurisdictional claims in published maps and institutional affiliations.

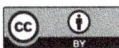

Copyright: © 2021 by the authors. Licensee MDPI, Basel, Switzerland. This article is an open access article distributed under the terms and conditions of the Creative Commons Attribution (CC BY) license (https://creativecommons.org/licenses/by/4.0/).

1. Introduction

A thoracic aortic aneurysm (thoracic AA) is increasing in prevalence and although it is less common than an abdominal aortic aneurysm (abdominal AA), it is more lethal; no screening programs are available [1] and treatment options are limited to surgical interventions. The most common form of thoracic AA occurs in the ascending aorta (ascending AA), which is the section of the aorta closest to the heart. Other forms of thoracic AA occur in the aortic arch and the descending aorta [2]. Surgical intervention in thoracic AA is needed before the ascending aorta reaches 4.5–5.5 cm, depending on the growth rate, possible risk factors, concomitant cardiac surgery, genetics and others [3,4]. The search for pharmaceutical agents and novel pharmaceutical targets for the prevention of an ascending AA is thus highly needed and has been fueled by the reduced prevalence of thoracic AA in patients with type 2 diabetes (T2D) [5,6], possibly related to the anti-diabetic therapy. Indeed, studies in animal models indicate that anti-diabetic incretin therapy, including glucagon-like peptide-1 (GLP-1) analogues and dipeptidyl peptidase-4 (DPP-4) inhibitors, may exert protective effects on ascending AA formation through anti-inflammatory and anti-oxidant effects, reduced intimal thickening, decreased matrix metalloproteinase-2 (MMP-2) and MMP-9 production and the suppression of macrophage infiltration [7–12].

Growing evidence supports an outside-in model where vascular inflammation is initiated in the adventitia, the outermost layer of the aortic wall [13–15]. Specifically, according to this model, exogenous cell types including macrophages and lymphocytes populate the adventitia, ultimately resulting in an increased local expression of cytokines and growth factors. This, in turn, may lead to an inflammatory response that propagates inward from the adventitia towards the media layer [16,17], causing medial degradation by MMPs, smooth muscle cell (SMC) loss and de-differentiation [13,15,18–20].

The cell surface proteoglycan syndecan-1 (Sdc-1) is a regulator of inflammation with a dual role in MMP activity, first as a regulator of the proteolytic activity and second as a substrate of proteases. It is mainly expressed on the surface of epithelial cells and non-circulating plasma cells but may be induced also in several other cell types including macrophages and SMCs. Sdc-1 may be proteolytically cleaved and shed from the cell surface by different MMPs such as MMP-2 and MMP-9 [21,22] in a process termed shedding. Shedding can be observed as a dramatic increase in the plasma concentrations of Sdc-1 ectodomains and occurs in response to different stimuli, e.g., inflammation, proteolytic activity and oxidative stress [23]. The aortic Sdc-1 expression protects from an abdominal AA formation in experimental models [24] where Sdc-1 knockout is associated with a reduced expression of the SMC differentiation markers and upregulated cytokine expression [25]. Its protective role is further indicated by the induction of Sdc-1 on infiltrating macrophages as a response to aneurysm formation where it provides an important counterbalance to T-cell-driven inflammation and proteolytic activity in the vascular wall by inhibiting the production of inflammatory markers [24]. The macrophage Sdc-1 expression is of particular interest, considering it is regulated by cAMP/protein kinase A (PKA) [26] and the recent availability of novel cAMP analogs, which explicitly target PKA. Interestingly, GLP-1 (and incretin therapy) target the cAMP/PKA pathway [27,28] and may contribute to a reduced prevalence of thoracic AA in T2D, in part through the induction of the Sdc-1 expression on infiltrating macrophages but also through an increased SMC and endothelial expression of Sdc-1. However, it is not known whether aortic Sdc-1 expression is increased in patients with T2D and the potential role for elevated fasting plasma GLP-1 (fpGLP-1) nor is it known whether a macrophage-specific expression of Sdc-1 is part of a response to aneurysm formation in patients.

Consequently, we set out to investigate whether the Sdc-1 expression is increased in association with T2D as well as if and how an elevated fpGLP-1 may contribute to this. Furthermore, we assessed the Sdc-1 expression and macrophage infiltration in the aortic tissue of patients with an ascending AA.

2. Materials and Methods

2.1. Patient Information

In this case-cohort study, the patients were recruited from a defined cohort (i.e., patients included in the Advanced Study of Aortic Pathology (ASAP) and Disease of the Aortic Valve, Ascending Aorta and Coronary Arteries (DAVAACA)) with suspected risk factors (aortic valve pathology). Two different disease groups (T2D/ascending AA) were compared with the same sub-cohort group of controls (patients without T2D and without an ascending AA) (Figure 1). Typically for a case-cohort study, the cases were not matched on calendar time or length of follow-up with the control. An ascending AA was defined as a diameter > 45 mm. A non-dilated aorta was defined by a diameter < 40 mm. Individuals with a diameter between 40–45 mm were excluded as were patients with both T2D and an ascending AA. Additional exclusion criteria were Type 1 diabetes, Marfan syndrome, monocuspid/bicuspid valves and atherosclerosis. During surgery, tissue biopsies were extracted from the proximal part of the ascending aorta. The intima-media layer was separated from the adventitia by an adventicectomy where the careful isolation of the vessel segment was performed with fine forceps and microscissors.

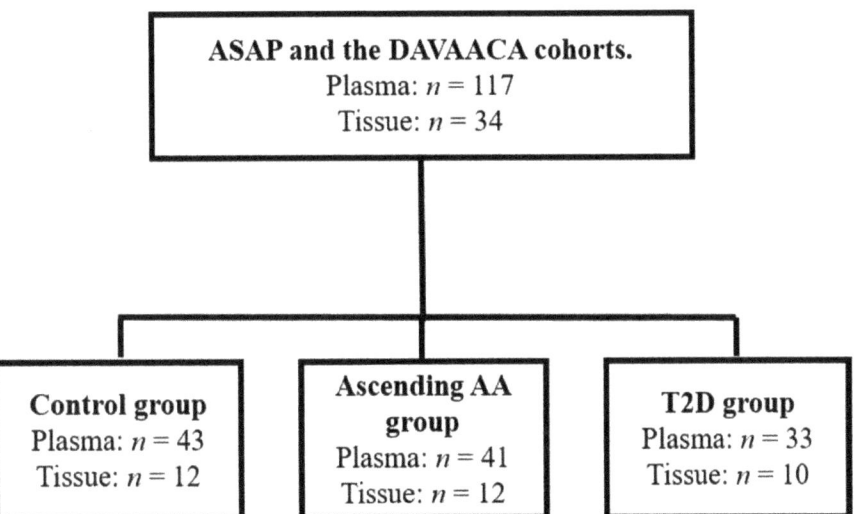

Figure 1. Study groups.

The patient characteristics can be found in Table 1. Ethical approval was received from the Stockholm Regional Ethical Committee (Dnr: 2006/784-31/1; approved: 15 September 2006 and Dnr: 2012/1633-31/4; approved 24 October 2012). All study participants provided written informed consent.

Table 1. Patient Information.

Patient Group	Number of Patients	Mean Age (± Standard error of Mean, SEM)	Gender (Male/Female)	Valve Pathology (Aortic Stenosis/Aortic Insufficiency) [1]
Control	43	67.6 ± 2.1	26/17	24/15
Ascending AA	41	65.3 ± 1.7	26/15	3/29
T2D	33	71.7 ± 0.94	27/6	30/1
Total Patients	117	62.1 ± 1.1	79/38	57/45

[1] For a few patients, information regarding the type of valve pathology (Aortic Stenosis/Aortic Insufficiency) was missing.

2.2. Measurement of the fpGLP-1

The patients were subjected to pre-operative fasting and plasma samples were collected before surgery, placed immediately on ice and transferred to −80 °C. The total GLP-1 (7–36 and 9–36) (Cat. No.: EZGLP1T-36K, Merck, Darmstadt, Germany) was measured according to the manufacturer's instructions.

2.3. Matrix Metalloproteinase-2 Activity Assay

The adventitia tissue was homogenized using a TissueLyser II in Tris HCl 50 mM with 0.1% Trition × 100, pH = 7–8. The proteolytic activity of MMP-2 was measured using the Human MMP-2 Activity Assay (Cat. No.: QZBmmp2Hv2, Quickzyme Biosciences, Leiden, The Netherlands) according to the manufacturer's protocol. The amount of endogenous active MMP-2 was directly proportional to the activity of a pro-enzyme substrate releasing a colored product detectable at 405 nm optical density. The absorbance data were normalized by the total amount of protein in the sample as measured by the Bio-Rad Laboratories (Hercules, CA, USA) detergent compatible (DC) protein assay (Cat. No.: 5000112).

2.4. Syndecan-1 Shedding

Sdc-1 was measured in the fasting plasma samples. The commercially available ELISA kit for Sdc-1 was utilized (Cat. No.: 950.640.096, Diaclone, Besançon cedex, France) according to the manufacturer's instructions. In brief, the heparin sulphate chains of Sdc-1 were allowed to bind to a capture antibody and then to a biotinylated secondary antibody. Following the addition of enzyme-conjugated streptavidin, a chromogen substrate was added for the color development. The reaction was terminated by the addition of an acidic stop solution and the absorbance was measured at 450 nm with a reference wavelength of 620 nm.

2.5. Cytokines

A multiplex ELISA Kit (Cat. No.: K15067L-1, Meso Scale Discovery, Rockville, MD, USA) was used according to the manufacturer's instructions for the analysis of seven cytokines; interleukin 1β (IL-1β), interleukin-6 (IL-6), interleukin-5 (IL-5), interferon-γ (IFN-γ), interleukin-4 (IL-4), tumor necrosis factor-α (TNF-α) and interleukin-12p70 (IL-12p70) in the fasting plasma samples.

2.6. Western Blot

The same samples used for the MMP-2 activity assay were also used to determine the expression of GLP-1R and Sdc-1 in the tissue. After determining the total protein concentration by a DC protein assay kit (Cat. No.: 5000112, Bio-Rad Laboratories), the samples were mixed with a sample buffer and boiled at 95 °C for 5 min. A 10% polyacrylamide gel was used for the sodium dodecyl sulphate–polyacrylamide gel electrophoresis followed by transference to a polyvinylidene fluoride membrane (Cat. No.: 1620177, Bio-Rad Laboratories). The membranes were blocked with 5% milk in tris-buffered saline and tween-20 (0.25 M Tris Base, 0.027 M KCl, 1.37 M NaCl and 0.1% Tween-20) prior to an overnight incubation with a primary antibody at 4 °C. The primary antibodies used were the recombinant anti-Sdc-1 antibody EPR6454 (Cat. No.: ab128936), the anti-GLP1R antibody (Cat. No.: ab186051) and the CD68 antibody (Cat. No.: ab213363), all from Abcam (Cambridge, UK). The secondary antibody (mouse anti-rabbit, Cat. No.: sc2357, Santa Cruz Biotechnology, Dallas, TX, USA) was added for 1 h at room temperature (RT) followed by a 5 min incubation with enhanced chemiluminescence reagents (Cat. No.: RPN2232, GE Healthcare, Chicago, IL, USA). Imaging and the quantification of data were performed using the ChemiDoc XRS+ v 4.6.5 (Bio-Rad Laboratories). The data were normalized to β-actin (Cat. No.: SC-47778, Santa Cruz Biotechnology) and the secondary antibody that was used was an anti-mouse antibody (Cat. No.: SC-2005, Santa Cruz Biotechnology) or with a Coomassie Brilliant Blue R-250 staining solution (Cat. No.: 1610436, Bio-Rad Laboratories).

2.7. Statistical Analysis

The data are presented as a mean ± SEM. The GraphPad Prism 6 (GraphPad Software, San Diego, CA, USA) was used for the analysis and for the graphs. A Pearson correlation and a linear regression analysis was used to evaluate the correlation between the selected variables. A Student's t-test or a Mann–Whitney was used, where appropriate, to compare two samples. A $p < 0.05$ was considered statistically significant. An analysis of covariance (ANCOVA) was performed using the R studio software version 4.0.3 (Boston, Massachusetts).

3. Results

3.1. Type 2 Diabetes Is Associated with Decreased Plasma Sdc-1 and Increased Expression of Sdc-1 in Aortic Tissue

We investigated whether an increased Sdc-1 expression was detected in the ascending aorta of T2D patients as this may contribute to the reduced prevalence of ascending AAs in T2D. Indeed, an increased expression of Sdc-1 was observed in the aortic adventitia of patients with T2D (0.78 ± 0.30 for T2D vs. 0.11 ± 0.03 procedure defined unit (p.d.u.) for the control, $p < 0.001$, Figure 2A,B). To determine the potential contribution of shedding to the increased protein expression of Sdc-1 in the adventitia in T2D patients, we assessed whether T2D was also associated with reduced adventitial MMP-2 activity and/or plasma Sdc-1 as well as any potential correlations to the increased adventitial Sdc-1 expression. The results demonstrated that T2D was not associated with significantly altered MMP-2 activity in the adventitia (1.04 ± 0.15 for T2D vs. 1.32 ± 0.38 ng/mL for the control, $p = 0.90$, Figure 2C) although plasma Sdc-1 levels were significantly lower in the T2D patient group compared with the control group (13.00 ± 1.22 for T2D vs. 19.41 ± 1.90 ng/mL for the control, $p < 0.01$, Figure 2D). However, no significant correlation between the adventitial Sdc-1 expression and plasma Sdc-1 levels was detected ($r = -0.0672$, $p = 0.89$, Figure 2E).

Hypothesizing that alterations to the relative Th1/Th2 balance of immune responses in association with T2D may contribute to the reduced shedding indicated, we continued by investigating the potential contribution of the IL-6/TNF-α ratio—a ratio associated with Th2-biased immune responses [29]—to the lower levels of plasma Sdc-1 detected in T2D patients. However, no significant correlation was observed between plasma Sdc-1 and the IL-6/TNF-α ratio and the significant decrease in plasma Sdc-1 associated with T2D remained after correcting for the IL-6/TNF-α ratio as a covariate ($p < 0.001$). The expression of Sdc-1 in the adventitia did not significantly correlate with an altered expression of any of the cytokines analyzed in the plasma except the IL-12p70 cytokine (Table 2 and graphical illustrations in Supplementary Data Figure S1A,B).

Table 2. Correlation of Sdc-1 Expression in the Adventitia and Different Cytokines.

Correlation With Sdc-1 in the Adventitia	IFN-γ (pg/mL)	IL-1β (pg/mL)	IL-4 (pg/mL)	IL-5 (pg/mL)	IL-6 (pg/mL)	IL-12p70 (pg/mL)	TNF-α (pg/mL)
r (T2D patients)	0.7136	−0.0811	0.0879	0.1359	0.0843	0.9201	0.1865
p value (T2D patients)	0.07	0.88	0.85	0.77	0.86	<0.01	0.66
r (control and T2D patients)	0.1270	−0.09170	0.1870	0.04293	0.03023	0.7263	−0.1046
p value (control and T2D patients)	0.6394	0.7657	0.5046	0.8700	0.9083	<0.01	0.6796

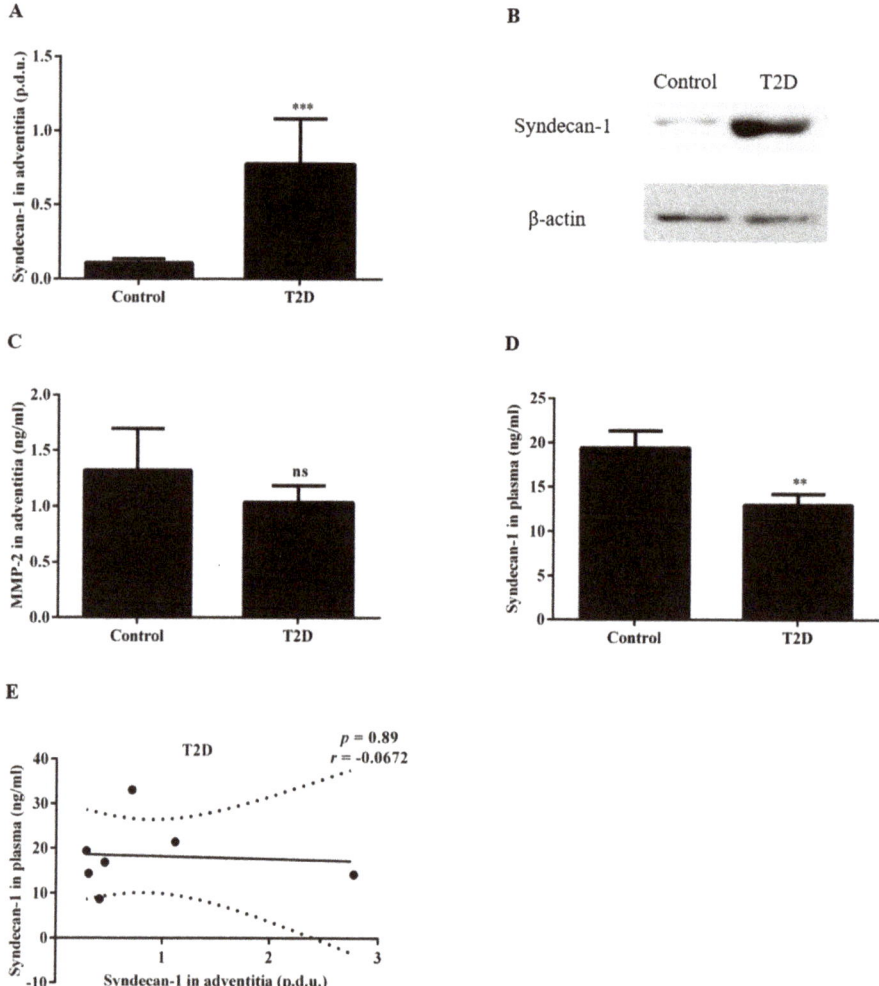

Figure 2. Type 2 diabetes was associated with decreased plasma Sdc-1 and an increased expression of Sdc-1 in the aortic tissue. The Sdc-1 expression in the adventitia was significantly increased in T2D patients (**A**) normalized data and (**B**) Western blot data (the full-length blot is provided in Supplementary Material Figure S3); (**C**) MMP-2 activity in the adventitia was not changed due to T2D; (**D**) The plasma Sdc-1 was significantly decreased in the same patient group. (**E**) The expression of Sdc-1 in the adventitia was not associated with Sdc-1 in plasma. Comparisons between the groups were made using an unpaired t-test or a Mann–Whitney. A Pearson correlation was used to assess the associations. For plasma, $n = 36$ for the control and $n = 30$ for T2D; for tissue, $n = 10$ for the control and $n = 9$ for T2D. ** $p < 0.01$, *** $p < 0.001$, ns = not significant.

3.2. Increased FpGLP-1 in T2D Is Not Significantly Associated with an Increased Sdc-1 Expression in the Adventitia of Patients with T2D

As GLP-1 has been shown to regulate processes that control Sdc-1 expression [23,26–28] and as the fpGLP-1 levels were upregulated in patients with aortic valve pathology in association with T2D [30] (Figure 3A), we investigated the possible contribution of fpGLP-1 to the increased adventitial expression of Sdc-1 in T2D patients. The expression of GLP-1R was, as expected, detected in the adventitia, facilitating the direct effects of GLP-1 (Figure 3B). However, no significant correlation was observed between Sdc-1 in the adventitia and fpGLP-1 ($r = -0.3129$, $p = 0.45$, Figure 3C) and the significant increase in the adventitial Sdc-1 expression in T2D remained also after controlling for fpGLP-1. Furthermore, fpGLP-1 was not associated with altered plasma Sdc-1 in patients from the T2D patient group ($r = 0.1548$, $p = 0.41$, Figure 3D). Interestingly, the Sdc-1 in plasma showed a strong positive correlation with the GLP-1R expression among patients from the T2D group ($r = 0.8348$, $p < 0.01$, Figure 3E).

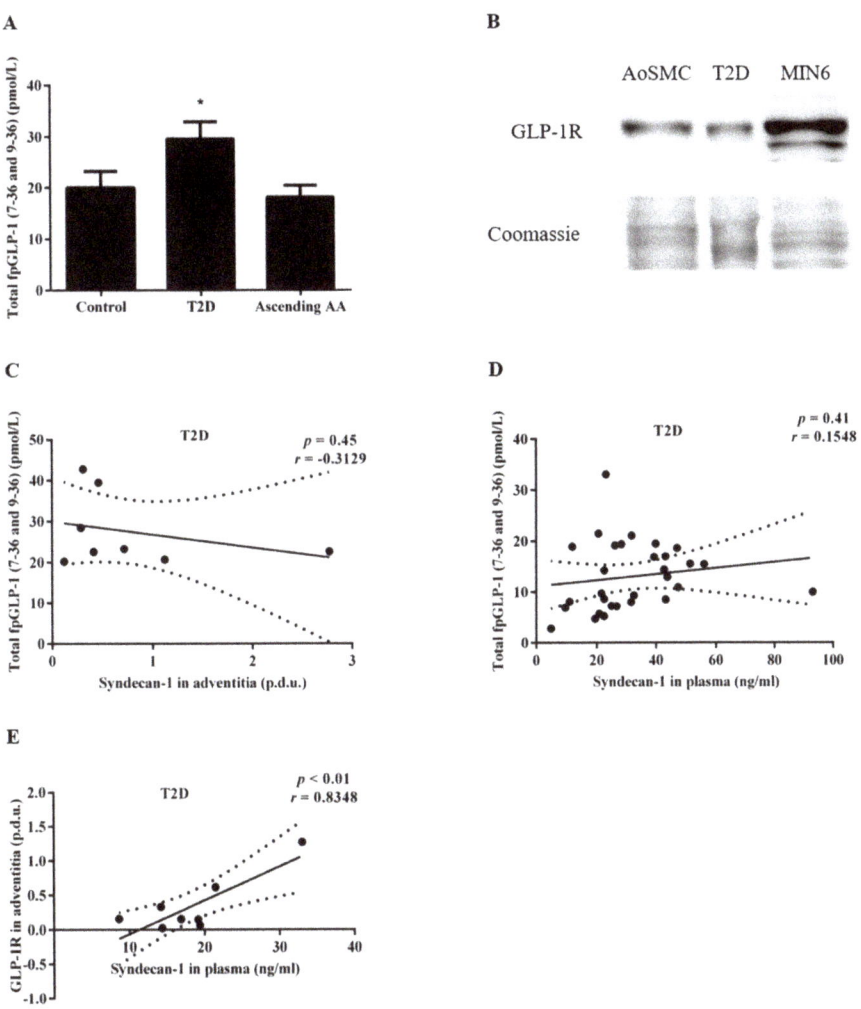

Figure 3. Increased fpGLP-1 in T2D was not significantly associated with the increased Sdc-1 expression in the adventitia of patients with T2D. (**A**) fpGLP-1 levels were upregulated in the T2D group of this study. (**B**) GLP-1R was detected in the adventitia of T2D patients. MIN6 cells and human aortic SMCs were used as a control and the bands were normalized with Coomassie Brilliant Blue (the full-length blot is provided in Supplementary Material Figure S3). (**C**) Sdc-1 in the adventitia was not associated with total fpGLP-1 in T2D patients and (**D**) the total fpGLP-1 was not associated with plasma Sdc-1 in patients with T2D. However, (**E**) the Sdc-1 in plasma was positively associated with GLP-1R in the adventitia ($n = 10$). A Pearson correlation was used to assess any potential associations. Comparisons between the groups were made using a one-sided unpaired t-test. For plasma, $n = 36$ for the control and $n = 30$ for T2D; for tissue, $n = 10$ for the control and $n = 9$ for T2D. * $p < 0.05$.

3.3. The Sdc-1 Is Increased in the Aortic Tissue of Patients with an Ascending AA

To determine whether the previously observed increased macrophage expression of Sdc-1 in the adventitia of rodent models of an abdominal AA could be identified in patients with an ascending AA [24], adventitia samples from the ascending aortic tissue of patients with and without an ascending AA were analyzed. Interestingly, the Sdc-1 expression in the adventitia was significantly increased in patients with an ascending AA compared with the controls (1.02 ± 0.27 vs. 0.11 ± 0.03 p.d.u. for the ascending AA and the control, respectively, $p < 0.001$, Figure 4A,B). Furthermore, a significant increase in the macrophage-specific marker CD68 was detected in the same adventitial samples (0.48 ± 0.17 vs. 0.02 ± 0.00 p.d.u. for the ascending AA and the control, respectively, $p < 0.05$, Figure 4C,D). No correlation between the Sdc-1 expression and MMP-2 activity in the adventitia ($r = 0.4803$, $p = 0.11$, Figure 4E) was observed nor was MMP-2 activity altered in the adventitia from ascending AA patients compared with the control patients (1.04 ± 0.19 vs. 1.32 ± 0.38 ng/mL for the ascending AA and the control, respectively, $p = 0.9$, Figure 4F). In addition, the expression of Sdc-1 in the adventitia did not correlate with the amount of Sdc-1 in plasma (Table 3) and no significant change in plasma Sdc-1 was detected in association with an ascending AA (17.62 ± 1.29 vs. 19.41 ± 1.90 ng/mL for the ascending AA and the control, respectively, $p = 0.43$, Figure 4G).

Table 3. Correlation of the Sdc-1 Expression in the Adventitia and Different Variants in Patients.

Correlation with Sdc-1 in the Adventitia	IFN-γ (pg/mL)	IL-1β (pg/mL)	IL-4 (pg/mL)	IL-5 (pg/mL)	IL-6 (pg/mL)	IL-12p70 (pg/mL)	TNF-α (pg/mL)	Sdc-1 in plasma (ng/mL)	FpGLP-1 (pmol/L)
r (ascending AA patients)	−0.2109	−0.1219	0.2103	−0.5401	−0.5252	−0.3461	0.3337	0.0983	−0.0590
p value (ascending AA patients)	0.65	0.77	0.62	0.13	0.15	0.45	0.38	0.82	0.87
r (control and ascending AA patients)	−0.2746	−0.1686	−0.0929	−0.3476	−0.1768	−0.1496	−0.0191	−0.0777	−0.2037
p value (control and ascending AA patients)	0.30	0.55	0.73	0.14	0.47	0.61	0.94	0.74	0.42

To determine whether altered systemic inflammation in an ascending AA characterized by a Th1 profile [31–34] could play a role in the increased adventitial Sdc-1 expression, we assessed the potential correlations between the Sdc-1 expression in the adventitia and the plasma expression of cytokines (Table 3 and graphical illustrations in Supplementary Data Figure S2A,B). However, the only significant correlation detected was a positive correlation between the adventitial Sdc-1 expression and the IL-4/IFN-γ ratio (often used to identify a Th2 shift [35]) ($r = 0.7224$, $p < 0.05$, Figure 4H). Finally, to investigate the potential role of fpGLP-1 in the adventitial Sdc-1 expression, we assessed whether fpGLP-1 levels correlated with an altered Sdc-1 expression in thoracic AA tissue. However, no significant association between fpGLP-1 and the Sdc-1 tissue expression was detected (Table 3).

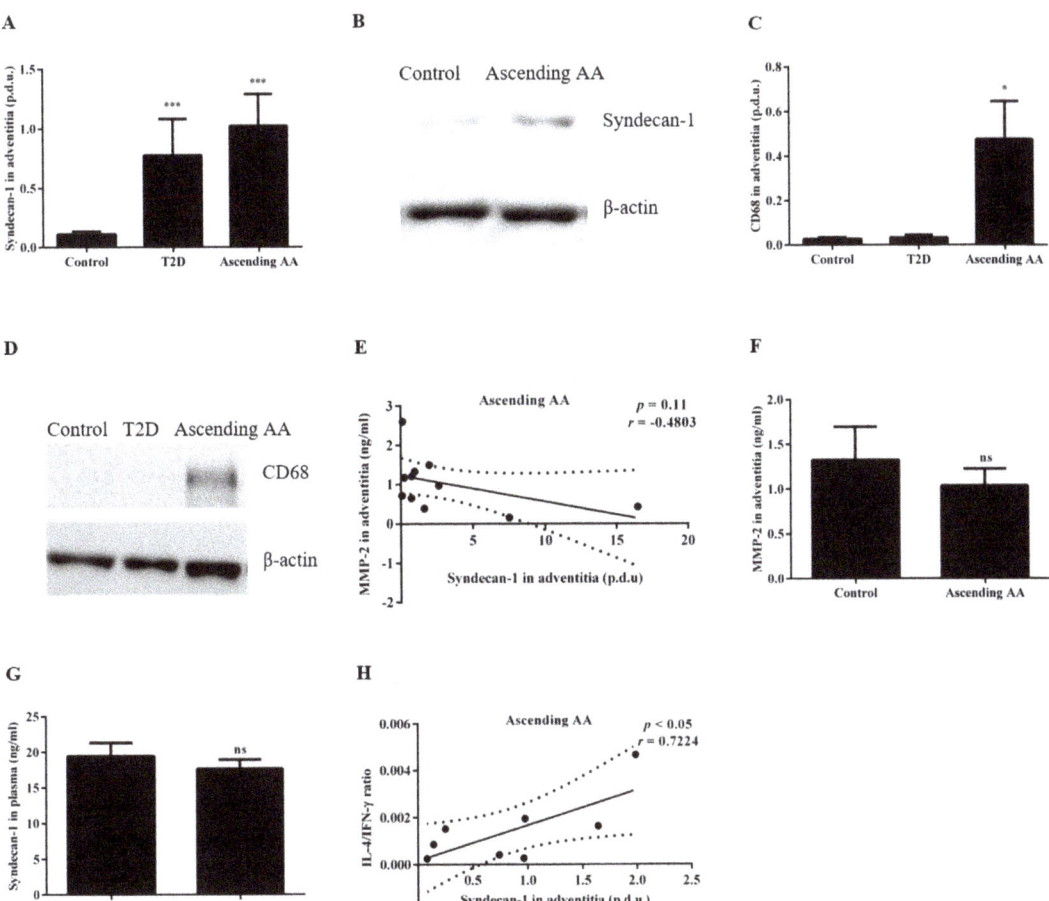

Figure 4. The Sdc-1 was increased in the aortic tissue of patients with an ascending AA. The Sdc-1 expression in the adventitia was higher in ascending AA patients compared with the control non-ascending AA patients, (**A**) normalized data and (**B**) Western blot data. The macrophage marker CD68 was increased in patients with an ascending AA compared with the control but no change of the same was noticed in the T2D patients, (**C**) normalized data and (**D**) Western blot data. (**E**) The MMP-2 activity in the adventitia was not associated with the Sdc-1 expression in the same tissue nor was MMP-2 altered in the ascending AA group (**F**). A Pearson correlation was used to assess the associations. (**G**) The plasma Sdc-1 was not changed in the ascending AA patients. (**H**) The Sdc-1 in the adventitia was positively correlated with the IL-4/IFN-γ ratio. Comparisons between the groups were made using an unpaired *t*-test or a Mann–Whitney. $n = 10$ for the control and $n = 10$ for the ascending AA. Pearson correlation analysis was performed to assess any associations. ns = not significant, * $p < 0.05$, *** $p < 0.001$. For (**B**,**D**) the full-length blot is provided in Supplementary Material Figure S3.

4. Discussion

Recent research using animal models of aneurysm development indicate an important role for Sdc-1 in preventing and counteracting aneurysm pathogenesis [24,25]. We hypothesized that increased fpGLP-1 and enhanced GLP-1 signaling in T2D contributed to a reduced shedding and an increased expression of Sdc-1 in the aortic tissue and that this played a role in the reduced prevalence of ascending AAs in T2D. Consequently, we investigated the Sdc-1 expression in the aortic tissue of patients with/without T2D as well as potential associations with fpGLP-1. Furthermore, as the macrophage Sdc-1 expression was induced in response to an aneurysm formation in experimental models counterbalancing the inflammatory processes ongoing during thoracic AA formation [24,36], we assessed whether the increased Sdc-1 expression could be detected also in patients with an established ascending AA as well as its potential association with increased macrophage infiltration and inflammation.

Throughout this study, aortic adventitial tissue was used because growing evidence supports that processes leading up to the medial degeneration observed in an ascending AA are initiated in the adventitia.

In line with the hypothesis, we detected reduced shedding and a significantly increased expression of Sdc-1 in the adventitia of T2D patients compared with the controls. The increased aortic tissue expression of Sdc-1 in T2D facilitates a potential role for an increased aortic Sdc-1 expression in the reduced prevalence of a thoracic AA in T2D [24]. Of potential interest here is that the knockdown of Sdc-1 inhibits pathways that upregulate the expression of importin-8 [37,38] and loss of function of importin-8 has been shown to cause a syndromic form of thoracic AA [39]. In addition, endothelial nuclear factor-κB (NF-κB) levels associate with a thoracic AA where NF-κB activation may trigger macrophage infiltration and inflammation in the adventitia and media [40] and Sdc-1 and GLP-1 alike have been shown to suppress NF-κB activation [41,42].

MMP-2 can proteolytically cleave and shed Sdc-1 from the cell surface [43] and reduced plasma Sdc-1 (shed Sdc-1) tended to correlate with a reduced local MMP-2 activity. However, the MMP-2 activity in the adventitia was not significantly altered in T2D. Taken together, these data indicate that a reduced Sdc-1 shedding in response to MMP-2 activity may not be a major contributor to the elevated adventitial expression of Sdc-1 in T2D. However, MMP-2 is not the only proteinase that sheds Sdc-1 from the cell surface; other proteases in and around the adventitia may serve to regulate Sdc-1 shedding (for example, disintegrin and MMP with thrombospondin motifs and MMP-9). There are also inhibitors of proteases that could affect the cleavage and shedding of Sdc-1 (for example, tissue inhibitors of MMPs) [44] and receptors that regulate the turnover of proteases and protease inhibitors (for example, low density lipoprotein receptor-related protein 1) [43,45]. Furthermore, although no significant association of plasma Sdc-1 and the adventitial Sdc-1 expression was observed, it should be considered that Sdc-1 from the ascending aorta is likely to be a small contributor to the plasma pool of Sdc-1. Specifically, altered shedding from the aorta localized to the site of the aneurysm could be masked by other larger contributors to Sdc-1 in plasma such as the liver, kidneys and/or digestive tract [46,47]. Consequently, the data obtained in the present report did not rule out that the increased aortic Sdc-1 expression in T2D resulted from a reduced local Sdc-1 shedding in the adventitia. No increase in macrophage-specific markers, indicating macrophage infiltration as a possible contributor to the increased Sdc-1 expression, was detected in the aortic tissue from the T2D group. Future studies should evaluate a potential relevance for the identified correlation between IL-12p70 and the expression of Sdc-1 in the adventitia as well as the trend toward a positive correlation between plasma IFN-γ and Sdc-1 in the adventitia within the T2D patient group. IFN-γ is known to cause shedding of Sdc-1 [48], which may imply that the tissue expression should be high when IFN-γ levels are low. However, plasma concentrations of IFN-γ may differ from the local adventitial expression of IFN-γ. Furthermore, the trend towards a positive correlation between IFN-γ and the adventitial Sdc-1 expression in T2D patients may be related to the fact that shed Sdc-1 in plasma binds and inhibits IFN-γ, resulting in less-detected IFN-γ under the conditions of increased shedding and a low Sdc-1 tissue expression [49,50]. However, this is purely speculative and if a positive correlation between IFN-γ and Sdc-1 is confirmed in larger observational studies, the underlying mechanisms should be further investigated.

The results presented herein did not support a role for elevated fpGLP-1 in the increased aortic expression of Sdc-1 associated with T2D. However, the total fpGLP-1 (7–36 and 9–36) was measured in this study and the differences between the groups in terms of enzymatic activity and the degradation of active GLP-1 could not be excluded.

Furthermore, the lack of association between fpGLP-1 and the aortic Sdc-1 expression may be due to the very small amount of fpGLP-1 reaching the GLP-1Rs at the site of the aneurysm and does not exclude the direct effects of incretin therapy on the aortic Sdc-1 expression. Specifically, GLP-1 has a half-life of only 1–2 min as it is rapidly degraded by DPP-4, resulting in approximately only 10% of active endogenous GLP-1 reaching systemic circulation [51,52].

In line with data from animal models of abdominal AAs, we report an increased expression of Sdc-1 in the adventitia after an ascending AA formation. The increased expression of Sdc-1 in the adventitia of patients with an established ascending AA was observed together with an increased expression of a macrophage-specific marker and not indicated to result from a reduced proteolytic cleavage or shedding by MMP-2 as local MMP-2 activity was not increased in association with an ascending AA and no association between the local MMP-2 activity and the Sdc-1 expression was detected. Unaltered MMP-2 activity in an ascending AA may seem contradictory to the reports of increased MMP-2 expression in thoracic AA patients [53,54]. However, one must consider the important difference between expression and activity and that these studies did not include patients with an ascending AA as they used specimens from the aortic arch. Furthermore, the stage of progression of the ascending AA could not be assessed at the time of the study, which may be of importance for analyses such as MMP-2 activity where increased MMP-2 levels are detected early in thoracic AA formation [55].

The amount of plasma Sdc-1 in the circulation was not significantly altered in an ascending AA nor was it associated with the expression of Sdc-1 in the adventitia. This indicated that the increased tissue expression of Sdc-1 was the result of factors other than altered shedding. Specifically, the positive correlation between the adventitial Sdc-1 expression and the increased detection of the macrophage-specific marker CD68 might indicate an induced expression on infiltrating macrophages in response to an ascending AA where the Sdc-1 expression counterbalanced the inflammatory processes ongoing [24,36]. Future studies should perform immunohistochemistry on an aortic cross-section for Sdc-1 and CD68 to confirm that Sdc-1 is localized to infiltrating macrophages as the positive correlation between CD68 and Sdc-1 indicates.

However, it is important to consider that we cannot rule out altered local Sdc-1 shedding as a contributor to the increased expression of Sdc-1 detected in the aortic tissue in association with an ascending AA. Particularly, as stated above, MMP2 is not the only protease to shed Sdc-1; the adventitial Sdc-1 from the ascending aorta is likely a small contributor to the plasma pool of Sdc-1.

The fact that the Sdc-1 in plasma was not increased in association with an ascending AA may seem contradictory to the known role of inflammation in an ascending AA as well as in the Sdc-1 shedding process [44,56,57]. However, we did not assess/compare the inflammatory profile of the patient groups in this study.

Although this type of cohort study can infer and interpret a causal relationship, it cannot establish one. Furthermore, due to the relatively low number of patients in each group for a few of the analyses, the patients could not be separated into subgroups depending on sex, type of valve pathology (i.e., aortic stenosis or aortic insufficiency) and anti-diabetic therapy. Future larger registry-based/multi-center studies should be undertaken to further our understanding of the role for GLP-1-based anti-diabetic therapy in the increased Sdc-1 expression in the adventitia of T2D patients and its potential relevance for the reduced prevalence of ascending AAs in T2D.

However, the present study presented novel and important information of an increased aortic expression of Sdc-1 in association with T2D while also indicting the infiltration of macrophages and an increased aortic Sdc-1 expression in response to an ascending AA. Considering that the local expression of Sdc-1 is indicated to protect from aneurysm formation [24], the increased aortic expression of Sdc-1 detected in T2D patients may contribute to a reduced prevalence of ascending AAs in T2D.

Supplementary Materials: The following are available online at https://www.mdpi.com/article/10.3390/biomedicines9060697/s1, Figures S1–S3.

Author Contributions: Conceptualization, C.K. and A.F.-C.; methodology, S.N.; software, S.N.; validation, S.N. and C.K.; formal analysis, S.N.; investigation, S.N.; resources, A.F.-C. and C.K.; data curation, S.N., L.M.T., H.M.B. and C.K.; writing—original draft preparation, S.N. and C.K.; writing—review and editing, S.N., L.M.T., A.F.-C., H.M.B. and C.K.; visualization, S.N.; supervision, C.K.; project administration, S.N. and C.K.; funding acquisition, C.K and A.F.-C. All authors have read and agreed to the published version of the manuscript.

Funding: This research was funded by the Wallenius Foundation, a private donation by Fredrik Lundberg, Mats Kleberg Stiftelse and Sven och Dagmar Saléns Stiftelser.

Institutional Review Board Statement: The study was conducted according to the guidelines of the Declaration of Helsinki and approved by the Stockholm Regional Ethical Committee (protocol code: 2006/784-31/1 and date of approval 15 September 2006 and protocol code: 2012/1633-31/4 and date of approval 24 October 2012).

Informed Consent Statement: Informed consent was obtained from all subjects involved in the study.

Data Availability Statement: The main data supporting the results of this study are presented in this paper or in the Supplementary Material. The amount of data generated for this study was quite large to be shared publicly but the raw data can be shared under a reasonable request.

Acknowledgments: The authors would like to thank Susanne Hylander and Karin Lång for their help with providing the samples and some of the patient information needed for this paper. They would also like to thank Susanna Eketjäll for allowing them to use the instrument for the multiplex analysis.

Conflicts of Interest: The authors declare no conflict of interest.

References

1. Kuzmik, G.A.; Sang, A.X.; Elefteriades, J.A. Natural history of thoracic aortic aneurysms. *J. Vasc. Surg.* **2012**, *56*, 565–571. [CrossRef] [PubMed]
2. Federle, M.P.; Rosado-de-Christenson, M.L.; Raman, S.P.; Carter, B.W.; Woodward, P.J.; Shaaban, A.M. Heart. In *Imaging Anatomy: Chest, Abdomen, Pelvis*, 2nd ed.; Federle, M.P., Rosado-de-Christenson, M.L., Raman, S.P., Carter, B.W., Woodward, P.J., Shaaban, A.M., Eds.; Elsevier: Amsterdam, The Netherlands, 2017; pp. 336–379.
3. Hiratzka, L.F.; Bakris, G.L.; Beckman, J.A.; Bersin, R.; Carr, V.; Casey, D., Jr.; Eagle, K.; Hermann, L.; Isselbacher, E.; Kazerooni, E. ACCF. *Circulation* **2010**, *121*, 1544.
4. Saliba, E.; Sia, Y.; Dore, A.; El Hamamsy, I. The ascending aortic aneurysm: When to intervene? *Int. J. Cardiol. Heart Vasc.* **2015**, *6*, 91–100. [CrossRef]
5. Tsai, C.L.; Lin, C.L.; Wu, Y.Y.; Shieh, D.C.; Sung, F.C.; Kao, C.H. Advanced complicated diabetes mellitus is associated with a reduced risk of thoracic and abdominal aortic aneurysm rupture: A population-based cohort study. *Diabetes/Metab. Res. Rev.* **2015**, *31*, 190–197. [CrossRef]
6. Prakash, S.K.; Pedroza, C.; Khalil, Y.A.; Milewicz, D.M. Diabetes and reduced risk for thoracic aortic aneurysms and dissections: A nationwide case-control study. *J. Am. Heart Assoc.* **2012**, *1*, e000323. [CrossRef]
7. Lu, H.Y.; Huang, C.Y.; Shih, C.M.; Chang, W.H.; Tsai, C.S.; Lin, F.Y.; Shih, C.C. Dipeptidyl peptidase-4 inhibitor decreases abdominal aortic aneurysm formation through GLP-1-dependent monocytic activity in mice. *PLoS ONE* **2015**, *10*, e0121077. [CrossRef]
8. Yu, J.; Morimoto, K.; Bao, W.; Yu, Z.; Okita, Y.; Okada, K. Glucagon-like peptide-1 prevented abdominal aortic aneurysm development in rats. *Surg. Today* **2016**, *46*, 1099–1107. [CrossRef] [PubMed]
9. Takahara, Y.; Tokunou, T.; Ichiki, T. Suppression of Abdominal Aortic Aneurysm Formation in Mice by Teneligliptin, a Dipeptidyl Peptidase-4 Inhibitor. *J. Atheroscler. Thromb.* **2018**, *25*, 698–708. [CrossRef] [PubMed]
10. Ikedo, T.; Minami, M.; Kataoka, H.; Hayashi, K.; Nagata, M.; Fujikawa, R.; Higuchi, S.; Yasui, M.; Aoki, T.; Fukuda, M.; et al. Dipeptidyl Peptidase-4 Inhibitor Anagliptin Prevents Intracranial Aneurysm Growth by Suppressing Macrophage Infiltration and Activation. *J. Am. Heart Assoc.* **2017**, *6*, e004777. [CrossRef]
11. Goto, H.; Nomiyama, T.; Mita, T.; Yasunari, E.; Azuma, K.; Komiya, K.; Arakawa, M.; Jin, W.L.; Kanazawa, A.; Kawamori, R.; et al. Exendin-4, a glucagon-like peptide-1 receptor agonist, reduces intimal thickening after vascular injury. *Biochem. Biophys. Res. Commun.* **2011**, *405*, 79–84. [CrossRef] [PubMed]
12. Bao, W.; Morimoto, K.; Hasegawa, T.; Sasaki, N.; Yamashita, T.; Hirata, K.; Okita, Y.; Okada, K. Orally administered dipeptidyl peptidase-4 inhibitor (alogliptin) prevents abdominal aortic aneurysm formation through an antioxidant effect in rats. *J. Vasc. Surg.* **2014**, *59*, 1098–1108. [CrossRef]

13. El-Hamamsy, I.; Yacoub, M.H. Cellular and molecular mechanisms of thoracic aortic aneurysms. *Nat. Rev. Cardiol.* **2009**, *6*, 771–786. [CrossRef]
14. Petit, C.; Mousavi, S.J.; Avril, S. Chapter 6—Review of the Essential Roles of SMCs in ATAA Biomechanics. In *Advances in Biomechanics and Tissue Regeneration*; Doweidar, M.H., Ed.; Academic Press: Cambridge, MA, USA, 2019; pp. 95–114.
15. Agaimy, A.; Weyand, M.; Strecker, T. Inflammatory thoracic aortic aneurysm (lymphoplasmacytic thoracic aortitis): A 13-year-experience at a German Heart Center with emphasis on possible role of IgG4. *Int. J. Clin. Exp. Pathol.* **2013**, *6*, 1713–1722. [PubMed]
16. Wu, D.; Choi, J.C.; Sameri, A.; Minard, C.G.; Coselli, J.S.; Shen, Y.H.; LeMaire, S.A. Inflammatory Cell Infiltrates in Acute and Chronic Thoracic Aortic Dissection. *Aorta* **2013**, *1*, 259–267. [CrossRef]
17. del Porto, F.; Proietta, M.; Tritapepe, L.; Miraldi, F.; Koverech, A.; Cardelli, P.; Tabacco, F.; de Santis, V.; Vecchione, A.; Mitterhofer, A.P.; et al. Inflammation and immune response in acute aortic dissection. *Ann. Med.* **2010**, *42*, 622–629. [CrossRef] [PubMed]
18. Dinesh, N.E.H.; Reinhardt, D.P. Inflammation in thoracic aortic aneurysms. *Herz* **2019**, *44*, 138–146. [CrossRef] [PubMed]
19. Lindsay, M.E.; Dietz, H.C. Lessons on the pathogenesis of aneurysm from heritable conditions. *Nature* **2011**, *473*, 308–316. [CrossRef]
20. He, R.; Guo, D.-C.; Estrera, A.L.; Safi, H.J.; Huynh, T.T.; Yin, Z.; Cao, S.-N.; Lin, J.; Kurian, T.; Buja, L.M.; et al. Characterization of the inflammatory and apoptotic cells in the aortas of patients with ascending thoracic aortic aneurysms and dissections. *J. Thorac. Cardiovasc. Surg.* **2006**, *131*, 671–678.e672. [CrossRef] [PubMed]
21. Endo, K.; Takino, T.; Miyamori, H.; Kinsen, H.; Yoshizaki, T.; Furukawa, M.; Sato, H. Cleavage of syndecan-1 by membrane type matrix metalloproteinase-1 stimulates cell migration. *J. Biol. Chem.* **2003**, *278*, 40764–40770. [CrossRef] [PubMed]
22. Brule, S.; Charnaux, N.; Sutton, A.; Ledoux, D.; Chaigneau, T.; Saffar, L.; Gattegno, L. The shedding of syndecan-4 and syndecan-1 from HeLa cells and human primary macrophages is accelerated by SDF-1/CXCL12 and mediated by the matrix metalloproteinase-9. *Glycobiology* **2006**, *16*, 488–501. [CrossRef]
23. Bernfield, M.; Götte, M.; Park, P.W.; Reizes, O.; Fitzgerald, M.L.; Lincecum, J.; Zako, M. Functions of cell surface heparan sulfate proteoglycans. *Annu. Rev. Biochem.* **1999**, *68*, 729–777. [CrossRef]
24. Xiao, J.; Angsana, J.; Wen, J.; Smith, S.V.; Park, P.W.; Ford, M.L.; Haller, C.A.; Chaikof, E.L. Syndecan-1 displays a protective role in aortic aneurysm formation by modulating T cell-mediated responses. *Arterioscler. Thromb. Vasc. Biol.* **2012**, *32*, 386–396. [CrossRef] [PubMed]
25. Chaterji, S.; Lam, C.H.; Ho, D.S.; Proske, D.C.; Baker, A.B. Syndecan-1 regulates vascular smooth muscle cell phenotype. *PLoS ONE* **2014**, *9*, e89824. [CrossRef]
26. Yeaman, C.; Rapraeger, A.C. Post-transcriptional regulation of syndecan-1 expression by cAMP in peritoneal macrophages. *J. Cell Biol.* **1993**, *122*, 941–950. [CrossRef]
27. Fehmann, H.C.; Goke, R.; Goke, B. Cell and molecular biology of the incretin hormones glucagon-like peptide-I and glucose-dependent insulin releasing polypeptide. *Endocr. Rev.* **1995**, *16*, 390–410. [CrossRef] [PubMed]
28. Drucker, D.J.; Philippe, J.; Mojsov, S.; Chick, W.L.; Habener, J.F. Glucagon-like peptide I stimulates insulin gene expression and increases cyclic AMP levels in a rat islet cell line. *Proc. Natl. Acad. Sci. USA* **1987**, *84*, 3434–3438. [CrossRef] [PubMed]
29. Angelone, D.F.; Wessels, M.R.; Coughlin, M.; Suter, E.E.; Valentini, P.; Kalish, L.A.; Levy, O. Innate Immunity of the Human Newborn Is Polarized Toward a High Ratio of IL-6/TNF-α Production In Vitro and In Vivo. *Pediatr. Res.* **2006**, *60*, 205–209. [CrossRef] [PubMed]
30. Krizhanovskii, C.; Ntika, S.; Olsson, C.; Eriksson, P.; Franco-Cereceda, A. Elevated circulating fasting glucagon-like peptide-1 in surgical patients with aortic valve disease and diabetes. *Diabetol. Metab. Syndr.* **2017**, *9*, 79. [CrossRef]
31. Treska, V.; Topolcan, O.; Pecen, L. Cytokines as plasma markers of abdominal aortic aneurysm. *Clin. Chem. Lab. Med.* **2000**, *38*, 1161–1164. [CrossRef]
32. Guo, D.C.; Papke, C.L.; He, R.; Milewicz, D.M. Pathogenesis of thoracic and abdominal aortic aneurysms. *Ann. N. Y. Acad. Sci.* **2006**, *1085*, 339–352. [CrossRef]
33. Juvonen, J.; Surcel, H.M.; Satta, J.; Teppo, A.M.; Bloigu, A.; Syrjala, H.; Airaksinen, J.; Leinonen, M.; Saikku, P.; Juvonen, T. Elevated circulating levels of inflammatory cytokines in patients with abdominal aortic aneurysm. *Arterioscler. Thromb. Vasc. Biol.* **1997**, *17*, 2843–2847. [CrossRef]
34. Batra, R.; Suh, M.K.; Carson, J.S.; Dale, M.A.; Meisinger, T.M.; Fitzgerald, M.; Opperman, P.J.; Luo, J.; Pipinos, I.I.; Xiong, W.; et al. IL-1beta (Interleukin-1beta) and TNF-alpha (Tumor Necrosis Factor-alpha) Impact Abdominal Aortic Aneurysm Formation by Differential Effects on Macrophage Polarization. *Arterioscler. Thromb. Vasc. Biol.* **2018**, *38*, 457–463. [CrossRef]
35. Gabrielsson, S.; Soderlund, A.; Nilsson, C.; Lilja, G.; Nordlund, M.; Troye-Blomberg, M. Influence of atopic heredity on IL-4-, IL-12- and IFN-gamma-producing cells in in vitro activated cord blood mononuclear cells. *Clin. Exp. Immunol.* **2001**, *126*, 390–396. [CrossRef]
36. Angsana, J.; Chen, J.; Smith, S.; Xiao, J.; Wen, J.; Liu, L.; Haller, C.A.; Chaikof, E.L. Syndecan-1 Modulates the Motility and Resolution Responses of Macrophages. *Arterioscler. Thromb. Vasc. Biol.* **2015**, *35*, 332–340. [CrossRef] [PubMed]
37. Hu, X.; Kan, H.; Boye, A.; Jiang, Y.; Wu, C.; Yang, Y. Mitogen-activated protein kinase inhibitors reduce the nuclear accumulation of phosphorylated Smads by inhibiting Imp 7 or Imp 8 in HepG2 cells. *Oncol. Lett.* **2018**, *15*, 4867–4872. [CrossRef] [PubMed]
38. Cui, J.; Jin, S.; Jin, C.; Jin, Z. Syndecan-1 regulates extracellular matrix expression in keloid fibroblasts via TGF-β1/Smad and MAPK signaling pathways. *Life Sci.* **2020**, *254*, 117326. [CrossRef] [PubMed]

39. Van Gucht, I.; Meester, J.A.N.; Bento, J.R.; Bastiaansen, M.; Bastianen, J.; Luyckx, I.; Van Den Heuvel, L.; Neutel, C.H.G.; Guns, P.J.; Vermont, M.; et al. A human importin-β-related disorder: Syndromic thoracic aortic aneurysm caused by bi-allelic loss-of-function variants in IPO8. *Am. J. Hum. Genet.* **2021**, *108*, 1115–1125. [CrossRef] [PubMed]
40. Saito, T.; Hasegawa, Y.; Ishigaki, Y.; Yamada, T.; Gao, J.; Imai, J.; Uno, K.; Kaneko, K.; Ogihara, T.; Shimosawa, T.; et al. Importance of endothelial NF-κB signalling in vascular remodelling and aortic aneurysm formation. *Cardiovasc. Res.* **2012**, *97*, 106–114. [CrossRef]
41. Zhang, Y.; Wang, Z.; Liu, J.; Zhang, Z.; Chen, Y. Suppressing Syndecan-1 Shedding Ameliorates Intestinal Epithelial Inflammation through Inhibiting NF-κB Pathway and TNF-α. *Gastroenterol. Res. Pract.* **2016**, *2016*, 6421351. [CrossRef]
42. Arakawa, M.; Mita, T.; Azuma, K.; Ebato, C.; Goto, H.; Nomiyama, T.; Fujitani, Y.; Hirose, T.; Kawamori, R.; Watada, H. Inhibition of monocyte adhesion to endothelial cells and attenuation of atherosclerotic lesion by a glucagon-like peptide-1 receptor agonist, exendin-4. *Diabetes* **2010**, *59*, 1030–1037. [CrossRef]
43. Manon-Jensen, T.; Itoh, Y.; Couchman, J.R. Proteoglycans in health and disease: The multiple roles of syndecan shedding. *FEBS J.* **2010**, *277*, 3876–3889. [CrossRef] [PubMed]
44. Fitzgerald, M.L.; Wang, Z.; Park, P.W.; Murphy, G.; Bernfield, M. Shedding of syndecan-1 and -4 ectodomains is regulated by multiple signaling pathways and mediated by a TIMP-3-sensitive metalloproteinase. *J. Cell Biol.* **2000**, *148*, 811–824. [CrossRef] [PubMed]
45. Deng, Y.; Foley, E.M.; Gonzales, J.C.; Gordts, P.L.; Li, Y.; Esko, J.D. Shedding of syndecan-1 from human hepatocytes alters very low density lipoprotein clearance. *Hepatology* **2012**, *55*, 277–286. [CrossRef] [PubMed]
46. Kind, S.; Merenkow, C.; Büscheck, F.; Möller, K.; Dum, D.; Chirico, V.; Luebke, A.M.; Höflmayer, D.; Hinsch, A.; Jacobsen, F.; et al. Prevalence of Syndecan-1 (CD138) Expression in Different Kinds of Human Tumors and Normal Tissues. *Dis. Markers* **2019**, *2019*, 4928315. [CrossRef] [PubMed]
47. Ledin, J.; Staatz, W.; Li, J.P.; Götte, M.; Selleck, S.; Kjellén, L.; Spillmann, D. Heparan sulfate structure in mice with genetically modified heparan sulfate production. *J. Biol. Chem.* **2004**, *279*, 42732–42741. [CrossRef]
48. Henry-Stanley, M.J.; Zhang, B.; Erlandsen, S.L.; Wells, C.L. Synergistic effect of tumor necrosis factor-alpha and interferon-gamma on enterocyte shedding of syndecan-1 and associated decreases in internalization of Listeria monocytogenes and Staphylococcus aureus. *Cytokine* **2006**, *34*, 252–259. [CrossRef] [PubMed]
49. Teng, Y.H.-F.; Aquino, R.S.; Park, P.W. Molecular functions of syndecan-1 in disease. *Matrix Biol.* **2012**, *31*, 3–16. [CrossRef]
50. Fritchley, S.J.; Kirby, J.A.; Ali, S. The antagonism of interferon-gamma (IFN-gamma) by heparin: Examination of the blockade of class II MHC antigen and heat shock protein-70 expression. *Clin. Exp. Immunol.* **2000**, *120*, 247–252. [CrossRef]
51. Araújo, F.; Fonte, P.; Santos, H.A.; Sarmento, B. Oral delivery of glucagon-like peptide-1 and analogs: Alternatives for diabetes control? *J. Diabetes Sci. Technol.* **2012**, *6*, 1486–1497. [CrossRef]
52. Holst, J.J.; Deacon, C.F. Glucagon-like peptide-1 mediates the therapeutic actions of DPP-IV inhibitors. *Diabetologia* **2005**, *48*, 612–615. [CrossRef]
53. Schmitt, R.; Tscheuschler, A.; Laschinski, P.; Uffelmann, X.; Discher, P.; Fuchs, J.; Kreibich, M.; Peyronnet, R.; Kari, F.A. A potential key mechanism in ascending aortic aneurysm development: Detection of a linear relationship between MMP-14/TIMP-2 ratio and active MMP-2. *PLoS ONE* **2019**, *14*, e0212859. [CrossRef] [PubMed]
54. Taketani, T.; Imai, Y.; Morota, T.; Maemura, K.; Morita, H.; Hayashi, D.; Yamazaki, T.; Nagai, R.; Takamoto, S. Altered patterns of gene expression specific to thoracic aortic aneurysms. *Int. Heart J.* **2005**, *46*, 265–277. [CrossRef] [PubMed]
55. Benjamin, M.M.; Khalil, R.A. Matrix metalloproteinase inhibitors as investigative tools in the pathogenesis and management of vascular disease. *Exp. Suppl.* **2012**, *103*, 209–279. [CrossRef] [PubMed]
56. Bartlett, A.H.; Hayashida, K.; Park, P.W. Molecular and cellular mechanisms of syndecans in tissue injury and inflammation. *Mol. Cells* **2007**, *24*, 153–166.
57. Day, R.M.; Mitchell, T.J.; Knight, S.C.; Forbes, A. Regulation of epithelial syndecan-1 expression by inflammatory cytokines. *Cytokine* **2003**, *21*, 224–233. [CrossRef]

MDPI
St. Alban-Anlage 66
4052 Basel
Switzerland
www.mdpi.com

Biomedicines Editorial Office
E-mail: biomedicines@mdpi.com
www.mdpi.com/journal/biomedicines

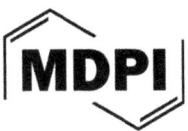

Disclaimer/Publisher's Note: The statements, opinions and data contained in all publications are solely those of the individual author(s) and contributor(s) and not of MDPI and/or the editor(s). MDPI and/or the editor(s) disclaim responsibility for any injury to people or property resulting from any ideas, methods, instructions or products referred to in the content.